Use newborn chapter
to demonstrate
diff bet original
— designs newborns

How will the designers
ing in this lit respond
to Strange Situation?

Attachment Disorganization

Attachment Disorganization

EDITORS

Judith Solomon
Carol George

THE GUILFORD PRESS
New York   London

Printed in the United States of America

This book is printed on acid-free paper.

Last digit is print number: 9 8 7 6 5 4 3 2

Library of Congress Cataloging-in-Publication Data

Attachment Disorganization / edited by Judith Solomon and Carol
  George.
     p. cm.
   Includes bibliographical references and index.
   ISBN 1-57230-480-4
   1. Attachment disorder in children. 2. Separation anxiety in
children. Attachment behavior in children. 4. Child
psychopathology. I. Solomon, Judith. II. George, Carol.
RJ507.A77A87   1999
618.92′89—dc21   99-23365
                                                        CIP

This book is dedicated with love and respect to the memory of

Mary D. Salter Ainsworth

About the Editors

Judith Solomon is a research associate at the Judith Wallerstein Center for the Family in Transition, Corte Madera, California. Attachment disorganization has been at the heart of her research for the past 15 years. Her original collaboration with Dr. Mary Main led to development of the indices of disorganization in infants. Dr. Solomon's recent work highlights disorganization in middle childhood, parental caregiving, and infants of divorce. Dr. Solomon has also contributed to the development of several new representational attachment measures, including classification systems for child doll play and a parental caregiving interview. In addition to her research activities, Dr. Solomon writes, lectures, and maintains a clinical practice with a focus on counseling divorcing families.

Carol George is Professor of Psychology at Mills College, Oakland, California. She became interested in attachment disorganization through her early work with abused infants and toddlers. Dr. George's recent work in child attachment has focused predominantly on middle childhood and parental caregiving. Dr. George has worked in collaboration with Dr. Solomon in the development of classification systems for child doll play and parental caregiving. She is also known for her work in adult attachment, including her coauthorship of the Adult Attachment Interview.

Contributors

Gwendolyn Atwood, EdD, Department of Psychiatry, Harvard Medical School, The Cambridge Hospital, Cambridge, MA

Marian J. Bakermans-Kranenburg, PhD, Center for Child and Family Studies, Leiden University, Leiden, The Netherlands

Douglas Barnett, PhD, Department of Psychology, Wayne State University, Detroit, MI

Marjolijn Blom, MA, School of Family Studies, University of Connecticut, Storrs, CT

Elisa Bronfman, PhD, Department of Psychiatry, Harvard Medical School, The Cambridge Hospital, Cambridge, MA

Christine M. Butler, MA, Department of Psychology, Wayne State University, Detroit, MI

Carol George, PhD, Department of Psychology, Mills College, Oakland, CA

Karin Grossmann, PhD, Institute of Psychology, University of Regensburg, Regensburg, Germany

Nancy Hazen, PhD, Child Development and Family Relationships, University of Texas, Austin, TX

Kelli Hill Hunt, MA, Department of Psychology, Wayne State University, Detroit, MI

Teresa Jacobsen, PhD, Department of Psychiatry, University of Illinois, Chicago, IL

Deborah Jacobvitz, PhD, Child Development and Family Relationships, University of Texas, Austin, TX

Melissa Kaplan-Estrin, PhD, Department of Psychology, Wayne State University, Detroit, MI

Giovanni Liotti, MD, Association of Cognitive Psychology, School of Cognitive Psychotherapy, Rome, Rome, Italy

Karlen Lyons-Ruth, PhD, Department of Psychiatry, Harvard Medical School, The Cambridge Hospital, Cambridge, MA

Robert S. Marvin, PhD, Department of Pediatric Psychology, Kluge Children's Rehabilitation Center, University of Virginia, Charlottesville, VA

John W. McCaskill IV, PhD, Department of Clinical and Health Psychology, College of Health Professions, University of Florida, Gainesville, FL

Laura J. Miller, MD, Department of Psychiatry, University of Illinois, Chicago, IL

Maria C. Morog, PhD, Curry School of Education, University of Virginia, Charlottesville, VA

Ellen Moss, PhD, Department of Psychology, University of Quebec at Montreal, Montreal, Quebec, Canada

Sophie Parent, PhD, School of Psychoeducation, University of Montreal, Montreal, Quebec, Canada

Odette Pettem, PhD, Foothills Hospital, Calgary, Alberta, Canada

Robert C. Pianta, PhD, Curry School of Education, University of Virginia, Charlottesville, VA

Sandra Pipp-Siegel, PhD, Department of Speech, Language, and Hearing Sciences, University of Colorado, Boulder, CO

Carlo Schuengel, PhD, Center for Child and Family Studies, Leiden University, Leiden, The Netherlands

Judith Solomon, PhD, Judith Wallerstein Center for the Family in Transition, Berkeley, CA

Gottfried Spangler, PhD, Institute of Psychology, University of Giessen, Giessen, Germany

Diane St-Laurent, PhD, Department of Psychology, University of Quebec at Montreal, Montreal, Quebec, Canada

Douglas M. Teti, PhD, Department of Psychology, University of Maryland, Baltimore County, Baltimore, MD

Marta Valenzuela, PhD, Institute of Family and Community Psychiatry, The Sir Mortimer B. Davis–Jewish General Hospital, Montreal, Quebec, Canada

Marinus H. van IJzendoorn, PhD, Center for Child and Family Studies, Leiden University, Leiden, The Netherlands

Everett Waters, PhD, Department of Psychology, State University of New York at Stony Brook, Stony Brook, NY

Malcolm West, PhD, Department of Psychiatry, University of Calgary, Calgary, Alberta, Canada

Preface

This book presents new research and theory on the topic of attachment disorganization, an area of investigation that is of increasing importance in the study of attachment, caregiving, and developmental and psychological risk throughout the lifespan. Disorganized attachment relationships were first formally identified by Mary Main and Judith Solomon on the basis of the anomalous but intriguing behavior of some infants during laboratory separations and reunions with the parent. Since that time, Main, Solomon, and a rapidly growing number of developmental and clinical researchers have established links between disorganized patterns of attachment and disturbed and disrupted patterns of caregiving, role reversal in the child–parent relationship, disorganization of representational processes, relationship violence, and later signs of psychopathology in children and adults, including conduct disorder and dissociative tendencies. Furthermore, because disorganized attachments are now known to be associated with the parent's own unresolved experiences of loss, separation, and trauma, they provide a direct link between the original concerns of attachment theory outlined by John Bowlby, the empirical study of early attachments pioneered by Mary Ainsworth, and contemporary problems in mental health and emotional development.

As with any vital area of scientific inquiry, there are also points of controversy and disagreement, definitional and methodological uncertainties, and questions of interpretation that must be addressed in order for progress to continue. The authors who have contributed to this volume were charged not only to present their newest findings, but to grapple with these challenges directly. They have risen to this task conscientiously, and with great originality. It is our hope that readers will find, as we do, the product of their collective labors informative, thought-provoking, and even profound.

Main and Solomon formally defined the disorganized classification (typically referred to in attachment research as the D group) on the basis of their analysis of the strange situation behavior of infants who would otherwise be judged "unclassifiable," that is, whose behavior would not qualify them for placement in any of Ainsworth's three standard attachment groups. In Main's normative middle-class sample, and in a selection of cases from high-risk samples, the unclassifiable cases had in common the absence of a coherent attachment strategy with respect to the parent. Absence of strategy and a breakdown in the smooth coordination of behavior manifested themselves in extremely diverse ways, including acute and sometimes bizarre approach–avoidance conflict behavior; interruption or misdirection of ongoing behavioral patterns by seemingly contradictory, incompatible, stereotyped, or irrelevant behaviors; disorientation and confusion; and fearfulness toward the parent. (A complete list of the indices of disorganization, from Main and Solomon's original publication of them, is included as the Appendix.)

The demarcation of this category immediately raised questions and even skepticism among experienced researchers. Main and Solomon believed, on theoretical grounds, that the breakdown or absence of organization in behavior would reveal important differences in infant–parent relationships, as had the coherent attachment patterns identified by Ainsworth. The next step in the evolution of the D classification was to extend attachment theory to include it as a classification and examine empirically the many questions that were emerging about it. Could the D group's pattern of attachment be added as a fourth to Ainsworth's secure, avoidant, and resistant patterns? Or, did it reflect a problem with the child, or some other factor, orthogonal to attachment security? Did the diverse behaviors that were characteristic of D children represent one or several subcategories? Were there long-term sequelae of disorganized patterns? Finally, and most important, was disorganized attachment related to distinct patterns of parent–infant interaction in the first year of life and beyond?

As empirical studies of this group have accumulated, these questions have been partially answered. Yet, as often happens with new findings in established fields, utilization of the disorganized category in the vast domain of attachment research remains very uneven. Many researchers, especially those working with clinical and high-risk samples, have found the D classification to be indispensable. This is because so many infant–parent dyads in such samples (up to 85% in maltreatment samples) are better placed in the new classification group than in the standard categories. On the other hand, many committed attachment researchers, especially those working with normative samples where D classifications comprise about 10–20% of the sample, still have not incorporated the new category into their studies or into their thinking. Furthermore, the concept of attachment disorganization has not been fully defined in adult attachment research; it is not clear that there is an entirely analogous phenomenon in adults. This has led to an uncomfortable and, ultimately, scientifically unsatisfactory state of affairs, in which researchers attempting to test and extend the same theoretical and empirical base risk diverging in their methodology, terminology, and in the interpretation of their findings.

The purpose of this volume, therefore, is twofold. First, it is the first collection of original papers on attachment disorganization, which together provide the reader with up-to-date information on current issues and advances in the area. Second, we hope to deepen attachment theory's engagement of this topic, to stimulate reflection and dialogue, both among the contributors to this volume and between the authors and our readers. To this end, we have solicited work from a broad cross-section of investigators who work with normative, high-risk, and atypical populations and who have diverse approaches to understanding the phenomenon of attachment disorganization across the lifespan. To ensure the quality of these contributions, the manuscripts underwent blind peer review in addition to our own editorial review. All of the papers that were accepted for this volume are the product of two or more painstaking revisions on the part of their authors.

The 14 chapters in this volume are organized in four sections. The first, on etiology, consists of four chapters that focus on the central questions of disorganized attachment: Does disorganization reflect specific patterns of interaction between caregiver and child? If so, what are they, and what are the psychological mechanisms responsible for causing both attachment and caregiving in these dyads to be disorganized? Ours is the first chapter in this section, and in it our goal is to place the phenomenon of attachment disorganization in the broader context of attachment theory as originally conceptualized by Bowlby. We propose that from this perspective, disorganized attachment behavior is neither unexpected or new. Rather, it provides a contemporary, empirical label for the phenomena of greatest interest to Bowlby—the responses of infants, children, and adults to the assaults on the attachment system represented by loss, separation, and the threat of these. In turn, some of Bowlby's most fundamental psychological constructs, especially that of segregated representational systems, may help us to understand both the etiology and the appearance of disorganized behavior and representation in children and caregivers.

In Chapters 2 and 3, the authors take on the important task of testing and expanding Main and Hesse's "frightening–frightened" hypothesis—currently, the most compelling and well-articulated explanation for both the etiology of disorganized attachment and the link between disorganization and the mother's lack of resolution with respect to attachment-related traumas. In Chapter 2, Karlen Lyons-Ruth, Elisa Bronfman, and Gwendolyn Atwood propose a relationship diathesis model that integrates Main and Hesse's focus on specific traumatic events in the caregiver's history with an appreciation of the underlying type of relationship that results in vulnerability to trauma. Their fine-grained observations of how infants classified as disorganized interact with their mothers indicate that frightening and frightened behavior on the part of the mother is embedded in pervasive patterns of disrupted communication in these dyads. This in turn is linked to mothers' earlier experiences of hostile or helpless relationships. In Chapter 3, Carlo Scheungel, Marian J. Bakermans-Kranenburg, Marinus H. van IJzendoorn, and Marjolijn Blom take a case-history approach and provide naturalistic observation narratives of infant–mother dyads in which the mother has experienced the earlier loss of an attachment figure. These descriptions are an especially important contribution because they capture so well the flavor of early interaction in these dyads. The findings in this chapter support Main and Hesse's "frightened–frightening" hypothesis but also indicate ways in which the hypothesis may need to be elaborated to explain the variability in organization and quality of maternal behavior associated with disorganized attachment classification. In Chapter 4, Gottfried Spangler and Karin Grossmann consider etiology from a different but equally important point of view. They present data that raise the intriguing possibility of neurological and temperamental contributions to the development of disorganized attachment. These are manifested in a child's having difficulty maintaining behavioral organization during neonatal assessment, having extreme physiological responses to separation, and in consistencies across children in their behavioral organization in the presence of their parents.

The second section, "Social and Cognitive Sequelae of Attachment Disorganization," provides stimulating and entirely new information showing an association between disorganized attachment and serious difficulties children have with peer relationships and cognitive and intellectual functioning in school. In Chapter 5, Deborah Jacobvitz and Nancy Hazen develop a framework for understanding the nature and extent of problems in peer interaction shown by children classified as disorganized. This framework emerges from their fascinating and unparalleled observations of mother–child interaction in the home, family processes, and the difficulties shown by children classified as disorganized in managing the give and take of peer relationships. In Chapter 6, Ellen Moss, Diane St-Laurent, and Sophie Parent, through the use of ingenious structured tasks, trace the effects of the noncontingent and role-reversed quality of interaction characteristic of disorganized children and their mothers on the children's metacognitive planning, self-esteem, and academic achievement.

The third section of this volume focuses on atypical populations with high levels of disorganized or "unclassifiable" attachments. These samples offer exceptional opportunities to investigate subgroups of the larger, heterogeneous disorganized attachment group, providing insights about the D category as a whole and various developmental pathways that may be associated with disorganization. In Chapter 7, Douglas Barnett, Kelli Hill Hunt, Christine M. Butler, John W. McCaskill IV, Melissa Kaplan-Estrin, and Sandra Pipp-Siegel report on their efforts to tease reliable signs of attachment disorganization out of indices of neurological compromise in a sample of toddlers with neurological disabilities. In answer to questions raised by earlier work in this area, their painstaking research suggests that even within this stressed population, truly disorganized attachments reflect relationship disturbances rather than child disability. This work also raises the possibility, however, that for some children disorganization may be associated with functional disorganization of the nervous system.

In Chapter 8, Douglas M. Teti takes on the challenge of integrating two different approaches to defining and measuring disorganized attachment in a sample of preschoolers with depressed mothers. Teti also compares the quality of mother–child interaction in dyads in which the preschooler has developed a controlling (role-reversed) attachment strategy with the mother—a common sequela to disorganized attachment in infancy—to that in dyads in which the child's attachment strategy is actually disorganized. Teti finds that relationships are more troubled for the disorganized subgroup than for the controlling subgroup, suggesting the continuing importance of the construct of attachment disorganization at later ages and the possibility that there may be "levels" of disorganization. In our own Chapter 9, we present longitudinal findings on disorganized attachment in separated and divorced families. Observations of mothers and their 2-year-olds in structured tasks before and after a laboratory separation support the conclusion that repeated overnight separations in the context of visitation with the father can lead to disorganized and unclassifiable attachment behavior in the strange situation.

In Chapter 10, Everett Waters and Marta Valenzuela examine the strange situation classifications of well-nourished as well as mild-to-moderately undernourished Chilean toddlers at 18 and 28 months of age. They report that disorganized attachment in the undernourished group is higher than for the well-nourished group at the first assessment, disorganization manifested especially as contradictory sequences of avoidant and resistant behavior. The authors place their specific findings within a control systems analysis of maternal behavior and in the broader and very stimulating discussion of attachment disorganization as an index of disturbance in the development of coping abilities.

The fourth and final section consists of chapters that apply observations and insights derived from the study of attachment disorganization in infants and young children to clinical and adult populations. In Chapter 11, Giovanni Liotti, building on Main's earlier proposal that disorganized infant behavior reflects dissociative states, expands his theory that disorganized attachment relationships create a vulnerability to later dissociative disorder. In contrast to a more traditional view that dissociation arises from the defensive exclusion of painful feelings and thoughts, Liotti proposes that dissociation is the direct product of failure to integrate experiences of irresolvable conflict in attachment relationships. In Chapter 12, Carol George, Malcolm West, and Odette Pettem describe the first empirical study in the field to explore attachment disorganization in adults. Their work is based on a new projective measure of adult attachment, the Adult Attachment Projective (AAP), which permits the assessment of mental representations of adult attachment in a form that can be compared directly with measures used with children. Their preliminary data indicate that AAP classifications are consistent with classifications based on the widely used Adult Attachment Interview, and that disorganization at the level of representation in adults shows strong parallels to the same phenomenon in children.

In Chapter 13, Teresa Jacobsen and Laura J. Miller compare the prevalence and the concomitants of organized and disorganized attachments in one of the most extreme, clinical samples investigated to date—mentally ill mothers who have lost custody of their very young children. Their findings suggest that both the child's foster placement experiences and the mother's capacity to appreciate her child as an individual contribute to the development of organized and disorganized child attachment. Furthermore, this work reminds us that removing a child from the mother's care can have an even more potentially dire outcome for the child than disorganized attachment: the failure of the child to experience any form of attachment to the mother at all. In Chapter 14, Robert C. Pianta, Robert S. Marvin, and Maria C. Morog approach disorganization from the perspective of current assaults on the caregiving system. Their findings demonstrate that the birth of a disabled child and the challenges of caring for one can be traumatic to parents, and therefore that such a child is risk for disorganized attachment if the parents are unable to resolve their reactions to the child's diagnosis. The ability of mothers to achieve resolution in these circumstances is independent of whether they have resolved past trauma. Thus, at least in the case of dealing with disability, and perhaps more generally, we can learn more about attachment disorganization by focusing on the mother's current experience of caring for her child than from her state of mind with respect to the past.

It has been both a privilege and a pleasure for us to work with the contributors to this volume—to make the acquaintance of some, and to deepen our collegial relationships with others in the give and take of the editorial and revision process. As editors, we have been fortunate to participate with our colleagues in the kind of dialogue about attachment disorganization that we envisioned 3 years ago when planning for this book began. The process has immensely enriched our own understanding of disorganized attachment. Many other researchers in the field also participated in these early conversations by reviewing, anonymously, the chapters of the contributing authors. We and the other authors are extremely grateful for their efforts and the depth of their commentary. The following individuals generously provided reviews: Lisa Capps, Susan Crockenburg, Judith Crowell, Diana Diamond, Mary Dozier, Judy Garber, Megan Gunnar, Carollee Howes, Russel Isabella, Barbara Ivins, Klaus Minde, Sandra Pipp-Siegel, Vivienne Roseby, Susan Spieker, Mary J. Ward, Malcolm West, Drew Westen, and Donna Weston. Dante Cicchetti, Michael Lynch, Miri Scharf, and Avi Sagi made important contributions to our thinking and this volume, and we would like to acknowledge their efforts here as well.

We also note with sincere gratitude the steady support, proficiency, and publishing wisdom of our editors, artist, publicists, and the staff at The Guilford Press. We have worked most closely with Paul Gordon, Carolyn Graham, Judith Grauman, Rowena Howells, Katherine Lieber, Bob Matloff, William Meyer, Kitty Moore, and Seymour Weingarten, receiving at every step the benefit of their guidance and equanimity. We also thank the many individuals who worked behind the scenes, but whose names we do not know, to whom we are in debt for their professional assistance. The preparation of this book now complete, we extend a warm welcome to the larger community of students, researchers, and mental health professionals to join with us in continuing this important scientific discussion.

JUDITH SOLOMON
CAROL GEORGE

Contents

Attachment Disorganization

PART 1

The Etiology of Attachment Disorganization

CHAPTER 1

The Place of Disorganization in Attachment Theory
Linking Classic Observations with Contemporary Findings

JUDITH SOLOMON
CAROL GEORGE

The identification of the disorganized/disoriented attachment group poses a number of challenges for attachment theory and research. The standard Ainsworth categories (Ainsworth, Blehar, Waters, & Wall, 1978) have behind them a substantial literature attesting to the construct and predictive validity of this straightforward approach to differentiating between secure and two types of insecure attachment relationships (Solomon & George, 1999). Although empirical validation for the new disorganized (D) category is beginning to accumulate (Lyons-Ruth & Jacobvitz, 1999; van IJzendoorn, Schuengel, & Bakermans-Kranenburg, 1999), it lags far behind what is available for the standard Ainsworth system, and many fundamental questions remain unanswered.

There are also important theoretical questions surrounding the phenomenon of attachment disorganization. Every new "discovery" within a field must be examined for its consistency with prevailing theory and knowledge, and for its potential to challenge, extend, or even disqualify theory. The ongoing task of establishing the construct validity of this category addresses this issue in terms of current measurement techniques. The same question must be posed conceptually: Does attachment theory as articulated by Bowlby encompass the phenomenon of attachment disorganization? If this is indeed the case, then the theory can be used to elucidate the phenomenon; in turn, the phenomenon of attachment disorganization can help to elucidate further the theory and even to extend its reach.

In this chapter, we examine attachment disorganization through the lens of Bowlby's attachment theory and the fundamental observations upon which this theory was built. We argue that one of the phenomena of greatest interest to him—the response of infants and children to separation—is the product of disorganization and dysregulation of the attachment system. We also suggest that the explanatory constructs developed by him to understand these responses can elucidate questions regarding both the appearance and the etiology of the disorganized attachment classification more generally.

We begin the chapter with an overview of the core constructs of attachment theory, emphasizing Bowlby's views about the nature and origins of segregated systems of attachment, the mechanism that he believed to be associated with the greatest attachment insecurity, and the adverse conditions that we describe below as "assaults to the attachment system." We next examine the classic observations of the responses of young children to prolonged separation from the primary caregiver and show how these responses both exemplify Bowlby's model of segregated systems and resemble the behaviors that currently define the disorganized attachment group. We go on to consider whether the construct of segregated systems can help us to understand the etiology of disorganized attachment and the quality and organization of attachment and caregiving representations of disorganized children and their mothers. We conclude with some thoughts about the place of disorganization in the study of attachment.

CORE CONSTRUCTS OF BOWLBY'S THEORY OF ATTACHMENT

Looking across the volumes of Bowlby's trilogy (*Attachment*, 1969/1982; *Separation*, 1973; *Loss*, 1980), it can be seen that attachment theory rests on three core constructs: behavioral systems, representational models, and defensive exclusion. All three are required to understand disorganized attachment in depth. In what follows, we briefly review Bowlby's understanding and use of each of these constructs.

The Attachment Behavioral System: A Control Systems Model of Attachment

Bowlby's model of the attachment behavioral system was based on an ethological analyses of behavior in terms of control systems theory (Bowlby, 1969/1982). The attachment system is viewed as an internal goal-correcting system that permits attachment behaviors (i.e., behaviors that promote proximity to the attachment figure) to be organized flexibly around a particular figure. Under certain conditions, the attachment system is activated strongly, leading the child to seek and to be satisfied with nothing less than close proximity to and contact with the attachment figure. These conditions include the *full range* of internal and external stressors or threats, for example, illness, fatigue, strange environments and persons, being alone, and the attachment figure's absence. When conditions are perceived to be nonthreatening, the child is free to pursue other goals and activities, although he or she continues to monitor the environment for possible sources of threat.

Emotion was relegated to a secondary role in Bowlby's model because of his conviction that emotion could not function as a first cause (activator) of attachment behavior. He emphasized, rather, situational cues and the primacy of perceptual or "appraisal" processes (of the self, the environment, and the attachment figure) in the chain of causality. Nevertheless, Bowlby viewed affective and emotional states as having an important place in the organization and expression of attachment. The child's affective states and emotional appraisals are expected to vary in accord with the activation of the attachment system. The absence of external or internal stressors and the accessibility of the attachment figure are associated with a low activation of attachment and with positive affect and feelings of being safe (Bowlby, 1969/1982; Sroufe & Waters, 1977). Activation of the attachment system increases as a function of internal stress or external threat; concomitantly, the individual's emotional state shifts progressively toward increasingly intense negative affect and emotional appraisals of anxiety, alarm, fear, or terror. In addition, when the attachment figure is appraised as inaccessible or unreliable, anger and sadness are also prepotent aspects of the child's affective state.

Representation

Beginning in late infancy, the child's attachment behaviors become increasingly organized at the representational, as well as the behavioral, level. The organization of these systems arises from the child's experiences with the attachment figure, especially experiences concurrent with the activation of the attachment system. Bowlby (1973) proposed that the child builds complementary representations of self and the attachment figure that he termed "internal working models." These models reflect the child's appraisal of, and confidence in, the self as acceptable and worthy of care and protection, and the attachment figure's desire, ability, and availability to provide protection and care. These models, in turn, organize appraisal processes, thought, memory, and feeling with regard to the attachment figure and serve to guide future behavior (Bowlby, 1973; Main, Kaplan, & Cassidy, 1985). Because these processes function largely outside consciousness, internal working models tend to be resistant to change. Bowlby (1980) stressed that under child-rearing conditions in which the child feels lovable and protected (mirrored by representations of the attachment figure as one who will and can provide care), representational models of self and attachment figure are reasonably aligned. Under conditions in which the child feels "unwanted and unlovable" (mirrored by representations of the attachment figure as one who cannot care for or rejects the child), representational models reflect a complex interplay of multiple representations of self and other that are to some degree incompatible and difficult to integrate. This condition results from the child's attempt to avoid negative appraisals of the self and other that might otherwise dominate consciousness and bring emotional pain if they were thought by the child to be accurate or "real" evaluations.

Defensive Exclusion

Bowlby conceived of the attachment system as a homeostatic system, that is, attachment functions to maintain the individual's state within certain limits necessary for overall functioning. Thus, Bowlby conceived of the attachment system as both analogous to and integrated with processes of physiological homeostasis. For the child, the caregiver is the first line of defense against environmental, physiological, and psychological stress of many kinds. Once a bond to this figure has been formed, her actual or threatened loss are, in and of themselves, an inevitable source of stress (and distress) that requires defensive strategies. When attachment behaviors such as searching, calling, and crying persistently fail to regain that figure, the child is forced to marshal defensive strategies that exclude this painful information from consciousness. Bowlby conceived of two qualitatively distinct forms of defensive exclusion—deactivation and disconnection—either of which might be expressed more or less completely.[1]

   Bowlby proposed that defensive exclusion of attachment becomes more or less complete when the child's attachment system and the feelings associated with it are strongly and chronically activated but not assuaged. Under these conditions, which we would term "assaults to the attachment system," the child is faced with the threat of affective, cognitive, and behavioral breakdown. Bowlby termed the defensive processes that emerged under these circumstances "segregated systems," defined as an extreme and potentially pathological form of exclusion that functions to separate attachment information from consciousness. He suggested that both extended separation from the attachment figure, loss, or being punished for the display of attachment behavior and feelings were circumstances in which segregated systems were most likely to develop.

Bowlby likened segregated systems to the psychoanalytic construct of repression. As with repression, although the child might normally be completely unaware of the segregated material, it is not actually lost, as in simple forgetting. Rather, memories and feelings may be evoked by attachment-relevant cues, sometimes quite idiosyncratic ones. The attachment behavior and feelings that emerge when inhibitory or "segregating" processes are circumvented are likely to seem dysregulated, that is, irrational, unpredictable, out of context, and out of control. Following Bowlby's argument then, evidence for the presence of segregated attachment systems derives from (1) the pronounced absence of attachment behavior in circumstances in which it is expected, especially when there is evidence of active suppression or "blocking" of attachment behavior, representation, and related affects such as fear and anger; (2) out-of-context and out-of-control attachment behavior, representation, and affect; or (3) the alternation of these two states.[2]

BEHAVIOR FOLLOWING PROLONGED SEPARATION

As a conscientious and rigorous scientific thinker, Bowlby was determined to derive his theory from a coherent and extensive body of observational data. For him, the "behavior to be explained" came from the detailed observations of children who had experienced major separations from the attachment figure (Bowlby, 1969/1982) and the behavior of children and adults who had lost an attachment or otherwise beloved figure through death. Although all students of attachment understand that the observations of young children who have been separated from their caregivers form the bedrock of attachment theory, extensive study of these observations is now rare. By returning to this source material, however, we may gain a deeper appreciation of Bowlby's inferential process and the theory itself. Equally important for the purpose of evaluating the place of disorganization in attachment theory, we see that the attachment behavior of young children in these circumstances was *disorganized*, in precisely the way we use this term today; that is, their behavior corresponds to Main and Solomon's (1990) criteria for judging a child as disorganized in the strange situation. This permits us to pose the question whether the same or similar mechanisms and conditions that Bowlby proposed to explain the classic separation findings may also be applied to an understanding of the disorganized/disoriented attachment category.

The behavior of toddlers who have been separated for 2 weeks or more falls into two broad categories corresponding to behavior seen directly upon reunion and its immediate aftermath, and behaviors that emerge more slowly after the child has returned home. When the conditions of separation were prolonged and stressful, the behavior observed upon reunion was termed "detached" (Bowlby, 1973) and has been considered by some attachment scholars to be in some ways analogous to the avoidance shown by infants in the strange situation (Main, 1981). Indeed, Ainsworth's familiarity with the separation literature alerted her to the importance of the avoidant and resistant patterns she saw in her early work with the strange situation (Ainsworth & Marvin, 1995). However, there are also important differences between detachment and avoidant behavior.

In the strange situation, avoidant infants are likely to avert their gaze from the mother and keep their distance from her. They are able to orient their attention flexibly to the environment, however, permitting them to play with toys, maintain distance interaction with the mother in the form of looks and smiles, and, often, within 2 minutes of reunion, to initiate interaction with her. Young children who have experienced separation of 1 or 2 weeks duration under highly supportive conditions, such as those provided by James and Joyce Robertson in their pioneering studies (Robertson & Robertson, 1989b), are also likely on first seeing the mother to engage very briefly in gaze aversion or redirection of their attention to the physical environment. This is usually followed by approach to the mother (e.g., as seen in the case of "Thomas"; Robertson & Robertson, 1990). Main (1981) has argued persuasively that this visual cutoff behavior is homologous to that shown by other vertebrates in approach–avoidance situations. As in other species, gaze aversion that is followed by "displacement" activities such as manipulation of objects in the environment is made possible by a shift of attention away from the source of conflict, that is, selective attention (Hinde, 1970). This behavior permits the organism to modulate arousal and to resolve conflicting behavioral tendencies. Brief cutoff behavior at the moment of reunion is a nearly ubiquitous feature of the early moments of reunion of infants in the strange situation, whatever their classification (A, B, or C). In the case of infants classified as avoidant, the conflict is resolved, temporarily, in favor of behavioral avoidance and attention to the environment. In the case of secure and ambivalent infants, the behavioral conflict is resolved in favor of attachment behavior or displays of anger toward the mother. Within Bowlby's framework, cutoff behavior, or gaze aversion, whether or not it is followed by more extensive avoidance of the mother, is one type of deactivating or inhibiting mechanism. To the extent that it results in only temporary withdrawal and is followed by organized and adaptive behavior (engagement with the environment or the mother), its appearance would not, in and of itself, be considered evidence of disorganization or segregated systems.

In contrast, when young children have been separated from primary caregivers for several weeks under adverse conditions, disturbances in reunion behavior go beyond brief moments of avoidance. Reunion behavior under these circumstances reveals profound disorientation to the current environment, a pervasive suppression of affect and behavior directed toward the mother, or conflicted variants of these states. The child's behavior is likely to seem extremely passive, disconnected, and bewildered. As noted by Heinicke and Westheimer (1965), and summarized by Bowlby (1973), the pervasiveness and persistence of this detached state is strongly linked to the length of the separation itself. This is revealed, for example, in Heinicke and Westheimer's description of Owen, a 30-month-old, who was separated from his mother for 4 months:

> Owen's sister, Sheila, who had been kept out of the way for twenty minutes or so to give him time to readjust, now rushed into the room full of happy anticipation. She called "Hello, Owen" and went to him. But Owen, who had till then been completely still in his chair, turned his head away from her. Passively he accepted her present of a toy bus. Sheila looked unhappy and bewildered. In a puzzled way she reiterated, "It's not Owen's face. It's a different face." (p. 141)

Family members often interpret this behavior as the child's failure to recognize the mother. In Owen's case, his behavior and affect were clearly so dampened and peculiar that his sister could not "recognize" him. Indeed, he seems almost to be in a trance-like or dissociated state. In many cases, the separated children clearly recognize other family members, suggesting that "forgetting" is selective. Furthermore, they certainly do not treat the mother as a stranger, that is, with casual interest and affiliative behavior. Considering these factors together, the inhibition of attachment behavior appears as if it is being maintained by a more active process than simple deterioration of memory. The quality of this inhibition differs from the simple avoidance described earlier in that the gating mechanism does not appear to be simply at the level of the receptors or of selective attention: Children in this state look but do not seem to "see" the mother. This suggests that additional, more profound exclusion processes have been enlisted, processes such as the defensive segregation of attachment-related material.

When separations have been briefer, the reunion behavior of young children may be aptly described as a behavioral combination of deactivating or inhibiting behaviors with attachment behaviors. The results of these combinations are, on the surface, incoherent and contradictory. They strongly resemble well-known types of conflict behavior observed in a variety of vertebrate species in approach–avoidance situations, but the exact nature of this conflict is not clear from the behavior itself. This is exemplified in the following two observations of children who had experienced prolonged separation. Laura, 33 months, upon reunion with her mother following the second of two long separations, ran with eager anticipation to the door of her house calling, "Mummy, Mummy." But when her mother appeared at the door, Laura abruptly went blank and seemed not to recognize her (Robertson & Bowlby, as cited in Heinicke & Westheimer, 1965, p. 283). Gillian, 19 months, initially rejected her mother quite pointedly on reunion (she refused to take her hand or to look at her), then broke into intense sobbing. Afterwards, "she lay across her mother's shoulder, still and motionless, with eyes brimming with tears and face averted from her mother. Indeed only once during the whole journey did she look at her mother" (Heinicke & Westheimer, 1965, p. 217). Behavioral sequences identical to these are "pathognomic" indicators for disorganized attachment in the Main and Solomon guidelines (1990, Appendix I) for identifying disorganized behavior. When compared to the more blanket inhibition shown by Owen, they are readily interpreted as indications of partial or incomplete deactivating or inhibitory processes through which attachment behavior has "broken through" or been simultaneously elicited.

Both at reunion and for sometime thereafter, separated children mix angry resistance to the mother with contact-maintaining behaviors. Somewhat later, such children are prone to show directly provocative and hostile behavior toward the mother as well. As with the insecure–avoidant patterns, Ainsworth's knowledge of this resistance to contact undoubtedly alerted her to similar behaviors shown by ambivalent children in the strange situation. Unlike the behavior of the ambivalent infant in the strange situation, however, separated children mixed distress and strong resistance or tantrum behavior with prolonged gaze aversion and efforts to run away from the mother. Our own observations of the Robertson's film of John's reunion (age 17 months) reveal that he alternated repeatedly between apparent attempts to flee from the mother (into the arms of other adults in the room), brief, close contact with the mother, during which he seemed almost to fall asleep, and strong tantrum behavior. When his father entered, he began to struggle away from mother, but rather than signaling clearly to his father for contact, John slumped limply over the arm of mother's chair like a rag doll (Robertson & Robertson, 1989a). The behaviors that emerge as delayed sequelae to detachment take the form of sudden, out-of-context, angry, provocative, or defiant behavior toward the mother, often mixed with approach, contact behaviors, or avoidance. For example, 6 days after reunion Dawn, 18 months, stomped her foot angrily at her mother for control of a sticky spoon. She was easily distracted, however, and "climbed over mother's lap in an affectionate way. Mother gladly put up with this until Dawn, for no apparent reason, smacked her" (Heinicke & Westheimer, 1965, p. 104).

We have seen quite similar patterns in our sample of infants who have undergone repeated separation from mother in divorcing families. Depending upon the particular behavior elements shown, infants who behaved like this were categorized as disorganized or unclassifiable (Solomon & George, 1999, and Chapter 9, this volume). More important for the present discussion, identical patterns of behavior are indices of attachment disorganization in the strange situation (Main & Solomon, 1990). These indices include (1) freezing, stilling, and slowed movements and expressions (e.g., Owen); (2) sequential display of contradictory behavior patterns (e.g., Laura); (3) simultaneous display of contradictory behavior patterns (e.g., Gillian); and (4) undirected, misdirected, incomplete, or interrupted movements and expressions (e.g., John, Dawn).

The parallels in the behavior of young children who have experienced prolonged separation and some children classified as disorganized in the strange situation demonstrate, at a minimum, that disorganization of attachment behavior in the latter context, although outwardly "strange" and "inexplicable" in terms of Ainsworth's classification criteria, was entirely familiar to early observers of attachment phenomena. Neither these observers nor Bowlby himself differentiated what we would now call disorganized behavior from other more coherent patterns. It is clear in retrospect, however, that it was *disorganized* attachment behavior, rather than the "organized" behavioral strategies of children judged insecure (avoidant and ambivalent) by Ainsworth's criteria that provided the strongest justification for Bowlby's theory.

Can the classic observations of children's behavior following separation clarify the meaning of disorganized attachment behavior in the strange situation? The answer to this question obviously will depend strongly on the information available to us about the child's experiences with his or her attachment figure, a topic we consider in the following section.

ANTECEDENT CONDITIONS FOR THE D CLASSIFICATION: FAILURE TO TERMINATE ATTACHMENT?

Although disorganized attachment classifications may sometimes be associated with the child's experience of prolonged or repeated separation from the caregiver (Chisolm, 1998; Solomon & George, 1999 and Chapter 9, this volume; Jacobsen & Miller, Chapter 13, this volume), there is no reason to believe that separations are a sole or necessary cause of this behavior. This raises the question of whether there are significant parallels in the experiences of separated children and other children who are assigned to the D category, and whether experiences that do not involve separation may also be understood in terms of the construct of segregated systems.

We have seen that for Bowlby, the underlying cause of segregated systems was failure to terminate strong or chronic activation of the attachment system; that is, activation was not followed by contact with, or reassurance by, the attachment figure. Whereas prolonged separation under adverse circumstances is clearly one circumstance that may result in failure to terminate attachment, Bowlby outlined others that might have a similar result. Foremost among these were strong parental rejection of the child's attachment behavior, and direct and implied threats to abandon or send the child away. These situations were viewed as potentially causing intense pain and suffering, because the parent's behavior both strongly activated the attachment system and prevented the child from achieving resolution. In the case of strong rejection, the child's attachment behavior is the very thing being rejected. In the case of the parent's threats to abandon or withdraw from the child, Bowlby proposed that both anxiety (fear) and anger are segregated because their display would likely alienate the attachment figure still further.

How well does Bowlby's formulation correspond to what is currently known about the etiology of the D classification? It has been established that the highest proportions of disorganized attachments (approximately 80%) are to be found in maltreatment samples (Carlson, Cicchetti, Barnett, & Braunwald, 1989). Disorganized attachment is also more common in samples of depressed and alcoholic mothers (DeMulder & Radke-Yarrow, 1991; Lyons-Ruth, Connell, Grunebaum, & Botein, 1990; O'Connor, Sigman, & Brill,1987; Teti, Gelfand, & Isabella, 1995), and in families with high marital conflict (Owen & Cox, 1997; Solomon & George, 1999). Bowlby (1973, 1980) specifically highlighted family alcoholism, depression, and marital conflict as predisposing factors for strong parenal rejection and threats to abandon the child. Although, surprisingly, he made no direct reference to physical and sexual abuse in his original work, abuse is easily accommodated by his hypothesis.

Currently, the major hypothesis advanced to account for disorganized attachment relationships is consistent with Bowlby's approach. Main and Hesse (1990) proposed that the disorganized/disoriented classification reflects the infant's experience of the parent as frightening or frightened. Because any cause for alarm will activate the attachment system, the child is compelled both to approach and withdraw from the same figure; thus, termination of the attachment system cannot be achieved. The frightening or frightened attachment figure is an inherently paradoxical stimulus, and Main and Hesse have proposed that the infant's unresolved (unresolvable) conflict is reflected in the conflict behavior that is at the core of most indices of disorganization. This hypothesis also easily encompasses the empirical association between disorganized attachment classifications and maltreatment, alcoholism, and some types of psychological disorder. It should be noted, however, that Bowlby's hypothesis is more general than that of Main and Hesse, since, in theory, segregated systems may arise in *any circumstance* in which the activation of the attachment system (e.g., illness, neglect) characteristically is not followed by clear resolution.

A problem for both Bowlby's and Main and Hesse's hypotheses is the fact that disorganized attachments, although most prevalent in high-risk samples, also occur in normative samples in which the mother appears to be functioning well psychologically and is also well disposed toward the infant or child (approximately 15% infants in middle-class samples are classified as disorganized). Indeed, home observations of maternal behavior in middle-class samples indicate that there is little that distinguishes these mothers from mothers of secure, avoidant, or ambivalent children (Spangler, Fremmer-Bombik, & Grossmann, 1996; Solomon, George, & Silverman, in press; Stevenson-Hinde & Shouldice, 1995). Based on close observations of mothers in the laboratory, Main and Hesse emphasize that the interactive behaviors leading to disorganization of attachment may be quite subtle and/or covert (Main & Hesse, 1990; Hesse & Main, in press). They suggest that some of these behaviors may be directly frightening (e.g., sudden looming into the infant's face, movements and postures that seem to be part of a pursuit–hunt sequence), others may arise from the mother's fear of the infant (e.g., parent moves hand away suddenly as if fearful of being hurt, flinching for no apparent reason), and still others may be sufficiently disturbing or inexplicable to frighten and, therefore, "disorganize" the infant (e.g., appearing to enter a trance-like state, unusual vocal patterns, such as simultaneously voicing and devoicing intonations).

Home and laboratory observation of mother–child interactions using the coding system that Main and Hesse developed to identify "frightened–frightening" behaviors provide some support for this view. Schuengel, Bakermans-Kranenburg, and van IJzendoorn (1999—middle-class mothers in their homes) and Lyons-Ruth, Bronfman, and Parsons (in press—high-risk mothers in the strange situation) found that mothers of infants who were classified as disorganized were significantly higher than mothers of organized A, B, or C infants in the intensity or frequency of "frightened–frightening" behavior. In the Schuengel et al. study, however, the overall effect was rather modest (see also Schuengel, Bakermans-Kranenburg, van IJzendoorn, & Blom, Chapter 3, this volume). In the Lyons-Ruth et al. study, "frightening" maternal behavior was associated with disorganization only if the infant's alternative (forced) classification was insecure (A). Maternal "frightening" behavior was not associated with disorganization if the child's alternative classification was secure, but mothers of infants in this group (D, alternate B) tended to behave in an inhibited or frightened manner. In both of these studies, however, the association between disorganization and "frightening–frightened" maternal behavior was attenuated by the fact that some mothers of D infants showed none of these behaviors and some mothers of organized infants sometimes did (see also Lyons-Ruth, Bronfman, & Atwood, Chapter 2, this volume).

Following Bowlby, we propose that one source of "noise" in these findings may arise from a failure to take into consideration the context in which "frightening–frightened" behaviors occurs. A key feature of this context should be whether or not the attachment figure engages in reparative behavior once she has, intentionally or inadvertently, frightened or distressed the child. The role of reparative behavior is implied in Main and Hesse's formulation, but this crucial interactive feature has previously not been incorporated into tests of the "frightened–frightening" hypothesis. Many mothers behave in ways that are alarming or even frightening to their young children, especially when they are annoyed, angered, distressed, or frightened. If the infant's or child's distress is modulated or reasonably quickly followed by maternal reassurance and reparation, the child's security is unlikely to be shaken; indeed, both the relationship and the infant's capacity for affect regulation may be strengthened (Birengen, Emde, & Pipp-Siegel, 1997; Tronick, 1989). Thus, mothers of disorganized children may be distinguished from mothers whose children's attachment behaviors are organized by their failure to correct or repair their errors as much as by the "errors" themselves. What may be most important is that mothers of disorganized children fail to "terminate" the attachment system.

Elsewhere, we have conceptualized this "failure to terminate" as an aspect of maternal abdication of caregiving (George & Solomon, 1999; Solomon & George, in press-b). Lyons-Ruth and her colleagues have also suggested that subtle or covert frightening or frightened behavior among D mothers is embedded in a more general maternal failure to respond to the infant's attachment signals or providing conflicting signals in response to them (see also Lyons-Ruth et al., Chapter 2, this volume). Paralleling our views, she has suggested that this behavior, whether or not it is inherently threatening or alarming, amounts to a failure to repair the relationship under stress.

To this point, we have highlighted the parallels in the experience of separated children and those classified as disorganized in the strange situation. Two fundamental and related questions remain that cannot be resolved given the present state of our knowledge. First, is strong activation of attachment a necessary condition for disorganization of attachment behavior in all contexts? Young children are clearly intensely distressed during prolonged separations in unfamiliar environments. These circumstances activate the attachment system strongly; by definition, the system cannot be terminated and the child's distress cannot be fully assuaged. The power of prolonged separation to elicit profound and severe defensive processes is apparent. To invoke the same or a similar mechanism as an explanation for disorganized attachment relationships in general, however, implies that D infants chronically or intermittently experience strong activation of attachment and intense distress, anxiety, or fear that are not terminated by the attachment figure. If strong activation of attachment is necessary, we may pose a second question: are the subtle and covert maternal behaviors that have been proposed by Main and Hesse as sources of fear or alarm sufficiently distressing in themselves to disorganize attachment behavior? Perhaps such behaviors, instead, are behavioral symptoms and concomitants that are related to the mother's tendency truly to frighten and fail to reassure the child when she is not being observed. The experience of the typical D infant may differ from the separated infant not just in the intensity of the "assault" to the attachment system; it may be chronically deficient. In this regard, Lyons-Ruth has noted that when a mother characteristically fails to repair the relationship (i.e., respond coherently to the infant's clear attachment signals) the infant cannot *develop* an organized or coherent attachment strategy in the first place (see also Waters & Valenzuela, Chapter 10, this volume).

In contrast to the "failure to terminate" hypothesis outlined earlier, Main and Hesse (1990; Hesse & Main, in press) have extrapolated backward from the immediate or concurrent effects of conflict on behavioral organization to long-standing etiological conditions. The emphasis here is on the infant's perception of the parent as simultaneously a source of alarm and safety, and the consequences this may have for a "collapse" of behavioral strategy and attention. This collapse of attention is believed to be the cause for behaviors sometimes seen in infants classified into group D, such as interrupted, undirected, or incomplete attachment behaviors, or dazed and "trance" behavior (which may be loosely described on the phenotypic level as "dissociated"). This perspective rests heavily on the influence of inherently conflicting or paradoxical information for cognitive processing; that is, the mother as a source of conflict cannot be assimilated cognitively and, therefore, attention and behavior cannot be integrated into coherent, goal-oriented patterns. Evidence of the power of cognitive conflict or confusion to disorganize behavior and thought can be found in both the clinical and developmental literatures (Haley, 1973; Hirshberg, 1990). Mildly frightening, frightened, or "inexplicable" behavior may thus be sufficient as immediate causes of disorganized attachment patterns, even if these behaviors are not particularly arousing. Whether such maternal behavior is also sufficient to compromise seriously the infant's sense of felt security and constitute a developmental risk factor is less certain.

There is obviously some overlap between the "failure to terminate" hypothesis we have articulated here and Main and Hesse's "conflict" hypothesis. Based on observations of mother–child interaction available at this time, it appears that either experience can evoke approach–avoidance conflict behavior.[3] In the following section, we present data on disorganized children and their mothers that allow us to examine these two hypotheses at the level of representation.

MENTAL REPRESENTATIONS OF ATTACHMENT AND CAREGIVING IN DISORGANIZED RELATIONSHIPS

According to Bowlby's view of the conditions that lead to the development of segregated systems, the disorganized infant or child is likely to experience him- or herself as both frightened or vulnerable, and without recourse or remedy, that is, as *helpless*.[4] Because, according to attachment theory, behavioral systems are inextricably tied to mental representation, these experiences should be reflected in the disorganized child's mental representation of *him- or herself* as vulnerable and helpless in the face of frightening events and the *attachment figure* as failing to provide protection and reassurance. Furthermore, mental representations of attachment should reflect severe forms of defensive exclusion, specifically, strong inhibition of attachment-related information or evidence of dysregulated (out-of-control) representational processes. Finally, given the reciprocal relation between attachment and caregiving, one would expect a high degree of complementary between the mother's and the child's representation of their mutual relationship (George & Solomon, 1996, 1999; Solomon & George, 1996; in press-b).

Over the last decade, we have undertaken a set of studies designed to investigate the nature of mothers' and children's mental representations of their mutual relationship (George & Solomon, 1989, 1996, 1998; Solomon, George, & De Jong, 1995). A central focus of much of this research has been on disorganized/controlling attachment in kindergarten-age children. We remind the reader that "controlling" was added to the designation of disorganization in this age group because this form of reunion behavior was shown by many children who had received the D classification in infancy (Main & Cassidy, 1988). To assess children's representations, we engaged the children in doll play, asking them to enact the endings to four attachment-related story stems. This procedure built upon representational assessments developed by Kaplan (Main et al., 1985) and Bretherton (Bretherton, Ridgeway, & Cassidy, 1990). Mothers were administered a semistructured, hour-long interview adapted from the work of Aber and Slade (Aber, Slade, Berger, Bresgi, & Kaplan, 1985) that asks the mother to provide detailed descriptions of her interaction with the child and her appraisals of those interactions both in everyday and exceptional circumstances. Using these measures, we have found that the attachment representations of disorganized/controlling children are qualitatively distinct from those of children classified into organized attachment groups (A, B, C). Similarly, the caregiving representations of the mothers of these children are also distinct from those of other mothers. What emerges when one compares children's play and mothers' reports is a picture of a relationship that is characterized by mutual feelings of helplessness and clear evidence of segregated or dysregulated representational processes in both mother and child (Solomon, 1998). Furthermore, analysis of mothers' representations as related to infant attachment parallel the patterns seen in the older sample (Solomon & George, in press-a).

The stories of children judged to be disorganized/controlling are of two distinct types. The first kind is characterized by the depiction of chaotic, frightening events leading to a separation, and often disintegration, of the family, as shown in the following excerpt:

> "And see, and then, you know what happens? Their whole house blows up. See. . . . They get destroyed and not even their bones are left. Nobody can even get their bones. Look. I'm jumping on a rock. This rock feels rocky. Aahh! Guess what? The hills are alive, the hills are shakin' and shakin'. Because the hills are alive. Uh huh. The hills are alive. Ohh! I fall smack off a hill. And got blowed up in an explosion. And then the rocks tumbled down and smashed everyone. And they all died."

In contrast, in the second kind of story, the child's helplessness is not depicted directly. Instead, the child demonstrates a startling absence and marked inhibition of play. It is as if the child is struggling to "flee" mentally from the situation as quickly as possible. As one child began,

> "Well, um of course something happens . . . but I can't show you because there's about a zillion different things that could . . . they're all . . . they're all good things to do with it, but I just, I can't do it. I don't know, I don't know what to pick. . . . "

We note that this mental struggle is usually accompanied by the child's attempts to avoid touching the doll play materials or remove him- or herself from the immediate vicinity of the doll house (e.g., scooting the chair back; sitting on hands; George & Solomon, 1998). Thus, in these types of stories, the child's attempts to inhibit play are intense.

At the level of content, the frightening and explosively angry themes depicted by many of the disorganized/controlling children are consistent with Bowlby's (1973) emphasis on the "dysfunctional" rage and immobiliz-

ing fear that would result when the attachment system was strongly activated but not assuaged. They are also consistent with Main and Hesse's
(1990) hypothesis that fear lies at the root of disorganization.

Disorganized/controlling children not only create stories in which
they are helpless to control the events around them, but they also reveal
themselves to be *helpless to control their own narratives*; that is, the discourse
features of their stories also suggest a quality of disorganization of representational process. These processes are consistent with what would be
expected for segregated representational systems, key aspects of which
include mental states that are actively and profoundly inhibiting, explosive
or out-of-control, or an alternation between the two extremes.These qualities are revealed in several different ways. First, children who create the
overtly chaotic stories appear to be *driven* to create their stories in a particular way, unable to control the final product. We have described these children as flooded by attachment-related affect and images. Disasters are literally explosive. Evil people, monsters, and witches arise suddenly, out of
nowhere, are vanquished, only to rise again and again. This nightmare
quality of the stories, especially the sudden and inexplicable transforma-
tions of commonplace characters into fantastical ones, is strongly reminiscent of dream material. This suggests that the doll play is relatively unpro-
cessed by higher cognitive integrative mechanisms, an impression that is
strengthened by the fact that some children abruptly stop the story to give
the administrator a more "rational" explanation of events, as though suddenly aware of the disturbing content of the stories.

In contrast, the inhibited type of stories seem to reflect a massive constriction of thought and, therefore, narrative. This profound and obviously
inflexible strategy may be the only option available to prevent these children from being flooded by unacceptable content. Some children say they
cannot think. Although this may simply be behavioral resistance, they
appear to be describing what is literally true. Again, looking more broadly
at their behavior, including nonverbal cues, their minds have appeared to
go quite blank in the moment.

Consistent with Bowlby's view of the processes revealed by segregated
systems, many children show a mixture of "flooded" and "constricted" processes. The majority of controlling children, even those whose stories are
flooded by fearful content, also become constricted in their thinking and,
like the globally inhibited children, try to quit the task or ask for an "easier" assignment. On the other hand, when a few of the inhibited children
finally gave in to friendly pressure from the task administrator or were sur-
prised by an untoward event, they produced frightening content identical
to that of the more flooded children (George & Solomon, 1998; Solomon
et al., 1995).

Turning now to the interviews with the mothers, they also describe themselves as helpless, in the sense of feeling themselves to be without strategies. When in this state, mothers are prone to abdicate care for the child, that is, they fail to provide caregiving that will terminate the child's attachment system. Maternal helplessness is revealed in two different kinds of caregiving themes. The first theme, one that on the surface is most obviously linked to abdication of care, is exemplified by the mother's explicit evaluation of herself as unable to manage the child, the situation, or her own behavior. Correlatively, the child is described as out of control, wild, unruly, or unmanageable. Significantly, neither mother nor child is able truly to resolve or extricate themselves from the conflict that arises in their relationship, resulting in the psychological defeat of one or both of them. This type of thinking is exemplified in the following interview excerpt:

> "She was going on a field trip and I needed to have her there by 11:30 . . . and I was on a really tight schedule . . . and 'Child' ran into the house and locked every door and locked everyone out and then sat there at the door and laughed and I lost it. I got in there and I know I whipped her more than she knew she needed to be whipped but I have never been so angry in my whole life. . . . "

The second theme is one of exceptional psychological closeness or merging between mother and child, with an emphasis on the child's special or precocious qualities. From these descriptions, it becomes clear during the interview that the mother believes her protection or control of the child is unnecessary. In some instances, this is exemplified by descriptions of the child as taking responsibility for the mother's emotions, for example, "cheering up" the mother or acting as a comedian or clown. Even though these relationships do not appear to be hostile or confrontational, the mother has still abdicated her role as caregiver; that is, she is not in the position of being the "older and wiser" figure, a role that Bowlby (1988) viewed as critical to attachment. In the following excerpt, merging and, therefore, abdication are revealed in the mother's choice of the words "close" and "funny" when she was asked to select specific words to describe her relationship with her child:

> " . . . the first one close because I feel . . . real physically . . . I mean we're really close, um, if not touching then, um . . . it's just . . . I don't know . . . with 'Child' . . . it's um . . . I feel . . . him in my space . . . and I think he does too, it's like a thing . . . I might just sort of put my hand out and suddenly he's holding my hand or . . . he . . . without looking. Sometimes, I just feel a very physical closeness with him.

Funny 'cause it's like . . . he's not always funny. I don't mean he's always cracking jokes, but he makes me smile."

These two distinctive themes frequently appear in the same interview, paralleling the joint occurrence of both flooded and constricted (inhibited) markers in the doll play of the children. Generally, however, we find that the predominance of the first theme is associated with punitive-type controlling child attachment, while the predominance of the second is associated with caregiving-type controlling child attachment (George & Solomon, 1998).[5] We have suggested elsewhere (George & Solomon, 1999; Solomon & George, 1996) that the child's experience of either kind of abdication is likely to evoke a feeling of being unprotected, vulnerable, or frightened.

Interviews with mothers in this group provide ample evidence both for Main and Hesse's frightened–frightening hypothesis and the more general proposition we have emphasized, that mothers of disorganized or controlling children are likely both to elicit attachment behavior and affect in their children and fail to "terminate" it. Marked rejection of the child is evident in the way some mothers describe themselves in these interviews as frequently or chronically punitive. Other mothers describe incidents in which they abandon the child to intense distress and fear, a state for which the mother is often directly or indirectly the cause. Below we provide several examples of the incidents or events described by the mothers (drawn from separate cases) to give readers a feel for the range of the phenomena. The first excerpt is taken from the interview of a mother of a punitive–controlling kindergarten child whose alternate (forced) classification was secure:

"If they're running around the department store and they slip and fall on their face or hurt their knee or something, I'll just say, 'Don't come to me with your problems. I said you shouldn't of been playing like that in the first place and . . . and I have no sympathy for you.' "[6]

The next excerpts are taken from the interviews of mothers of caregiving–controlling kindergarten children whose alternate classifications were ambivalent and secure, respectively:

"Her hamster [died] . . . she wanted 'Hamster' back now and that she was going to see him. . . . So . . . I showed her a dead skunk in the road . . . and I said . . . this is what dead is. And if this happens to you, you'll never come back."

" . . . he wasn't getting his teeth brushed and he was complaining, he wanted company brushing his teeth. . . . Finally it just snapped . . . I

just say, 'This is it. I can't take it! "Child"!' . . . and then I end up just
. . . out of proportion. . . . And I got mad so fast. . . . [Interviewer: So
how would you say you handle your angry feelings?] I have to leave
. . . 'cause I know I'm just gonna . . . it's not gonna help."

The final excerpt is taken from the interview of a mother of a disorganized 18-month-old infant whose alternate classification was avoidant:

"When I would get 'Baby' back from his Dad . . . he was incredibly
fussy and I couldn't handle it. . . . I remember just leaving 'Baby' in
his room for a while and I'd shut the door and [say] 'Fine.' "

There are three points to be noted about these examples relating to
our earlier discussion about whether mothers of D children are definitely
or only subtly alarming to their children. First, among mothers who
described the details of their experiences with their children, all presented
incidents quite similar to those we have excerpted. By mothers' own admis-
sion, these incidents represent common events in the relationship. Second,
in our view, there is nothing particularly subtle or ambiguous about the
mothers' frightening behavior, strong rejection, or abandonment of the
child. Third, in none of these incidents do mothers describe reparations of
their relationship with their child; in some instances, mothers describe
conscious decisions on their part not to repair the situation. The failure to
repair is another clear, unambiguous source of alarm for the child. We note
that there is no indication in our samples that these relationships are tech-
nically abusive.

These interactive episodes may well be embedded in a broader context
of more subtly hostile, frightened, or "inexplicable" behavior, such as that
reported by other investigators (Lyons-Ruth et al., in press, Lyons-Ruth &
Jacobvitz, 1999; Lyons-Ruth et al., Chapter 2, this volume; Main & Hesse,
1990; Schuengel et al., 1998; Schuengel et al., Chapter 3, this volume). Nevertheless, we believe that the mothers' descriptions of their behavior when
they and their children are highly aroused become defining moments in
the relationship. As such, they are sufficient cause for the disorganization
of attachment in infancy and for the later development of controlling
behavior.

Although mothers are frank in the course of the interviews about the
common crises in the relationship with their children, they are unlikely to
succumb to these states in the presence of observers. Furthermore, many
structured observation situations are not sufficiently challenging to evoke
these out-of-control states in either mother or child (but see Jacobvitz &
Hazen, Chapter 5, this volume; Solomon & George, Chapter 9, this volume). Based on the evidence from the interviews, then, we suggest that

what most observers using microanalytic techniques have identified as frightening behavior, and the like, reflects leakage of mothers' dysregulated feelings of anger and helplessness toward the child. These behaviors may be symptomatic of mothers' difficulties with the modulation and integration of thoughts and feelings about the relationship but are not necessarily causal in themselves.

This leads us to our final point about the maternal interviews: The vignettes reveal something of the mothers' defensive processing of caregiving-related events. Paralleling what we have seen in the children's doll play, mothers describe themselves as alternately out of control, rigidly controlling distress and arousal, or alternating between these strategies (see also George, West, & Pettem, Chapter 12, this volume). Just as their children do in doll play, all of the mothers describe incidents of intense, sudden, and inexplicable emotion with respect to the child. At these times, they experience themselves as helpless to regulate their internal experience or to select appropriate strategies for containing or reassuring the child.

Notably, our recent analyses of the interviews show that mothers of children who are constricted in doll play also reveal tendencies toward constriction, reporting that they are literally compelled to walk away from the child, shut the child away, or psychologically abandon the child in order to maintain fragile control over their own behavior. Paradoxically, in their attempt to protect the child, they threaten him with abandonment by leaving in the "heat of the fray." These behaviors require the child to inhibit strongly his or her own very intense affect in order to be permitted to approach the mother once again. They are associated with "caregiving–controlling" attachment classifications (George & Solomon, 1999; Solomon et al., 1995).

We have also found that mothers whose children are flooded in doll play fail completely to protect the child from their anger. They reveal tendencies to be flooded by emotion themselves, reporting confrontation, screaming, throwing objects, and no hesitancy at all to "take on" the child. These mothers model hostility and confrontation as a response to conflict in the relationship. Their children, who tend to be classified as "punitive" controlling, in turn, use their own anger to capture the mother's attention and control her behavior.

CONCLUSIONS

Our purpose in this chapter has been to explore the links between Bowlby's theory of attachment and the phenomenon of attachment disorganization. We have presented three sets of ideas:

1. *The observations upon which attachment theory was founded–the behavior of young children following prolonged separation–reflect disorganization of attachment behavior rather than avoidance or resistance as defined in Ainsworth's standard classification system.* This insight places the phenomenon of attachment disorganization in historical perspective, permitting us to see it as central to a complete understanding of attachment relationships. The disorganized and disoriented behaviors noted in the classic observations of the reunion behavior of separated toddlers overlap with several (but not all) of the categories of indices presently used to identify disorganized attachments in the strange situation (Main & Solomon, 1990), including (a) behavioral stilling and slowed movements; (b) undirected, misdirected, incomplete, and interrupted movements; (c) simultaneous display of contradictory behavior patterns; and (d) sequential display of contradictory behavior patterns. Similarities in behavior cannot, in themselves, be taken as evidence for similarities in etiology or mechanisms. Nevertheless, we have suggested, for heuristic reasons, that Bowlby's construct of segregated systems and his view of the antecedent conditions that give rise to them may elucidate behavior and representational processes of infants and children classified as disorganized upon reunion with that figure.

2. *Disorganized attachment behavior and representations may reflect "segregated systems," that is, a profound failure to integrate attachment-related behavior, feelings, and thoughts.* Bowlby used the construct of segregated systems to describe the severest form of defensive exclusion of information, a mental process by which painful and distressing feelings associated with attachment are maintained outside of awareness. He proposed that the presence of segregated systems could be inferred from (a) the marked absence of attachment behavior in situations in which it would be expected, along with evidence of attempts to "block" stimuli that might activate the attachment system from awareness; (b) the appearance of dysregulated, that is, out-of-context and out-of-control behavior, affect, and thought; or (c) alternations (combinations) of these extremes. We have argued that all three of these indices can be discerned in the behavior of children who have experienced prolonged and/or distressing separations, and in the behavior of children classified as disorganized in the strange situation, as described earlier. They can also be observed in the symbolic representations of attachment situations shown by kindergarten-age children classified as controlling or disorganized during laboratory reunions with the mother. Such children are unable to construct attachment narratives, are flooded by frightening and chaotic images and affect, or show combinations of these extremes. Finally, the mothers of such children describe similar dichotomous states and vacillations between them in their *own* behavior and feelings toward the child in the home, including overwhelming states of rage

and helplessness toward the child, marked physical withdrawal from the child, and combinations of these.

3. *Disorganized children may experience a chronic failure on the part of the caregiver to terminate the attachment system and to assuage attachment-related fear and distress.* Bowlby proposed that segregated systems arise in three sets of circumstances—separation from or loss of the attachment figure, or the threat of these, in the form of strong parental rejection of attachment behavior and threats to abandon the child. Although the disorganized classification has been associated in some cases with difficult separation experiences, we have suggested that in the majority of cases, the infant's or child's experience has been more similar to the last condition, threats of separation. Our analysis of mothers' interviews suggest that these mothers are capable of (1) exacerbating the child's attachment-related anxieties and fears by rejecting or frightening the child at the very moment when the child is distressed and in need of consolation, and (2) simultaneously activating the child's attachment system with threatening or angry behavior followed by rejection or withdrawal. These conditions prevent the infant from developing an organized attachment strategy and subject the child to an extreme state of fear that overwhelms his or her capacity for flexible defense, affect regulation, and adaptation. We propose that these conditions exist, in the extreme, in maltreating families, where disorganized attachments are most prevalent, but are also evident, in attenuated form, in normative, middle-class families in which the infant or child has been classified as disorganized or controlling.

Bowlby's model is consistent in many ways with Main and Hesse's hypothesis that the disorganized child has been frightened by overtly or covertly threatening, alarming, or confusing behavior on the part of the caregiver. It directs our attention somewhat differently, however. Whereas Main and Hesse have emphasized the role of cognitive conflict and confusion in the organization of attachment behavior, Bowlby's approach leads us to focus on the quality of the mother's response to strong activation of the child's attachment system and the powerful emotions that are evoked. It suggests that, with regard to disorganization, what is most important is the mother's capacity to assuage and repair versus heighten or even precipitate the child's distress. Ultimately, both views may be necessary for a full understanding of the developmental and immediate causation of disorganized attachment behavior.

What are the implications of our analysis of attachment disorganization for the study of attachment? Bowlby developed attachment theory as an alternative to the contemporary psychoanalytic models of his day to explain the development of behavior that was rooted in extreme forms of relationship-based anxiety. The phenomena of interest included the

responses of young children, adolescents, and adults to experiences of prolonged separation, threats of separation, and loss. These responses
included a range of psychological symptoms previously attributed to
overdependency and regression, and include chronic anxieties, phobias,
depression, rage, chronic mourning, and manifestations of the absence or
suppression of these states in the form of psychological detachment, denial
of personal vulnerability, and failure to mourn.

As a clinician, Bowlby was naturally interested in the more pathogenic
or extreme manifestations of attachment insecurity. Furthermore, at the
time he began to construct his theory, the normative information available
to him was sparse and largely couched in terms of the psychoanalytic and
behaviorist models he hoped to revise (Ainsworth, 1969). Indeed, although
Bowlby had a firm intuitive grasp of the meaning of attachment security
and healthy responses to loss, he defined security merely as the *absence* of
insecurity, that is, as the state of being "free from care, apprehension or
alarm" (1973, p. 182). It was Ainsworth's genius to translate Bowlby's
insights into a measurement approach and to provide an operational definition of attachment security and insecurity within a normative developmental framework. The result was a paradigm shift in the study of early
relationships.

Developmentalists and clinicians, including Bowlby himself, quickly
assimilated his original construct of insecurity to Ainsworth's avoidant and
ambivalent insecure attachment groups (Bowlby, 1969/1982; Sroufe, 1997;
Rutter, 1997). The disorganized/disoriented classification was identified
after a decade and a half of research with Ainsworth's instrument in normative populations, and its application to various at-risk groups indicated
that the original insecure categories did not capture the full range of
attachment insecurity. Research in the last 15 years now suggests that it is
this group rather than the "organized" insecure groups that is most closely
linked to pathological outcomes (Carlson, 1998; Lyons-Ruth, 1996; Lyons-
Ruth & Jacobvitz, 1999). It is our conviction that the D category more
nearly corresponds to the type of insecure attachment that was the original
focus of Bowlby's interest.[7] If we are correct, this category will provide an
important tool for understanding Bowlby's observations, for reexamining
traditional questions with current knowledge and methodology, and
understanding new findings in the light of Bowlby's pioneering insights.

NOTES

1. In deactivation, information and affective appraisals that are linked to the
activation of the attachment system are excluded from consciousness. Behaviors
such as looking, turning, or moving away from an activating stimulus (including the

mother herself) may be deactivating, as would failure to evoke or "recall" attach-ment-relevant information. In cognitive disconnection, information about a situa-tion or individual that is experienced as painful is cognitively "disconnected" from awareness. The person is unaware of the reasons for his or her behavior or feelings, but especially when disconnection is partial, feelings associated with the activation of attachment gain limited access to consciousness.

Bowlby failed to spell out clearly the conditions related to partial or complete forms of exclusion. We would suggest that the degree of exclusion is likely to be associated with the intensity and persistence of the child's experience of the parent as able versus failing to provide protection and care.

2. Bowlby analogized the process of segregation to hypnotic phenomena, especially evidence of some individuals' capacity to generate a "hidden observer" while hypnotized (Hilgard, 1977/1986). More recently, Spiegel (1990) has argued that both repression and "hidden observers" are a function of dissociative pro-cesses, which by definition imply divided or parallel access of information to con-sciousness. Synthesizing these influences, Main and colleagues (Hesse & Main, in press; Main & Hesse, 1990; Main & Morgan, 1996) proposed that disorganized attachment behavior and its analogues in the mother's state of mind (lack of resolu-tion with respect to mourning or trauma of her own attachment relationships) and behavior are the result of dissociative processes. When the term "dissociative" is understood in this broad sense as reflecting a failure of "integrative processes of identity, memory, or consciousness" (American Psychiatric Association, 1994; see also Liotti, 1992, and Chapter 11, this volume), it may serve as a synonym for the construct of segregated systems. Many features of dissociative states, for example, trance states and amnesia, may *also* be seen as extreme examples of defensive exclu-sion, resulting in both the inhibition of behavior and the elimination of affect and thought from consciousness. On the other hand, Bowlby's construct and the range of phenomena associated with attachment disorganization should not be confused with or assimilated to dissociative disorders as they are usually understood in clini-cal diagnostic terms. Frank dissociative disorder does not appear to be a universal correlate of disorganized attachment or unresolved mourning (Scheungel et al., 1999) and there is likely to be a range or family of processes responsible for the evi-dence of inhibition versus flooding of thought, feeling, and behavior that are asso-ciated with the disorganized classification (e.g., Horowitz, Markman, Stinson, Fridhandler, & Ghannan, 1990). The display of "out-of control" attachment behav-ior and affect seems to reflect the breakdown of defensive exclusion or the circum-vention of inhibitory controls due to the simultaneous strong activation of the attachment system. The emergence of such behavior, therefore, may be taken as a mark of the partial or complete *failure* of inhibitory processes, dissociative or oth-ers, and echoing Bowlby's homeostatic model of attachment, the dysregulation of the attachment system. Ultimately, it may be possible to understand these interre-lated processes at the neurophysiological level as the products of failed integration of brain functioning (e.g., Davidson, 1992; Fox, 1994; Gunnar & Barr, 1998; Perry, Pollard, Blakeley, Baker, & Vigilante, 1995; Schore, 1997).

3. In practice, it may be difficult to disentangle cognitive and affective pro-cesses. We note, for example, that Erickson gave his well-known "paradoxical injunctions" while at the same time intentionally evoking intense, usually painful

affect in his patients. There is reason to believe that the one potentiated the other in inducing hypnotic states (Haley, 1973). On the other hand, observations of young children during prolonged separation indicate that they experience considerable anger toward the mother and toward *themselves* in her absence (Heinicke & Westheimer, 1965). As a result, upon reunion, the mother is indeed an object of conflict, although, obviously, she has not actually behaved in a threatening manner. The experience of mourning following the death of a loved one also entails a cognitive working through of conflicting mental attitudes or states toward that individual, which in turn, may be associated with emotional appraisals of fear or anxiety. This state of affairs is illustrated in the exceptionally beautiful and articulate ruminations on this experience by C. S. Lewis (1961):

> No one ever told me that grief felt so like fear. I am not afraid, but the sensation is like being afraid. (p. 1) . . . I think I am beginning to understand why grief feels like suspense. It comes from the frustration of so many impulses that had become habitual. Thought after thought, feeling after feeling, action after action, had H. for their object. Now their target is gone. I keep on through habit fitting an arrow to the string; then I remember and have to lay the bow down. So many roads lead thought to H. But now there's an impassable frontier-post across it. So many roads once; now so many *culs de sac.* (p. 39)

4. We have used this term in previous publications (e.g., George & Solomon, 1996; Solomon et al., 1995) and have noted some confusion about our meaning in the way others have cited this work. The *American Heritage Dictionary* (1976) provides three meanings of the term: (a) unable to manage by oneself, dependent; (b) lacking power or strength; and (c) incapable of (beyond) remedy. Our use of this term corresponds most closely to the third meaning; that is, we suggest that both D children and their mothers tend to perceive themselves as unable to improve or remedy distressing or frightening events in the environment and/or their own internal state. This may in some circumstances result in dependent or childlike behavior, but other strategies of desperation may also result from this state of mind, including rages and aggression on the one hand, or frozen withdrawal on the other.

5. We have not developed formal classification guidelines to identify the two types of caregiving representations, and the correspondence between maternal representations of the relationship and the type of controlling child attachment (punitive vs. caregiving) is not always clear-cut. It is our impression, however, that overall descriptions of directly coercive parent–child relationship are associated with the punitive subtype of controlling attachments, while those in which psychological merging is salient are associated with the caregiving subtype. Additionally, some relationships generally characterized by a great deal of struggle between mother and child (i.e., similar to the coercive caregiving representations) are also associated with controlling–caregiving attachments. In these cases, however, the mother seems to view the child particularly vulnerable or especially sensitive or reactive, rather than as a direct threat.

6. The parallel between this example and the conditions for "reckless" attachment disturbances described by Lieberman and Pawl (1990) is striking.

7. We emphasize, however, that while the D classification appears to reflect higher risk for psychopathology than the other classifications, it does not in itself constitute an attachment disorder.

REFERENCES

Aber, L., Slade, A., Berger, B., Bresgi, I., & Kaplan, M. (1985). *The Parent Development Interview.* Unpublished manuscript, Barnard College, Columbia University, New York.

Ainsworth, M. D. S. (1969). Object relations, dependency, and attachment: A theoretical review of the infant–mother relationship. *Child Development, 40,* 969–1025.

Ainsworth, M. D. S., Blehar, M., Waters, E., & Wall, S. (1978). *Patterns of attachment.* Hillsdale, NJ: Erlbaum.

Ainsworth, M. D. S., & Marvin, R. S. (1995). On the shaping of attachment theory and research: An interview with Mary D. S. Ainsworth. In E. Waters, B. E. Vaughn, G. Posada, & K. Kondo-Ikemura (Eds.), Caregiving, cultural, and cognitive perspectives on secure-base behavior and working models. *Monographs of the Society for Research in Child Development, 60*(203, Serial No. 244), 3–12.

American Heritage Dictionary (2nd college ed.). (1976). Boston: Houghton Mifflin.

American Psychiatric Association. (1994). *Diagnostic and statistical manual of mental disorders* (4th ed.). Washington, DC: Author.

Birengen, Z., Emde, R. N., & Pipp-Siegel, S. (1997). Dyssynchrony, conflict, and resolution: Positive contributions to infant development. *American Journal of Orthopsychiatry, 67,* 4–19.

Bowlby, J. (1969/1982). *Attachment and loss: Vol. 1. Attachment.* New York: Basic Books.

Bowlby, J. (1973). *Attachment and loss: Vol. 2. Separation.* New York: Basic Books.

Bowlby, J. (1980). *Attachment and loss: Vol. 3. Loss.* New York: Basic Books.

Bowlby, J. (1988). *A secure base.* New York: Basic Books.

Bretherton, I., Ridgeway, D., & Cassidy, J. (1990). Assessing internal working models of attachment relationships: An attachment story completion task for 3-year-olds. In M. T. Greenberg, D. Cicchetti, & E. M. Cummings (Eds.), *Attachment in the preschool years* (pp. 273–308). Chicago: University of Chicago Press.

Carlson, E. A. (1998). A prospective longitudinal study of attachment disorganization/disorientation. *Child Development, 69,* 1107–1128.

Carlson, V. Cicchetti, D., Barnett, D., & Braunwald, K. (1989). Finding order in disorganization. In D. Cicchetti, & V. Carlson (Eds.), *Child maltreatment: Theory and research on the causes and consequences of child abuse and neglect* (pp. 494–528). New York: Cambridge University Press.

Chisolm, K. (1998). A three year follow-up of attachment and indiscriminate friendliness in children adopted from Russian orphanages. *Child Development, 69,* 1092–1106.

Davidson, R. J. (1992). Anterior cerebral asymmetry and the nature of emotion:

Implications for the study of individual differences and psychopathology. *Brain and Cognition, 20,* 121–151.

DeMulder, E. K., & Radke-Yarrow, M. (1991). Attachment with affectively ill and well mothers: Concurrent behavioral correlates. *Development and Psychopathology, 3,* 227–242.

Fox, N. A. (1994). Dynamic cerebral processes underlying emotion regulation. In N. A. Fox (Ed.), The development of emotion regulation. *Monographs of the Society for Research in Child Development, 59*(2–3, Serial No. 240), 152–166.

George, C., & Solomon, J. (1989). Internal working models of caregiving and security of attachment at age six. *Infant Mental Health Journal, 10,* 222–237.

George, C., & Solomon, J. (1996). Representational models of relationships: Links between caregiving and attachment. *Infant Mental Health Journal, 17,* 198–216.

George, C., & Solomon, J. (1998, July). *Attachment disorganization at age six: Differences in doll play between punitive and caregiving children.* Paper presented at the meeting of the International Society for the Study of Behavioural Development, Bern, Switzerland.

George, C., & Solomon, J. (1999). Attachment and caregiving: The caregiving behavioral system. In J. Cassidy & P. R. Shaver (Eds.), *Handbook of attachment: Theory, research, and clinical applications* (pp. 649–670). New York: Guilford Press.

Gunnar, M., R. & Barr, R. G. (1998). Stress, early brain development and behavior. *Infants and Young Children, 11,* 1–14.

Haley, J. (1973). *Uncommon therapy: The psychiatric techniques of Milton H. Erickson, M.D.* New York: Norton.

Heinicke, C. M., & Westheimer, I. J. (1965). *Brief separations.* New York: International Universities Press.

Hesse, E., & Main, M. (in press). Frightened behavior in traumatized but non-maltreating parents: Previously unexamined risk factor for offspring. *Psychoanalytic Inquiry.*

Hilgard, E. R. (1977/1986). *Divided consciousness: Multiple controls in human thought and action.* New York: Wiley.

Hinde, R. A. (1970). *Animal behavior: A synthesis of ethology and comparative psychology* (2nd ed.). New York: McGraw-Hill.

Hirshberg, L. M. (1990). When infants look to their parents: II. Twelve-month-olds' response to conflicting parental emotional signals. *Child Development, 61,* 1187–1191.

Horowitz, M. J., Markman, H. C., Stinson, C. H., Fridhandler, B., & Ghannan, J. H. (1990). A classification theory of defense. In J. L. Singer (Ed.), *Repression and dissociation* (pp. 61–84). Chicago: University of Chicago Press.

Lewis, C. S. (1961). *A grief observed.* New York: Seabury Press.

Lieberman, A. F., & Pawl, J. H. (1990). Disorders of attachment and secure base behavior in the second year of life: Conceptual issues and clinical intervention. In M. T. Greenberg, D. Cicchetti, & E. M. Cummings (Eds.), *Attachment in the preschool years* (pp. 375–398). Chicago: University of Chicago Press.

Liotti, G. (1992). Disorganized/disoriented attachment in the etiology of the dissociative disorders. *Dissociation, 5,* 196–204.

Lyons-Ruth, K. (1996). Attachment relationships among children with aggressive behavior problems: The role of disorganized early attachment patterns. *Journal of Consulting and Clinical Psychology, 64,* 64–73.

Lyons-Ruth, K., Bronfman, E., & Parsons, E. (in press). Maternal disrupted affective communication, maternal frightened or frightening behavior, and disorganized attachment strategies. In J. Vondra & D. Barnett (Eds.), Atypical patterns of infant attachment: Theory, research and current directions. *Monographs of the Society for Research in Child Development.*

Lyons-Ruth, K., Connell, D. B., Grunebaum, H., & Botein, S. (1990). Infants at social risk: Maternal depression and family support services as mediators of infant development and security of attachment. *Child Development, 61,* 85–98.

Lyons-Ruth, K., & Jacobvitz, D. (1999). Attachment disorganization: Unresolved loss, relational violence, lapses in behavioral and attentional strategies. In J. Cassidy & P. R. Shaver (Eds.), *Handbook of attachment: Theory, research, and clinical applications* (pp. 520–554). New York: Guilford Press.

Main, M. (1981). Avoidance in the service of attachment: A working paper. In K. Immelman, G. Barlow, L. Petrinovich, & M. Main (Eds.), *Behavioral development: The Bielefeld interdisciplinary project* (pp. 651–693). New York: Cambridge University Press.

Main, M., & Cassidy, J. (1988). Categories of response to reunion with the parent at age 6: Predictable from infant attachment classifications and stable over a 1-month period. *Developmental Psychology, 24,* 1–12.

Main, M., & Hesse, E. (1990). Parents' unresolved traumatic experiences are related to infant disorganized attachment status: Is frightened and/or frightening parental behavior the linking mechanism? In M. T. Greenberg, D. Cicchetti, & E. M. Cummings (Eds.), *Attachment in the preschool years* (pp. 161–182). Chicago: University of Chicago Press.

Main, M., Kaplan, N., & Cassidy, J. (1985). Security in infancy, childhood, and adulthood: A move to the level of representation. In I. Bretherton & E. Waters (Eds.), Growing points in attachment theory and research. *Monographs of the Society for Research in Child Development, 50*(1–2, Serial No. 209), 66–104.

Main, M., & Morgan, H. (1996). Disorganization and disorientation in infant strange situation behavior: Phenotypic resemblance to dissociative states? In L. Michelson & W. Ray (Eds.), *Handbook of dissociation: Theoretical, empirical, and clinical perspectives* (pp. 107–138). New York: Plenum.

Main, M., & Solomon, J. (1990). Procedures for identifying infants as disorganized/disoriented during the Ainsworth Strange Situation. In M. T. Greenberg, D. Cicchetti, & E. M. Cummings (Eds.), *Attachment in the preschool years* (pp. 121–160). Chicago: University of Chicago Press.

O'Connor, M., Sigman, M., & Brill, N. (1987). Disorganization of attachment in relation to maternal alcohol consumption. *Journal of Clinical and Consulting Psychology, 51,* 831–836.

Owen, M. T., & Cox, M. J. (1997). Marital conflict and the development of infant–parent attachment relationships. *Journal of Family Psychology, 11,* 152–164.

Perry, B. D., Pollard, R. A., Blakley, T. L., Baker, W. L., & Vigilante, D. (1995). Childhood trauma, the neurobiology of adaptation, and "use dependent" development of the brain: How "states" become "traits." *Infant Mental Health Journal, 16,* 271–291.

Robertson, J., & Robertson, J. (1989a). *John.* New York Library Film Series.

Robertson, J., & Robertson, J. (1989b). *Separation and the very young child.* London: Free Association Books.

Robertson, J., & Robertson, J. (1990). *Thomas.* New York Library Film Series.

Rutter, M. (1997). Clinical implications of attachment concepts: Retrospect and prospect. In L. Atkinson & K. J. Zucker (Eds.), *Attachment and psychopathology* (pp. 17–46). New York: Guilford Press.

Schuengel, C., Bakermans-Kranenburg, M. J., & van IJzendoorn, M. H. (1999). Attachment and loss: Frightening maternal behavior linking unresolved loss and disorganized infant attachment. *Journal of Consulting and Clinical Psychology, 67,* 54–63.

Schore, A. N. (1997). Early organization of the nonlinear right brain and development of a predisposition to psychiatric disorders. *Development and Psychopathology, 9,* 595–632.

Solomon, J. (1998, August). Security, defense, and dysregulation: Understanding the links between disorganized attachment and childhood behavior disorders. In L. Atkinson (Chair), *Attachment and behavior disorders.* Symposium conducted at the annual meeting of the American Psychological Association, San Francisco, CA.

Solomon, J., & George, C. (1996). Defining the caregiving system: Toward a theory of caregiving. *Infant Mental Health Journal, 17,* 183–197.

Solomon, J., & George, C. (1999). The measurement of attachment security in infancy and childhood. In J. Cassidy & P. R. Shaver (Eds.), *Handbook of attachment: Theory, research, and clinical applications* (pp. 287–316). New York: Guilford Press.

Solomon, J., & George, C. (1999). The development of attachment in separated and divorced families: Effects of overnight visitation, parent, and couple variables. *Attachment and Human Development.*

Solomon, J., & George, C. (in press-a). The caregiving behavioral system in mothers of infants: A comparison of divorcing and married mothers. *Attachment and Human Development.*

Solomon, J., & George, C. (in press-b). Toward an integrated theory of caregiving. In J. Osofsky & H. E. Fitzgerald (Eds.), *World Association of Infant Mental Health handbook of infant mental health.* New York: Wiley.

Solomon, J., George, C., & De Jong, A. (1995). Children classified as controlling at age six: Evidence of disorganized representational strategies and aggression at home and school. *Development and Psychopathology, 7,* 447–464.

Solomon, J., George, C., & Silverman, N. (in press). Maternal caregiving Q-sort: Describing age-related changes in mother–infant interaction. In E. Waters, B . Vaughn, & D. Teti (Eds.), *Patterns of attachment behavior: Q-sort perspectives in secure base behavior and caregiving in infancy and childhood.* Hillsdale, NJ: Erlbaum.

Spangler, G., Fremmer-Bombik, E., & Grossmann, K. (1996). Social and individual determinants of infant security and disorganization. *Infant Mental Health Journal, 17,* 127–139.

Spiegel, D. (1990). Hypnosis, dissociation, and trauma: Hidden and overt observers. In J. L. Singer (Ed.), *Repression and dissociation* (pp. 121–142). Chicago: University of Chicago Press.

Sroufe, L. A. (1997). Psychopathology as an outcome of development. *Development and Psychopathology, 9*, 251–268.

Sroufe, L. A., & Waters, E. (1977). Attachment as an organizational construct. *Child Development, 48*, 1184–1199.

Stevenson-Hinde, J., & Shouldice, A. (1995). Maternal interactions and self-reports related to attachment classifications at 4.5 years. *Child Development, 66*, 583–596.

Teti, D., Gelfand, D., & Isabella, R. (1995). Maternal depression and the quality of early attachment: An examination of infants, preschoolers, and their mothers. *Developmental Psychology, 31*, 364–376.

Tronick, E. Z. (1989). Emotions and emotional communication in infants. *American Psychologist, 44*, 112–119.

van IJzendoorn, M. H., Schuengel, C., & Bakermans-Kranenburg, M. J. (1999). Disorganized attachment in early childhood: Meta-analysis of precursors, concomitants, and sequelae. *Development and Psychopathology, 11*, 225–249.

CHAPTER 2

A Relational Diathesis Model of Hostile–Helpless States of Mind

Expressions in Mother–Infant Interaction

KARLEN LYONS-RUTH
ELISA BRONFMAN
GWENDOLYN ATWOOD

Main and Solomon (1990) chose the term "disorganized/disoriented" to describe the array of fearful, odd, and/or contradictory infant behaviors sometimes observed around separation–reunion sequences. In their view, these behaviors represented a breakdown in organized strategic behavior for maintaining access to the attachment figure when under stress. Recent studies of stress responses mediated by the hypothalamic–pituitary–adrenocortical axis have supported this view of disorganized attachment strategies as ineffective coping strategies in that infants displaying disorganized attachment behaviors have exhibited sustained elevations in cortisol levels following brief stressors. In animal models, elevated cortisol levels are associated with the animal's helplessness to find an effective strategy to cope with a stressor (Spangler & Grossmann, 1993; Hertsgaard, Gunnar, Erickson, & Nachmias, 1995). Disorganized infants appear to be unable to maintain the strategic adjustments in attachment behavior represented by organized avoidant or ambivalent attachment strategies, with the result that both behavioral and physiological dysregulation occurs.

In addition to this central construct of contradictory tendencies governing the infant's attachment behaviors, discontinuity or dissociation of mental contents occurs at the level of mental representation among parents of disorganized infants. This discontinuity appears as a lapse in the monitoring of reasoning or discourse on the Adult Attachment Interview (AAI; George, Kaplan, & Main, 1984/1985/1996; Main & Goldwyn, 1985/1991/1994/1998). In this dissociative process, contradictory mental contents are maintained in parallel organizations that are not well integrated with one another. This mental segregation might be said to occur in mild forms in dismissing/avoidant or preoccupied/ambivalent states of mind. In the "unresolved" and "cannot classify" AAI categories associated with infant disorganization, however, contradictory mental organizations become elaborated enough to be explicitly stated in discourse without apparent monitoring and without mobilizing apparent defensive attempts to cover up or undo the contradiction.

Finally, research in this area documents the emerging bimodality of the behavioral profiles associated with disorganization in childhood. For example, during the first 2 years of life, infants within the disorganized spectrum may combine disorganized behavior either with behavior that preserves the outlines of a secure attachment strategy or with behaviors characteristic of an insecure–avoidant or ambivalent strategy. With the increasing cognitive capabilities of the preschool and school-age child, the disorganized infant reorganizes attachment behavior toward the parent into a controlling attachment strategy, a strategy reoriented away from seeking comfort and protection around the child's own needs and toward maintaining engagement with the parent on the parent's terms (Main & Cassidy, 1988). Again, controlling behavior can take one of two behaviorally distinct forms, becoming either controlling–caregiving or controlling–punitive. Caregiving attachment behavior is further associated with inhibited doll play, while punitive attachment is associated with chaotic play (Solomon, George, & De Jong, 1995; George & Solomon, 1998). In adulthood, this bimodality of behavioral profiles is also reflected in Main and Hesse's (1990) hypothesis that parents may display either frightened or frightening behavior toward the child (or both).

Thus, across the lifespan, the disorganized attachment category is characterized by contradictory behavioral strategies and unintegrated mental contents. These contradictions are observed within the individual and they are also observed in the composition of the disorganized group, where such sharply contrasting behavioral stances as punitive versus caregiving, or frightened versus frightening, have been united in a single classification. One question raised by these findings is how to account for the bimodality of behavioral presentations within the spectrum of disorganized attachment patterns. In the first section of this chapter, we outline a relational diathesis framework that seems capable of providing an integrative model to account for these discontinuities. In the second section of the chapter, we present new data describing the hostile or helpless maternal stances observed within the disorganized group in infancy.

A second question arising from the accumulated literature on attachment disorganization that needs further consideration is how an unresolved state of mind has developed in the parent of a disorganized infant. Initial work on disorganized attachment relationships reported an association between loss of a parent by death in the caregiver's childhood and the display of a disorganized attachment strategy by her infant (Main, Kaplan, & Cassidy, 1985; Lyons-Ruth, Repacholi, McLeod, & Silva, 1991). It soon became apparent, however, that most caregivers who had experienced parental death in childhood did not have disorganized infants and that many caregivers who had suffered a variety of less significant losses did have infants with disorganized strategies (e.g., Ainsworth & Eichberg, 1991). What characterized the members of both groups whose infants became disorganized was the presence of lapses of reasoning or discourse in the interview context. This led to the realization that it was the caregiver's unresolved loss or trauma, not loss or trauma per se, that predicted the infant's display of a disorganized strategy. Despite the apparent central etiological role of lack of resolution, however, the question of why some experiences of childhood loss or trauma become resolved and others do not has received little attention in the literature to date. A relational diathesis model also offers specific hypotheses about the relational processes that should be related to resolution of loss. The implications of a relational diathesis model for the resolution of loss or trauma are spelled out in the first section of the chapter.

A third aspect of the literature on disorganization that needs to be addressed concerns a paradox at the heart of the theory regarding how intergenerational transmission of disorganized forms of attachment occurs. In the model to date, caregivers are viewed as developing unresolved states of mind in relation to specific experiences of loss or trauma, experiences usually occurring later than the first few years of life (and often much later). Infants are viewed as developing disorganized attachment strategies through exposure to the caregiver's unintegrated fear (Main & Hesse, 1990). This leads to the conundrum that if a disorganized infant grows up without loss or trauma, then, by definition, he or she will not be judged as unresolved on the Adult Attachment Interview. Do we assume, then, that all disorganized infants grow out of disorganized forms of attachment behavior unless further unresolved loss or trauma occurs? Or is the caregiver's frightened or frightening behavior sufficient in itself to lead to intergenerational transmission of disorganized attachment behavior, regardless of whether the child also experiences later loss or trauma? A relational diathesis model can contribute to the resolution of this intergenerational paradox, as also outlined in the first section of the chapter.

THE CONTRIBUTION OF THE RELATIONAL DIATHESIS TO DISORGANIZED ATTACHMENT PATTERNS

We now turn to the first question, which is how to account for the bimodality of behavioral presentations within the spectrum of disorganized attachment patterns. In prior literature, the term "diathesis," meaning vulnerability or predisposition, has been used to refer to genetic predisposition. However, inadequate early caregiving regulation constitutes a second source of vulnerability to later stressors. For example, Nemeroff (1996) has shown that neonatal rats subjected to repeated brief separations from their caregivers exhibited permanent increases in stress hormone production as adults. Similarly, infant macaques whose mothers were subjected to an uncertain food supply were ignored by their mothers and became less likely to explore and more fearful in novel situations. In adulthood, they also exhibited marked increases in stress hormone production. Similarly, Kraemer and Clarke (1996) reported that peer-reared monkeys who had no available adult attachment figure displayed exaggerated fear responses and elevated stress hormone levels as adults (see also Clarke, 1993). In humans, Cadoret et al. (1996) have demonstrated that the genetic diathesis in adoptees with alcoholic biological parents interacts with disturbed behavior exhibited by the adoptive parents to predict depression in adulthood among female offspring.

Attachment theory has advanced the primary conceptual model for understanding the relational contribution to the regulation of fearful arousal in early life. The infant comes equipped with a preadapted set of attachment behaviors that are activated by fear or distress and serve to signal to the caregiver the infant's need for proximity or close bodily contact. Close bodily contact, in turn, functions to mediate "felt security," that is, to reduce the infant's sense of fear or threat, with its associated physiological arousal (Bowlby, 1973; see also Solomon & George, Chapter 1, this volume). The attachment behavioral system functions as what might be called the "psychological immune system," in its role of buffering the effects of psychological stressors and maintaining psychophysiological arousal within acceptable limits. Vulnerability to stress-related dysfunction, then, should be a joint function of at least three factors: (1) the characteristics of the threat or stressor, (2) the genetic vulnerability to stress, and (3) the capacity of the attachment relational system to reduce arousal to acceptable levels. In such a model, the impact of traumatic attachment-related events is mediated in part by the degree of comfort and soothing available in close relationships.

A central argument of this chapter is that a core problem in disorganized attachment relationships lies in the hostile–helpless working model of attachment that is transmitted intergenerationally from the parent to the infant. We propose that hostile–helpless dyadic models are actualized in unbalanced parent–infant relationships in which one partner's initiatives are elaborated at the expense of the other's. Such unbalanced hostile–helpless relationships are those relationships least likely to offer the adequate protection and soothing needed to resolve a sense of threat, loss, or trauma, and are those most likely to contribute to the development of contradictory behavioral and mental processes. This model is elaborated below.

The Role of Unresolved Parental Fear in Parent–Infant Affective Communication

In their hypothesis regarding the etiology of infant disorganization, Main and Hesse (1990) have proposed that the result of a caregiver's unresolved fear related to past loss or trauma is frightened or frightening behavior toward the infant. This frightened or frightening behavior, in turn, creates fear of the caregiver in the infant, which disorganizes the infant's propensity to seek proximity to the caregiver as a solution to fear. A relational diathesis perspective elaborates more fully some of the ways in which the caregiver's unresolved fear impairs the attachment relational system, transmitting unintegrated mental and behavioral strategies intergenerationally.

For the infant's attachment strategy to become disorganized by a caregiver's frightened or frightening behavior, as hypothesized by Main and Hesse (1990), the caregiver's unresolved fear either must be pervasive enough to be repeatedly communicated to the infant or must be profound enough to traumatically impact the infant when occurring in isolated instances. On further reflection, it is apparent that such continuing exposure and/or periodic traumatic eruption must occur in ways that are not monitored and repaired by the caregiver. It is likely that many infants experience frightening events at the hands of their caregivers that do not become disorganizing, for example, when a parent trips on a stone and drops her 9-month-old infant headfirst onto the sidewalk. If the caregiver is not herself disorganized by the infant's fear and pain, she will continue to serve as a reliable source of comfort and soothing for the infant, both by seeing the child through her distress and pain at the time and by acting to guard against such events in the future.

If the caregiver has not experienced such comfort and soothing in relation to her own past losses or fear-evoking experiences, however, the infant's pain and fear will evoke her own unresolved fearful affects, as well as her helplessness to know how to find comfort and resolution in relation to them (see also Fraiberg, Adelson, & Shapiro, 1975; George & Solomon, 1999). Thus, there is an inherent, although not one-to-one, relation between the experience of unresolved fear and the openness of the caregiving system to hear, to respond to, and to help modulate fear-related affects. It is apparent that a caregiver who is repeatedly provoking fear in her infant by her own behavior is also unlikely to be able to recognize and respond adequately to her infant's fear-related attachment cues. If she were able to do so, she would be aware of the effect of her fear-evoking behavior on the infant. Therefore, when the attachment figure herself is evoking fear in the infant repeatedly, some impairment in her ability to monitor and respond to the infant's attachment-related affective states exists almost by definition.

This view of the ramifications of unresolved fear on the process of caregiver–infant affective communication leads to an important further postulate. If the parent must restrict her conscious attention to the infant's fear-related cues in order not to evoke her own unresolved fearful experiences, the parent's fluid responsiveness to the infant's attachment-related communications becomes restricted. The more pervasive these restrictions on the parent's conscious attention and responsiveness, the more the parent's need to regulate her own negative arousal will take precedence over the infant's concomitant need for a soothing response to his or her attachment-related communications. To the extent that the parent's regulation of affect related to her own unresolved fearful experiences guides her deployment of attention at the expense of flexible attention to the child's current states, the interaction between parent and child becomes less balanced and less mutually regulated to meet the needs of both partners.

Such unbalanced or nonmutual relational processes provide a conceptually powerful construct that can explain many additional aspects of the findings regarding disorganized attachment patterns. Both Bowlby (1980) and his forebears in psychoanalytic scholarship emphasized that mental representations of relationships are inherently dyadic. What is represented is not only the individual's way of participating in the relationship, for example, as the coercively controlled child, but also the entire dyadic relational pattern of controlled child–controlling parent. The more skewed these relational roles become, that is, the more one partner's initiatives are ignored or overridden by the other, the more discontinuous and self-contradictory are the internalized models that accommodate both relational possibilities (e.g., I should accept external control and take no initiative/I should control the other by overriding the other person's initiative).

In addition to self-contradictory internal models, highly unbalanced relational processes offer at least two contradictory and unintegrated behavioral possibilities that might become actualized in any given relational transaction. For example, if an early victim–victimizer model is never reevaluated, an abused child may become both a battered spouse and a battering parent by actualizing opposite poles of a single dyadic model in different relationships. Only if the underlying unresolved fear is acknowledged, and the old dyadic patterns found wanting, can new ways of being in relationship to others be constructed, and new and more responsive behavior toward the attachment-related needs of both the self and the other emerge.

These unbalanced relational processes can be observed in a broad range of relational patterns. A dominant–submissive pattern in which the parent coercively opposes and counters the initiatives of the child is the most obvious example of an unbalanced relational pattern (for examples, see Hann, Castino, Jarosinski, & Britton, 1991; Jacobsen & Miller, 1998). However, overriding the initiatives of the child can occur in much more subtle forms that on the surface appear helpless rather than powerful. Profound withdrawal and unresponsiveness is an obvious example in which the unresponsive parent may look depressed and helpless rather than hostile and coercive, and yet the end result of the unresponsive stance is to defeat the attempts of the child to jointly regulate the attachment relationship. In one example of parental control by withdrawal, described by Fraiberg and colleagues (1975), in the context of a home-visiting program, the home visitor observed long bouts of an infant crying at home, with no response from the mother of the baby. The clinical team posed the question, "Why can't this mother hear her baby cry?" The baby's mother was later discovered to have been a victim of incest and neglect in her own childhood.

The extreme end of unbalanced attachment-related interaction due to withdrawal occurs in cases of prolonged infant separation or loss of the parent. Kraemer and Clarke (1996) have described the extremely fearful behavior, alternating with discontrolled aggression, that characterizes the behavior of infant rhesus monkeys raised with peer companionship but no adult attachment figure. The disregulated fear appears to be a consequence of the absence of early maternal soothing responses to the infant's attachment behaviors. This evidence indicates that infant fearful and disorganized behavior can result from profound lack of response, as well as from specifically frightened or frightening behavior (see also Solomon & George, Chapter 1, this volume). In a related set of observations on film, Robertson and Robertson (1969) have documented the progressive disorganization of the child's organized attachment behaviors over time in the context of a prolonged parental absence of 9 days, during which kindly but inadequately available nurses engaged in routine care. Thus, infant fear without resolution can come about through a variety of caregiving conditions that result in inadequately specific and balanced responses to the infant's attachment initiatives.

More subtle variants of such unbalanced relational patterns occur when a parent (or marital partner) is active in the relationship but is acting primarily to call attention to his or her own attachment needs or to express his or her own concerns and directions, without reference or response to the attachment-related needs or initiatives of the child or partner. Zahn-Waxler and Kochanska (1990) give a compelling description of unbalanced interaction of this more active kind when a depressed parent was asked to feign sadness before her 2-year-old in a laboratory assessment of child empathy. The parent began expressing sadness about what she was reading but quickly generalized the source of her sadness to her own child's misbehaviors and how sad they made her, especially when she was already having such a difficult time struggling with her problems. She had trouble bringing the elaboration of her sadness to a close. Neither in this case of parental self-reference nor in the case of parental withdrawal was there a balanced sharing of initiative and response between parent and child. However, neither hostile nor frightening behavior was displayed in either case, and one can easily sympathize with the struggle of an ill or traumatized parent in attempting to manage her own painful states while also dealing with the constant emotional demands of an infant or young child. Other subtle but pervasive imbalances occur when the parent or partner responds to the other's needs only when they coincide with and are expressing the needs of the self. For example, the parent may respond only to behaviors that are enhancing to the parent's self-esteem, such as a child's precocious achievements, or to behaviors through which the parent's needs may be vicariously expressed, such as a child's physical symptoms requiring extensive medical visits (see Lyons-Ruth, Kaufman, Masters, & Wu, 1991).

All of these more subtle variants are well-documented in the clinical literature but are only beginning to be systematically conceptualized and researched by developmental psychopathologists. However, in one early pathbreaking study of a large cohort of school-aged children of depressive, manic–depressive, and non-ill parents, Baldwin et al. (1982) demonstrated that a pattern of balanced initiatives in the observed interaction between parent and child was one of the best predictors of child functioning at school and was a much stronger predictor of child functioning than parental diagnosis.

To be relevant to the attachment system, however, such relational imbalances must necessarily involve the child's attachment-related initiatives and communications. Current studies are only beginning to explore the point at which the relational imbalance around the child's attachment-related initiatives might become severe enough to create a disorganized attachment relationship rather than merely an insecure one. Conceptually, however, such a point should exist, since some degree of parental protection and responsiveness is presumably required for an organized infant attachment strategy to work well enough to be sustained over time. Bowlby's (1969/1982) descriptions of the collapse of organized attachment strategies in cases of prolonged parental absences, captured on film as well as in text, speak to this point, albeit from the vantage point of imbalance due to absence rather than imbalance due to the lack of response of a physically present caregiver. Such serious disruptions in balanced attachment-related communication and their relation to unresolved parental fear are only beginning to receive systematic attention in infancy (but see Hann et al., 1991; Lyons-Ruth, Bronfman, & Parsons, in press; Main & Cassidy, 1988; Main, Kaplan, & Cassidy, 1985; Moss, Parent, Gosselin, Rousseau, & St. Laurent, 1996; Strage & Main, 1985, for relevant evidence). However, such imbalances become much more visible in the controlling attachment patterns of preschoolers, in which clear role reversal has occurred between parent and child and the child is attending disproportionately to the parent's affective states. In addition, Strage and Main (1985) have related dysfluency in parent–child communication at age 6 to the child's classification as disorganized in infancy. Their definition of dysfluency included some indicators of relational imbalance as defined here, such as nonresponse to a partner's communication, as well as other aspects of speech, such as stammering or trailing off in midsentence.

Inherent in a model of unbalanced relationships is an asymmetry of power in which one partner's (attachment-related) goals or initiatives are elaborated at the expense of the other's goals or initiatives. By definition, then, one partner is more helpless in the relationship and the other more controlling of the relationship, whether or not the control is exerted through active aggression or through the more covert mechanisms of withdrawal, guilt-induction, or self-preoccupation. Thus, a helpless versus hostile–controlling dyadic model of relationship roles should be especially evident among individuals in disorganized attachment relationships and may partially account for the bifurcation into punitive or caregiving stances that occurs among disorganized infants during the preschool period. This also accords well with George and Solomon's (1996) description of mothers of controlling children as having a helpless state of mind in which the child is viewed as beyond the parent's control, either because of the unmanageability of the child or because of the child's perceived special or "larger-than-life" qualities.

In support of a hostile–helpless model of the relational diathesis, Lyons-Ruth and Block (1996) demonstrated that mothers with serious trauma histories were much less likely to engage in balanced and positive verbal and physical interaction with their infants at home, regardless of the type of trauma or abuse. However, they also found that mothers with childhood histories of abuse might be either very withdrawn in their interactions with their infants or quite negative and intrusive. These two stances, in turn, were differentially associated with the type of the mother's early abusive experiences, with hostile mothers more likely to have experienced violence or physical abuse in childhood (with or without associated sexual abuse) and withdrawn mothers more likely to have experienced sexual abuse without associated physical abuse. Lyons-Ruth and Block speculated that the option to deal with helplessness by identifying with the controlling stance of the aggressor may be more accessible to female victims of physical abuse than to female victims of sexual abuse, for whom the role of sexual aggressor is not so easily adopted. These two opposite maternal stances in the aftermath of trauma, that is, helplessness or hostile control, again point to the presence of an unbalanced, helpless versus hostile–controlling relational template accompanying aggressor–victim relationships.

A RELATIONAL DIATHESIS MODEL OF THE DEVELOPMENT OF DISORGANIZED/UNRESOLVED STATES OF MIND IN ADULTHOOD

We now turn to the second and third questions raised earlier, which both concern how disorganized attachment patterns are carried into adulthood. First, why do some experiences of loss or trauma in childhood become resolved and others do not? Second, if no loss or trauma occurs, do disorganized infants grow out of disorganized attachment patterns by adulthood?

From a relational diathesis perspective, the ability to resolve a loss or trauma should be a function of at least two factors: (1) the qualities of the loss or trauma itself, such as its suddenness, developmental timing, involvement of central attachment figures, and horror-inducing aspects; and (2) the quality of ongoing comfort, communication, and protection regarding fear-evoking experiences available in important attachment relationships. According to this hypothesis, in cases where characteristics of the loss or trauma make the experience unusually difficult to integrate (e.g., the murder of a sibling or the crib death of an infant), lack of resolution of the trauma may occur even in the face of an otherwise secure attachment history. In cases where the circumstances of the losses have not been unusual or particularly fear inducing, however, one would expect lack of resolution to be associated with a less adequate attachment relationship in childhood.

The concept of a relational diathesis, or vulnerability to disorganization in the face of trauma, is foreshadowed in Bowlby's (1980) discussion of the conditions affecting the course of mourning. He states that "adults whose mourning takes a pathological course are likely before their bereavement to have been prone to make affectional relationships of certain special, albeit contrasting, kinds" (p. 202). He lists the three classes of affectional relationships as those "suffused with overt or covert ambivalence," those in which "there is a strong disposition to engage in compulsive caregiving," and those in which "there are strenuous attempts to claim emotional self-sufficiency and independence of all affectional ties" (p. 202). A similar point was made by Freud (1917/1957), who described persons prone to pathological mourning as those who experienced marked but consciously unacceptable ambivalence toward the lost person. In short, the more insecure the underlying attachment, the more difficult it becomes mentally to resolve a loss.

In our view, however, organized dismissing or preoccupied attachment relationships should provide sufficient protection and soothing in response to the heightened attachment stress that accompanies normative, uncomplicated experiences of loss to allow integrated mental functioning (see also George & Solomon, 1999; George & Solomon, 1996; Stevenson-Hinde & Shouldice, 1995). Only if the loss or traumatic experience falls well outside the norm, or if the degree of comfort, communication, and protection available from the parent falls outside the spectrum associated with organized attachment strategies, would we expect to see the kinds of behavioral and mental lapses that herald a process of intergenerational transmission of disorganization. As noted earlier, Lyons-Ruth and Block (1996) demonstrated that severity of trauma in the mother's childhood was associated with very misattuned caregiving behavior toward the infant at home, caregiving of either a hostile–intrusive or helpless–withdrawn type. The type and degree of parental withdrawal or negative–intrusive behavior observed at home went beyond the cool rejection of attachment behavior observed among parents of infants classified as avoidant (Ainsworth, Blehar, Waters, & Wall, 1978; Cassidy & Kobak, 1988; Main, Tomasini, & Tolan, 1979) or the delayed and inconsistent but reasonably tender responding described among parents of infants classified as ambivalent (Ainsworth et al., 1978; Cassidy & Berlin, 1994; for related hostile–helpless clinical descriptions, see Fraiberg et al., 1975). Therefore, we propose that lack of resolution should occur most frequently among children with disorganized early relationships rather than avoidant or ambivalent relationships alone. Unfortunately, using the AAI, there is no way currently to distinguish disorganized states of mind stemming from early disorganized relationships from disorganized states generated by later loss or trauma.

However, from a relational diathesis viewpoint, there should also be a group of adults who have not experienced childhood loss or abuse whose experience of unintegrated fearful affects is rooted in the relationship with a hostile or helpless caregiver. Lyons-Ruth and Block (1996) have hypothesized that such seriously misattuned caregiver responses to attachment behaviors in infancy will constitute a source of fear to the infant by themselves because the infant will experience little sense of reliable influence over the behavior of the attachment figure when under stress. In such cases, early attachment figures would have been unable to provide adequate protection and soothing around fearful affects aroused in early attachment relationships, including both fears related to separation and lack of protection, and fears evoked by parental helpless or hostile behavior that did not necessarily qualify as abusive. According to this hypothesis, in these cases, no later loss or trauma would be necessary for the sequence of infant disorganization, childhood controlling behavior, and adult unintegrated mental states to occur. However, it should also be noted that in a caregiving context where the caregiver is systematically misattuned to the infant's attachment cues, the infant is both more likely to be exposed to later trauma and is also less likely to be able to rely on attachment figures to help resolve the trauma-related fear and mentally integrate the traumatic experience. So, in practice, deviant early caregiving is likely to potentiate the occurrence of later loss or trauma, as well as to increase the likelihood that the trauma will not be resolved. These multiple influences of a relational diathesis on the intergenerational transmission of disorganized attachment patterns are modeled in Figure 2.1.

Examining the fear-modulating resources available in caregiving relationships may also help to explain why severe loss or trauma in some cases is not associated with unresolved states of mind, while in other cases, losses of relatively peripheral persons yield high scores for lack of resolution of loss on the AAI. If unresolved states of mind must be a joint product of

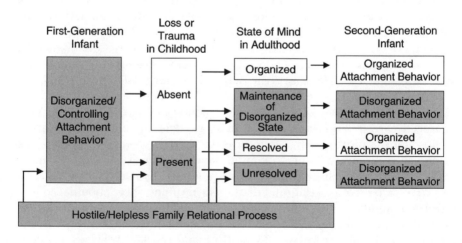

FIGURE 2.1. Proposed contributions of a relational diathesis.

both fear-inducing experience and the quality of comfort and communication around that experience available over time (as well as other sources of influence), children or adults in less secure attachment relationships would be more likely to fail to resolve fearful affects related to more minor fear-evoking experiences or relationship disruptions. In particular, children experiencing disorganizing early caregiving might manifest unresolved fear generated in the early caregiving relationship itself in relation to very minor later losses as well, even though the later loss per se was not the original cause of the unintegrated state of mind.

Therefore, a hostile–helpless infant–caregiver relationship should be viewed as a primary source of dysregulated fearful arousal for the infant, one that holds little promise of resolution over time in the absence of significant changes in the caregiving environment or significant new relationships (e.g., Egeland, Jacobvitz, & Sroufe, 1988). The early existence of such a hostile–helpless diathesis should predict intergenerational transmission of disorganized attachment patterns whether or not later loss or trauma occurs in the infant's life, as was modeled in Figure 2.1. If such an unbalanced hostile–helpless relational diathesis contributes to the emergence of a disorganized attachment relationship in infancy, we would also predict that such hostile–helpless states of mind could be identified on the AAI independent of indices of lack of resolution of loss or trauma. Work is currently underway in our lab to describe hostile–helpless indicators on the AAI, and pilot results indicate that these indicators significantly predict infant disorganization (Atwood, 1995; Lyons-Ruth & Atwood, in press). To some extent, these descriptors represent elaborations of the Main and Goldwyn (1985/1991/1994/1998) categories labeled preoccupied/overwhelmed by trauma (E3) and cannot classify (CC), which have not as yet received detailed treatment in the AAI coding system. Theoretically, however, this work ties both categories to a postulated hostile–helpless internal working model and to the transmission of disorganized attachment patterns, rather than to the ambivalent attachment pattern thought to be associated with the preoccupied/overwhelmed by trauma subgroup.

Indicators of lack of resolution of loss or trauma on the AAI have probably served reasonably well to date to capture the subgroup of adults who have experienced primary hostile–helpless relationships, because this subgroup should be at heightened risk for also experiencing later loss or abuse and for failing to integrate and resolve those experiences. These three hypotheses—(1) that hostile–helpless relationships in infancy should predict intergenerational transmission in the absence of later loss or trauma, (2) that hostile–helpless relationships in infancy should predict increased incidence of later loss or trauma (for related data, see Ogawa, Sroufe, Weinfield, Carlson, & Egeland, 1997), and (3) that hostile–helpless relationships in infancy should predict lack of resolution of later-occurring trauma—are all testable hypotheses. However, such testing will require more basic descriptive work identifying the hostile–helpless caregiving behaviors that fall outside the spectrum consistent with organized attachment strategies in infancy and will also require longitudinal attachment data from infancy to adulthood.

In the next section of the chapter, we present emerging data that point to the existence of both hostile and helpless caregiving stances among mothers of disorganized infants. These two caregiving stances, in turn, are correlated with different profiles of disorganized infant attachment behaviors.

THE RELATIONAL DIATHESIS: HOSTILE–HELPLESS RELATIONAL STANCES IN PARENT–INFANT COMMUNICATION

Following a relational diathesis model, we would predict that both helpless and hostile relational stances would be evident in infancy in interactions between many disorganized infants and their mothers. Evidence is emerging in support of this hypothesis. In this section of the chapter, we present recent work suggesting that at least two distinct behavioral subgroups are evident among both infants and mothers in disorganized dyads. The first part of the section reviews earlier data indicating that separable profiles of infant behavior exist within the disorganized spectrum. The second part reviews recent data regarding frightened, frightening, and other atypical behaviors of mothers of disorganized infants. The third section presents new data describing a profile of maternal behavior termed helpless–fearful of attachment.

Profiles of Infant Disorganized Behavior: Description, Family Correlates, and Longitudinal Outcomes

Disorganized Subgroups in Infancy

In the 1980s, before the coding criteria for disorganized infant behavior were formalized, two infant behavioral profiles were described among high-risk samples that did not fit established coding criteria for secure, avoidant, or ambivalent behavior. These two groups were roughly captured by the labels "pseudo-secure" and "avoidant/resistant" or "A/C" (Radke-Yarrow, Cummings, Kuczynski, & Chapman, 1985; Crittenden, 1985; Egeland & Sroufe, 1981; Gaensbauer & Harmon, 1982). When Main and Solomon (1990) published comprehensive guidelines for coding disorganized infant behavior, they acknowledged these subgroups by recommending that all disorganized infants also be assigned a subclassification of secure, avoidant, or ambivalent to identify the closest-fitting attachment organization underlying the disorganized behavior. This established the current convention of labeling the disorganized (D) subgroups as D/secure, D/avoidant, or D/ambivalent. We use these terms in the remainder of this chapter but collapse the D/avoidant and D/ambivalent subgroups into a single D/insecure grouping due to the small numbers of infants displaying the ambivalent pattern (van IJzendoorn, 1995).

Infants in the "pseudo-secure" or D/secure subgroup preserve the outlines of a secure attachment strategy in that they often protest or cry when the parent leaves the room but also resolve their distress when the parent returns. Infants in this group also show very little avoidant behavior or angry, resistant behavior toward the parent. However, these infants show other problematic behaviors rare in low-risk cohorts, such as wandering aimlessly in the vicinity of the parent, backing up sharply when the parent first approaches, stopping to huddle on the floor when crawling toward the parent, looking fearful when the parent enters the room, appearing limp and unresponsive when held, freezing or stilling when near the parent, or displaying other confused, depressed, apprehensive, or inexplicable behaviors in the parent's vicinity. These behaviors are often not displayed when the infant is alone or with a stranger, so they do not appear to be characteristic of the infant more generally.

Disorganized infants in the D/insecure subgroup combine confused and contradictory behavioral sequences toward the parent with more marked avoidance of contact and/or with angry, resistant behavior. In our own sample of socially at-risk infants, infants in this subgroup most often displayed marked distress while the mother was out of the room, only to shift abruptly to pointed avoidance when she entered. This sudden shift was often shocking to the observer. The infant's avoidant behavior was often combined with angry resistance to contact, passive behaviors, and other apprehensive or conflict behaviors in the presence of the parent.

Differing Family Correlates of the Two Infant Profiles

In a previous paper on the family correlates of disorganization in infancy, we called attention to the significantly different family characteristics associated with these two disorganized subgroups (Lyons-Ruth, Repacholi, McLeod, & Silva, 1991). First, in the literature on disorganization as a whole, disorganized infants in samples without social risk factors were more likely to display the D/secure pattern of behavior. Proportions of D/secure infants in the disorganized group ranged from 62% D/secure among infants from predominantly low-risk families, reported on by Main and Solomon (1990), to 27% D/secure in the low-income sample of Carlson, Cicchetti, Barnett, and Braunwald (1989), one-half of whom were maltreated. Second, in our own low-income sample, the type of loss experienced in the mother's childhood was different for mothers of D/secure and D/insecure infants. Among mothers of D/secure infants (n = 17), 59% had experienced loss of a parent by death, separation, or divorce during childhood, compared to only 12% of mothers of D/insecure infants (n = 26). In contrast, 27% of mothers of D/insecure infants had experienced periods of out-of-home care during childhood, compared to only 6% of mothers of D/secure infants. Finally, the severity of concurrent maternal psychosocial problems was different for the two infant subgroups, with mothers of D/insecure infants having elevated rates of depressive symptoms, psychiatric hospitalization, or documented maltreatment, while no significant elevation in maternal psychosocial problems was evident among mothers whose infants were in the D/secure subgroup (Lyons-Ruth, Repacholi, et al., 1991).

Similar Maladaptive Outcomes for the Two Infant Profiles

Based on these different maternal correlates for D/secure and D/insecure behavior, we had speculated that infants in the D/secure subgroup might have more favorable outcomes than infants in the D/insecure subgroup. However, these predictions were not borne out in our follow-up studies at ages 5 and 7. At age 5, both D/secure and D/insecure infants were at elevated risk for hostile–aggressive behavior toward peers in preschool, with 50% of D/secure infants and 42% of D/insecure infants rated over clinical cutoff points, compared to 9% of secure infants and 25% of avoidant infants (Lyons-Ruth, Alpern, & Repacholi, 1993). (All ambivalent infants were also cross-classified as D in this cohort.) Again, at age 7, both disorganized subgroups displayed elevated rates of externalizing behavior at school, with 25% of each D subgroup rated over clinical cutoffs, compared to 5% of children who were secure in infancy and no children who were avoidant. In addition, at age 7, both D subgroups were at equal risk for even higher rates of general maladjustment to the school environment as rated by teachers, with 50% of both D subgroups rated over clinical cut-off points, compared to 20–21% of secure and avoidant infants. Therefore, with socioeconomic status controlled, the two infant subtypes appear to carry comparable risk. In addition, the higher rate of overall maladjustment (50%) as compared to the rate of externalizing behavior alone (25%) suggests that conventional symptom checklists do not capture all the maladaptive behaviors later displayed by children classified as disorganized in infancy. The only behavior that was not equally elevated among both subgroups of disorganized infants by age 7 was internalizing symptoms. D/insecure infants, who displayed a great deal of avoidance in this sample, were at risk *both* for internalizing and externalizing symptoms, while D/

secure infants were at risk only for externalizing symptoms. Therefore, the patterning of the outcome data for the two subgroups of disorganized infants suggests that the two subgroups are associated with comparable long-term risks of maladaptive social behavior (for related data on later behavior problems of disorganized infants, see Goldberg, Gotoweic, & Simmons, 1995; Moss, Rousseau, Parent, St-Laurent, & Saintonge, 1998; Shaw, Owens, Vondra, Keenan, & Winslow, 1996).

Are the Two Infant Profiles Precursors to the Two Profiles of Controlling Behavior?

Disorganized infants have previously been shown to reorganize their behavior by the end of the preschool period into one of two forms of controlling behavior toward the parent, termed either punitive or caregiving (Main & Cassidy, 1988; Wartner, Grossmann, Fremmer-Bombik, & Suess, 1994). Again, these two forms of behavior can look very different, with controlling–caregiving children attempting to entertain, direct, organize, or reassure the parent, while controlling–punitive children are involved in coercing, attacking, or humiliating the parent (Main et al., 1985). No studies to date have attempted to explore whether a particular infant subtype is a precursor to a particular type of controlling behavior in preschool. However, similar to infants in the two disorganized subgroups, children in both of the controlling subgroups appear to be at risk for elevated externalizing behavior problems during the preschool and early school-aged periods (Moss et al., 1996, 1998; Greenberg, Speltz, DeKlyen, & Endriga, 1991; Solomon et al., 1995; Speltz, Greenberg, & DeKlyen, 1990; van IJzendoorn, Schuengel, & Bakermans-Kranenburg, 1999).

Profiles of Disrupted Affective Communication among Mothers of Infants in the Disorganized Group

Frightening, Hostile–Intrusive, and Role-Reversed Behaviors of Mothers of Disorganized/Insecure Infants

Recently, two groups of researchers have examined the relation between infant disorganized attachment and parent–infant interaction, focusing on the fear-related parental behaviors hypothesized by Main and Hesse (1990) to be particularly associated with the disorganization of infant attachment strategies. Schuengel, Bakermans-Kranenburg, and van IJzendoorn (1999) and Lyons-Ruth, Bronfman, and Parsons (in press) both tested aspects of Main and Hesse's (1990) hypothesis regarding the role of frightened or frightening parental behavior in the genesis of disorganized infant attachment strategies. Schuengel et al. (1999) and Jacobvitz, Hazen, and Riggs

(1997) also examined the relation between maternal fear-related behavior and the mother's classification as unresolved in regard to loss or trauma on the AAI (see also Schuengel, Bakermans-Kranenburg, van IJzendoorn, & Blom, Chapter 3, this volume).

According to Main and Hesse's (1990) hypothesis, disorganized infant attachment behavior arises from experiencing the caregiver herself as frightened or frightening. In this formulation, a frightened or frightening caregiver presents an inherent paradox to the infant. Fear activates the attachment system and the infant feels compelled to seek proximity to and comfort from the attachment figure. However, the caregiver herself is associated with increased infant fear, and the infant then contradicts the tendency to approach. In the words of Main and Hesse (1990), the attachment figure is "at once the source of and the solution to its alarm" (p. 163). This paradox results in a collapse of the infant's attempt to organize a consistent secure, avoidant, or ambivalent strategy toward the caregiver. The parent's frightened or frightening behavior is viewed as stemming from the activation of parental unresolved fear related to the parent's own past traumatic experiences. Main and Hesse (1992, 1995) have developed a coding instrument for frightened or frightening behavior, which includes criteria for coding frightened, frightening, dissociative, and sexual/spousal behaviors. The symbol FR refers to the codes for frightened or frightening behavior only; FR+ refers to all four codes.

Coding 4 hours of videotaped naturalistic observation among 85 middle-income mothers and their 10-month-old infants at home, Schuengel et al. (1997, 1999) found a relationship between maternal unresolved loss on the AAI and maternal display of frightened or frightening behaviors toward the infant. However, a significant association occurred only among the subgroup of mothers classified as both unresolved and insecure (U/Ds or U/E) on the AAI. Mothers classified unresolved and *secure* (U/F) displayed significantly less frightened or frightening behavior than did mothers classified unresolved and *insecure* (U/E or U/Ds). However, in a more puzzling finding, mothers classified unresolved and secure (U/F) displayed significantly *less* frightened or frightening behavior than did mothers judged fully secure (F). This finding suggests some overall behavioral inhibition on the part of mothers classified as unresolved and secure (U/F), since the fully secure–autonomous (F) mothers displayed more frightened or frightening behavior than did the U/F group.

Schuengel et al. (1997, 1999) also tested Main and Hesse's hypothesis that a mother's frightened or frightening behavior would be associated with a disorganized attachment pattern on the part of her infant. Maternal frightened or frightening behavior was marginally related to infant disorganization, $p < .04$, one-tailed. However, dissociated behavior, as well as a broader set of maternal "disorganized" behaviors that included the frightened or frightening behavior codes, predicted disorganized infant behavior more strongly than did the frightened or frightening behaviors alone (Schuengel et al., 1997) Maternal behavior was not analyzed separately in relation to the two disorganized infant subgroups as it had been in relation to the two analogous unresolved maternal subgroups on the AAI. Based on these AAI results, however, these data lend support to the hypothesis that mothers in the D/secure subgroup may organize their behavior toward the infant differently than mothers in the D/insecure group, who exhibited elevated rates of frightened or frightening behavior.

Jacobvitz et al. (1997) also tested the link between prenatal maternal AAI responses and maternal frightened or frightening behavior assessed at home 8 months after the child's birth in a middle-income cohort of 113 families. They found a marginally significant difference in maternal behavior among unresolved mothers based on whether the secondary classification was secure or insecure, with unresolved/insecure mothers showing the most elevated rates of frightened or frightening behavior. In contrast to Schuengel et al.'s (1999) results, however, unresolved/secure mothers also displayed significantly more frightened or frightening behavior than mothers judged resolved on the AAI. This difference in results could stem from the fact that Jacobvitz et al. (1997) required the mothers to interact with their infants in a series of structured tasks, while Schuengel et al. (1999) relied on naturalistic observation. If mothers in the unresolved/ secure group attempt to withdraw from the infant and inhibit their frightened or frightening behavior, forcing more interaction at home or observing interaction in the strange situation where the infant's attachment behaviors are elicited (see below) may provide a more revealing window on the structure of the mother's behavior in the unresolved/secure subgroup.

Lyons-Ruth et al. (in press) observed mother–infant interaction in the strange situation among a low-income cohort of 65 mothers and infants. Sixty-six percent of the mothers were supported by government assistance and 45% were single parents. Infants were 18 months of age. In addition to Main and Hesse's (1992) frightened or frightening behaviors, a broader spectrum of maternal behavior was coded, indexing disrupted affective communication between mother and infant. Lyons-Ruth et al. (in press) reasoned that, in addition to displaying directly frightened or frightening behavior, a parent who is experiencing a continuing state of fear around attachment needs is likely to experience competing tendencies both to respond to and to avoid the infant when the infant's attachment needs are aroused, similar to the disorganized infant's display of competing and contradictory strategies toward the parent. Contradictory caregiving tendencies to both elicit and reject infant attachment affects would constitute one type of disrupted affective communication between parent and infant.

Lyons-Ruth et al. (in press) also reasoned that the maintenance of an organized infant attachment strategy depends on a minimal level of parental appropriate responsiveness to the infant's attachment-related cues in order for the infant to modulate fear and maintain some sense of felt security. Very disrupted maternal responsiveness should impede the infant's capacity to draw upon the strategies of deactivation or heightened activation of attachment-related cues that avoidant and ambivalent infants employ in order to maintain a minimal level of proximity and parental accessibility (Main, 1990). The failure of either deactivation or heightened activation of attachment cues to maintain minimally adequate parental responsiveness should lead to infant fear and a breakdown of behavioral strategies. This repeated lack of appropriate responsiveness to the intention conveyed in the infant's communications could take many forms, including antagonism, withdrawal, intrusive overriding of the infant's cues, or role-reversing focus on the parent's needs rather than the infant's needs. The five behavioral dimensions that were coded as indices of such disrupted maternal affective communication are displayed in Table 2.1.

Mothers of disorganized infants displayed elevated rates of disrupted affective communication with their infants (Lyons-Ruth et al., in press). The most important dimension of the overall disrupted communication score was the subscore for affective communication errors, which was also significantly elevated. However, the means for all subscores were in the predicted direction and contributed to the overall finding. When analyzed separately rather than as part of the total disrupted communication score,

TABLE 2.1. Dimensions of Disrupted Maternal Affective Communication

1. Affective errors
   a. Contradictory cues; for example, invites approach verbally then distances.
   b. Nonresponse or inappropriate response; for example, does not offer comfort to distressed infant.
2. Disorientation (items from Main & Hesse, 1992)
   a. Confused or frightened by infant; for example, exhibits frightened expression.
   b. Disorganized or disoriented; for example, sudden loss of affect unrelated to environment.
3. Negative–intrusive behavior (including frightening items; Main & Hesse, 1992)
   a. Verbal negative–intrusive behavior; for example, mocks or teases infant.
   b. Physical negative–intrusive behavior; for example, pulls infant by the wrist.
4. Role confusion (includes items from Sroufe et al., 1985; Main & Hesse, 1992)
   a. Role reversal; for example, elicits reassurance from infant.
   b. Sexualization; for example, speaks in hushed, intimate tones to infant.
5. Withdrawal
   a. Creates physical distance; for example, holds infant away from body with stiff arms.
   b. Creates verbal distance; for example, does not greet infant after separation.

the mother's frightened or frightening behaviors alone also predicted disorganized infant attachment behaviors. However, with all frightened or frightening behaviors excluded from the total score for disrupted communication, disrupted communication still significantly predicted infant disorganization. Disorganized infant attachment behavior, then, was related to a broader context of maternal fear-related behavior than the behaviors captured by the frightened or frightening codes alone.

Lyons-Ruth et al. (in press) also examined separately the behaviors of mothers whose infants were classified D/secure and D/insecure. Paralleling the AAI findings of Schuengel et al. (1999) and Jacobvitz et al. (1997), mothers whose infants were classified D/insecure were significantly more likely to display both disrupted communication and frightening behavior than were mothers whose infants were classified D/secure, Eta = .44, p < .025. Mothers in the D/insecure subgroup were also significantly more likely than D/secure mothers to display role confusion and negative–intrusive behavior toward the infant. In contrast, D/secure mothers were more likely to display withdrawing behaviors. Scores for role confusion and negative–intrusive behavior were also strongly correlated in this sample, r = .53.

Given these large differences in patterns of maternal behavior *within* the disorganized group, both D/secure and D/insecure subgroups were compared separately to mothers in the organized group. Again, paralleling the AAI findings of Schuengel et al. (1999), only mothers in the D/insecure subgroup differed significantly from mothers of infants with organized attachment strategies, both on measures of frightened or frightening behavior and on the broader disrupted affective communication measures.

We interpret the pattern of findings in which D/insecure mothers displayed both role confusion and negative–intrusive behavior as evidence for the display of contradictory attachment strategies among mothers in the D/insecure subgroup. In the larger attachment literature, role-reversing behavior has been associated with the ambivalent category and viewed as part of an involving strategy to turn the child's attention toward attachment relationships; hostile, rejecting behavior has been associated with avoidant attachment patterns and viewed as part of a strategy to decrease attention to attachment relationships (Main, 1990). In summary, two significantly different patterns of maternal behavior occurred among mothers of disorganized infants. Mothers in the D/insecure subgroup exhibited high rates of affective communication errors, role confusion, negative–intrusive behavior, and frightening behavior, while mothers in the D/secure subgroup displayed elevated rates of withdrawal from the infant compared to D/insecure mothers.

Frightened and Withdrawing Behaviors of Mothers of Disorganized/Secure Infants

Lyons-Ruth et al. (in press) also hypothesized that there might be separable subgroups of predominantly frightened mothers and predominantly frightening mothers, and that these maternal behavior patterns might have different correlates in infant behavior. This possibility had received some support in that frightening, dissociative, and sexual/spousal behaviors were significantly intercorrelated, rs = .32 to .38, all p < .01, while frightened behavior was independently distributed, rs = 0 to .16, all n.s. However, because many mothers who displayed *frightened* behavior also displayed *frightening* behavior, a subject-based pattern analysis across all four Main and Hesse (1992) behavior codes at once (frightened, frightening, dissociated, sexual-spousal) was necessary to identify mothers whose behavior could be characterized as predominantly frightened, but not also frightening, dissociated, or role-reversed.

The first pattern analysis compared the infant attachment behaviors of mothers displaying (1) no FR+ behaviors of any kind (n = 20), (2) frightened behavior only (n = 7), (3) frightening behavior only (n = 5), (4) frightened and frightening behavior only (n = 10), or (5) frightened and frightening behavior plus other types of FR+ behavior (n = 8). The small numbers of mothers showing only one type of FR behavior resulted in small cell sizes and omission from the analysis of 15 mothers with other mixed behavior patterns. Nevertheless, the direction of the findings was clear. Among the 20 mothers who exhibited no FR+ behavior, 65% had secure infants. Among the three subgroups of mothers who displayed any frightening behavior (n = 23), 50–87% had infants with D/insecure behavior. In contrast, among mothers who displayed frightened behavior only, no infant displayed D/insecure behavior. However, only 29% were secure while 43% exhibited D/secure behavior patterns. In comparison, D/secure behaviors were only shown by 10% of infants of mothers with no FR+ behavior, and by 9% of infants whose mothers were in one of the three frightening behavior categories. Thus, the data suggested that mothers displaying frightened behavior only were more likely to have infants who displayed D/secure forms of attachment behavior, while mothers who displayed frightening behavior were more likely to have infants who displayed D/insecure behavior, Fisher's exact test (n = 30), p < .07, phi = .39.

Based on these results, the categorization criteria were broadened to include mixed patterns of maternal behavior, allowing all mothers to be categorized. The broadened criteria were also designed to reflect previous quantitative results indicating that *high* frequencies of all types of FR+ behavior, including frightened behavior, were associated with infant D/insecure behavior.

Results of the broadened classification criteria are displayed in Figure 2.2. Mothers of D/secure infants were more likely than other mothers to exhibit frightened behavior at moderate but not extreme levels and without associated elevations in frightening, dissociated, or role-reversed behavior. This was termed a frightened–inhibited pattern. Fifty percent of mothers of D/secure infants displayed this pattern of behavior, compared to 17% of mothers of organized infants and 10% of mothers of D/insecure infants, as shown in Figure 2.2. Consistent with previous linear analyses, higher levels of frightening behavior, as well as higher levels of frightened, dissociated or role-reversed behaviors, were displayed by mothers of D/insecure infants, as also shown in Figure 2.2.[1] Because of small expected cell sizes, the data in Figure 2.2 were collapsed into two orthogonal two-way tables for Fisher's exact tests. The two tests evaluated, first, whether mothers of D/secure infants were more likely to be in the frightened–

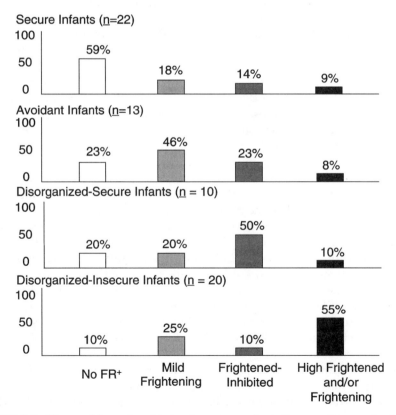

FIGURE 2.2. Maternal fear-related behavior patterns by infant attachment classification.

inhibited group than mothers of organized infants and, second, whether mothers of D/secure infants were more likely to be in the frightened–inhibited group than mothers of D/insecure infants. Both analyses were significant, D/secure versus organized, Fisher's exact test ($n = 45$), $p < .05$, phi = .32; D/secure versus D/insecure, Fisher's exact test ($n = 30$), $p < .03$, phi = .44.

In order to better understand and characterize this frightened–inhibited behavior pattern shown by many mothers of D/secure infants, additional statistical and descriptive analyses have been carried out since the Lyons-Ruth et al. (in press) report. These analyses have resulted in a much clearer picture of the behavior patterns of D/secure mothers. These additional analyses are presented in the remainder of this section.

Given the strength of this subject-based, pattern-analysis approach to classifying maternal behavior, a subject-based analysis was also carried out on the five dimensions of maternal behavior contributing to the disrupted affective communication rating. As already noted, D/secure mothers did not differ significantly from mothers of secure infants on any of these variables considered singly. As also reported earlier, however, separate analyses of variance on each of the five dimensional scores had revealed that D/secure mothers differed significantly from D/insecure mothers in being less negative and role reversing but more withdrawn in interaction with their infants. We reasoned that the combination of these behaviors into a pattern of maternal nonhostile withdrawal from the infant might provide more powerful discrimination of D/secure mothers than analyses evaluating each variable separately.

To operationalize this analysis, a withdrawal score consistent with the mean of the D/secure group but above the mean of the secure group (≥ 4) was chosen as a cutoff point indicating a withdrawing stance. A negative–intrusive score well below the mean of the D/insecure group (≥ 2) but consistent with the means of all other groups was chosen as a cutoff point indicating a nonhostile stance. The proportion of mothers displaying nonhostile withdrawal for each infant attachment group is displayed in Figure 2.3. Mothers of D/secure infants were significantly more likely to display nonhostile withdrawal in attachment-related interactions with their infants than either mothers of organized infants or mothers of D/insecure infants, D/secure versus organized, Fisher's exact test ($n = 45$), $p < .02$, phi = .40; D/secure versus D/insecure, Fisher's exact test ($n = 30$), $p < .02$, phi = .45.

Clearly, the frightened–inhibited pattern, yielded by the FR codes alone, and the pattern of nonhostile withdrawal, yielded by the broader disrupted communication codes, had some behavioral similarity. In addition, both the withdrawal and negative–intrusive scores included some behaviors from the Main and Hesse (1992) FR inventory. It seemed possible that both analyses were identifying the same subset of D/secure moth-

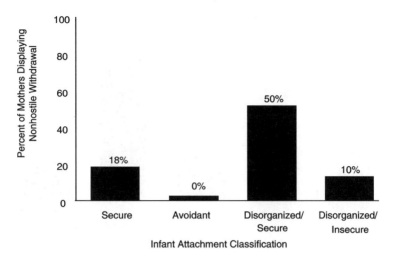

FIGURE 2.3. Percentage of mothers displaying nonhostile withdrawal by infant attachment classification.

ers. To examine whether the two analyses were redundant, we combined into a single group mothers who displayed frightened–inhibited behavior and mothers who displayed nonhostile withdrawal. In fact, the two patterns were not highly overlapping. Only 20% of mothers of D/secure infants displayed both fearful–inhibited behavior and nonhostile withdrawal; 30% displayed fearful–inhibited behavior without nonhostile withdrawal; and 30% displayed nonhostile withdrawal without fearful–inhibited behavior. However, combining the two patterns strengthened the relation to infant D/secure behavior, with 80% of mothers of D/secure infants displaying one of these two patterns, as shown in Figure 2.4. Thus, fearful maternal behaviors and nonhostile withdrawing maternal behaviors appear to represent alternative manifestations of a single underlying parental stance that we termed "helpless/fearful of attachment," an underlying stance that was strongly related to infant D/secure attachment behavior, D/secure versus organized, Fisher's exact test ($n = 45$), $p < .005$, phi = .44; D/secure versus D/insecure Fisher's exact test ($n = 30$), $p < .005$, phi = .58.

Helpless/Fearful of Attachment: Narrative Description of Maternal Fearful–Withdrawn Behavior

In light of these statistical findings, we reviewed our videotapes to create a narrative description of how these mildly fearful, inhibited, and withdrawn maternal behaviors were organized in relation to the infant's attachment behaviors. First, it is important to note that mothers in the D/secure group

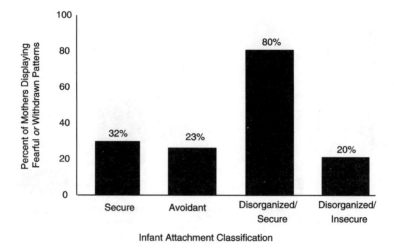

FIGURE 2.4. Percentage of mothers displaying fearful *or* withdrawal patterns by infant attachment classification.

were neither the most withdrawn nor the most fearful mothers in the sample. Consistent with previous findings, the most immediately salient aspect of the behavior of mothers of D/secure infants was that they appeared reasonably active and responsive in relation to the infant. Mothers who were unable to make any overtures in response to clear infant cues, or who were so fearful as to appear disoriented and disorganized, were more likely to have infants who mixed avoidance and resistance with their disorganized behavior and were therefore classified in the D/insecure subgroup. However, in the reunion behaviors of most mothers in the D/secure group, there was at least one moment of tension between mother and baby, when the baby clearly wanted more satisfying contact with the mother and the mother appeared reluctant to comply. The mother's reluctance was usually signaled by hesitation or subtle physical distancing rather than by a more active and negative countering of the infant's cue, however, and if the infant persisted, the mother usually complied, at least briefly. She often seemed somewhat tense, uncomfortable, or hesitant, however, and directed the infant away from herself as soon as possible. Some mothers in this group seemed particularly gentle, timid, or fragile, while others were more active but awkward and distancing. The fearful behavior most often coded in this group was a high, tense, quavering voice tone as the mother entered the room and greeted the infant, although recoiling from the infant's movements and subtle deferential behaviors toward the infant were also noted. Some mothers countered this apparent underlying fearful tension with a forced, somewhat overbright immediate approach and kiss for the infant upon reentry into the room, but most remained distanced and attempted to go around the infant or to direct the infant's attention immediately back to the toys. If the infant persisted in asking for contact, however, mothers in this group ultimately complied, and the infant's distress was quieted. On first viewing, these interactions had appeared adequate. However, closer inspection revealed that the infant was carrying undue responsibility for initiating or maintaining the comforting contact. Some mothers in this group also appeared to be in a generally deferential position in relation to the infant, being unable to refuse a bid from the infant for contact, even though they were reluctant or uncomfortable. Parents in this group seemed generally uncomfortable displaying forceful or directly negative behavior themselves, however, so they resisted the infant's bids passively or indirectly, or gave in quickly in response to the child's negative signals. While the infant's signals for contact were entirely appropriate, the mother's behavior raised the possibility that she might find it difficult to counter inappropriate behavior of the child as well, a problem that might not become more evident until toddlerhood. This stance in turn might contribute to the increasingly controlling behavior of the child toward the parent that has been demonstrated among disorganized infants as they develop into the preschool years. In these controlling patterns, the child apparently takes over responsibility for fashioning a semblance of an attachment relationship by directing, entertaining, and organizing the parent, or alternatively, by becoming more punitive and coercive. These data indicate, however, that any issues that emerge over limit setting in later toddlerhood are likely to be preceded by the mother's hesitancy and fearfulness in initiating and responding to appropriate attachment-related behaviors.

In contrast to mothers of D/secure infants, mothers of avoidant infants were much more likely to maintain a parental stance in relation to the infant. While not offering a lot of physical affection or contact, they remained in charge of the interaction, often approached and greeted the infant, asserted themselves, took initiative, and interacted verbally with the infant, at times with a degree of command or intrusiveness that elicited avoidant behavior in return. They did not generally appear hesitant or fearful in relation to the infant, nor did they appear frightening. We could not compare mothers of D/secure infants with mothers of organized–ambivalent infants because all ambivalent infants in this sample also displayed disorganized behavior.

The superficially responsive behavior of mothers of D/secure infants to the infants' concerted overtures might appear to contradict a relational diathesis hypothesis for this subgroup. Perhaps these are mothers who have suffered particularly acute trauma or loss in the context of otherwise adequate attachment relationships. We feel that an equally likely hypothesis, however, is that mothers of D/secure infants are drawn disproportionately from among women who developed controlling–caregiving adaptations to a sense of helplessness experienced in their own early attachment relationships. Theoretically, we would suggest that the D/secure mother's hesitant and fearful but ultimately compliant stance toward the infant's attachment bids may reflect an unresolved fearful and helpless stance toward a hostile attachment figure in the past. Therefore, the outlines of appropriate caregiving behavior were developed and are displayed in adulthood. However, caregiving control is viewed theoretically as an anxious adaptation to a failure of the attachment system, erected in the face of profound dysphoria, attachment disorganization, and fear on the part of the child. Therefore, we would predict that mothers of D/secure infants would show more appropriate caregiving behavior when the child's attachment system is *not* aroused, and would become more fearful, hesitant, inappropriate, or withdrawn when the infants' fearful and distressed attachment affects are more directly aroused and expressed.

At such times, one would expect the mother's own underlying sense of helplessness to become more pronounced. As the infant begins to react with conflict and apprehension to the mother's hesitancy and fear in responding to attachment affects, the mother's sense of helplessness would be likely to increase, which might lead to more obvious dysregulation in the relationship and compensatory controlling behavior on the part of the child by the time the child is seen during the preschool period.

The following three examples illustrate some of the variability in the maternal behavior patterns occurring among mothers in the D/secure group. In the first case, the baby was whimpering and crying throughout the first brief separation. The mother returned and stood across the room from the crying infant saying, "What? . . . What?" as the infant began to crawl toward her. When the infant was halfway to her mother, her mother took one step backward. The infant immediately stopped crawling forward, began to circle in place, then leaned her body onto the floor and rubbed her cheek against the rug. When it became apparent that the infant was not going to continue to approach, her mother came over to her, picked her up briefly until she stopped crying, and then moved her to the center of the toys, where she sat her down and heaped all the toys around her before moving away. This was all done silently. However, the mother was not abrupt, rough, or awkward, and the infant did not continue to fuss after the brief pick up.

In the second mother–infant pair, the mother's behavior was more active and apparently positive, though strained. However, a similar moment of hesitation to reciprocate her infant's attachment behavior occurred at the second reunion. At the first reunion, as the mother entered, she said, "Hi, there," but her son did not look up at her. She then said, "I love you," in a high voice that wavered with a frightened quality as she picked him up and hugged him. He remained somewhat flaccid and unresponsive to her. She then carried him to the toys and placed him on her lap on the floor, with his back to her. He slid sideways halfway off her lap and remained in this awkward position as she pulled various toys over for his attention. At the second reunion, as soon as he saw her, he held out his arms to be picked up. She kneeled in front of him, saying, "I love you," again in a high, strained voice, and hugged him. She then stood him up, away from her, and asked, "Did you have fun while I was gone? What did you play?" He looked down at the floor and did not respond, apparently in disappointment at being put off of her lap, and as she sat back away from him, he gave an exclamation of protest and lifted both arms out to her again. She ignored his signal and repeated, "What did you play?" He continued to hold out his arms and vocalized again. Instead of responding to his repeated signal, however, she cocked her head sideways in a coy posture that had a deferential air, pursed her lips, and withheld a response, imitating his vocalization in a teasing manner. He dropped his arms and head and looked away, scowling. She asked him again if he had fun and tickled him under the chin. He turned back to her, smiled, raised his arms again, and fell into her arms as she hugged him and asked, "Did you miss me? I missed you, too." One's impression in observing the session was that neither mother nor child felt comfortable and fluent in responding to the other's initiatives for close affectionate contact.

In the third example, at the end of the first separation period, the infant was undistressed but stood fingering the door. His mother opened the door and entered silently, as the infant drew in his breath with a frightened sound and backed up with his head down to make room for his mother. Both mother and infant stood silently in this posture until the stranger left. The infant then held up his arms, walked up to her, and put his upstretched hands on her abdomen. When he touched her, she said, "Hi," and looked down and rubbed the top of his head. She then picked him up awkwardly by his upper arms and kissed him on the cheek as he looked and pointed at the door. She put him down, facing him away from her, toward the toys, while she walked in a semicircle around the toys to face him, with the toys between them. He was still for a moment, then abruptly threw down the toy he was holding. She knelt and pointed to a toy, saying, "Look," but he ignored her overture and went to the door, whining. When she finally did engage him with a toy, she withdrew to sit in the chair.

During the second separation, he was distressed throughout. At the second reunion, mother again entered silently and stopped, and stood at the door. He immediately stood up and started hurriedly toward her through the toys but tripped and fell. His mother did not speak or move while he got himself onto all fours and crawled the rest of the way to her. As he reached her, wailing, she said, "What's the matter?" then bent to pick him up. She held him, saying in a comforting tone, "Aw, stop that. Stop it." His wailing subsided and he pointed to the door. She patted his head and said, "Yeah," a couple of times, then bent down to the toys with him on her knee. He slid onto the floor and as soon as he became interested in a toy, she went to sit in the chair.

Through all these examples, the mother's momentary withdrawal, hesitation, or inaction when approached by the infant was notable. Her eventual compliance with the infant's attachment overtures was also notable, although this sometimes occurred only after clear, angry signals or dysphoric behavior on the part of the infant. The full set of D/secure maternal behaviors that emerged from both statistical analyses and subsequent descriptive tape review is summarized in Table 2.2.

DISCUSSION AND CONCLUSIONS

In this chapter, we have elaborated a model of a hostile–helpless caregiving diathesis that is proposed to contribute to the emergence of disorganized attachment behaviors in infancy. Our view of the role of highly unbalanced relational processes in parent–infant interaction began with our data on the severity of trauma in the mother's childhood and its relation to her interactive behaviors with her infant at home. Those data revealed that the severity of trauma in the mother's childhood predicted her increased withdrawal from responsive affective engagement with her infant when observed at home. In addition to the emotional withdrawal noted among mothers with more severe trauma, a second finding specifically related

TABLE 2.2. Fearful of Attachment: Attachment-Related Behaviors of Mothers of Disorganized/Secure Infants during Reunions

1. Withdrawal (e.g., sits in chair; interacts from a distance; steps back as infant approaches).
2. Directs infant away from self to toys quickly after reunion.
3. Cursory responding (e.g., gives quick hug then moves away).
4. Delayed responding, but eventual compliance to infant cues (e.g., greets or hugs infant only after persistent bids by infant).
5. Little or no hostility or intrusion.
6. Subtle fearful, hesitant, or deferential behavior toward the infant (e.g., high frightened voice on entry; hesitates with arms out before embracing infant).

physical violence or abuse in the mother's childhood to increased covert hostility and intrusive behavior toward her infant. This increased subtle hostility and interference was not displayed by mothers who had experienced sexual abuse without associated physical abuse. Those mothers displayed only emotional withdrawal. Because extended clinical treatment of sexual abuse survivors clearly reveals both the underlying fear and anger of those who have been victimized (see Terr, 1991), sexually abused mothers appeared more likely to manage these negative affects by withdrawing from interaction with the infant, while mothers who had been physically abused appeared to handle their trauma-related negative affects by identifying with an aggressive style of interaction.

Our thinking about hostile–helpless dyadic representations took fuller shape when we began to explore the difficult-to-classify adult attachment interviews from the same cohort of mothers. Again, the bimodality of the internal working models of attachment associated with infant disorganization was notable (Atwood, 1995; Lyons-Ruth & Atwood, in press).

Finally, in the work presented in this chapter, we found that mothers' attachment-related interactions with their infants presented a converging picture of at least two significantly different maternal stances within the disorganized spectrum. These different organizations of maternal behavior, in turn, related to long-noted differences in the organization of infant behavior within the disorganized spectrum, differences captured in the secondary classifications of secure and insecure (avoidant or ambivalent) assigned to all disorganized infants.

In conjunction with the partially converging data from Schuengel et al. (1997, 1999), we have tentatively labeled these two distinct organizations of parent–infant behavior "hostile" or "helpless" in relation to attachment. In the helpless–fearful subgroup, disorganized infants combine approach behaviors, relative absence of avoidance or resistance, and abatement of distress, with indicators of conflict, apprehension, or dysphoria, and mothers combine nonhostile and superficially responsive behavior with subtle indicators of fearfulness, withdrawal, and disrupted affective communication around the infant's attachment goals. In the hostile subgroup, infants display disorganized forms of avoidant and/or ambivalent behavior, and mothers combine elevated rates of frightening and total FR+ behaviors with disrupted affective communication and contradictory hostile–rejecting and role-reversed caregiving strategies.

Lyons-Ruth and Atwood (in press) have developed coding conventions for hostile versus helpless states of mind on the AAI, both of which our pilot work suggests are related to infant disorganization. We have speculated, in turn, that these two parental stances may reflect alternative expressions of a single unbalanced victim–aggressor relationship prototype experienced in the parent's own attachment history. As a single dyadic prototype, we would expect that individuals displaying disorganized strategies or unresolved states of mind would have access to both the hostile and helpless aspects of this single representational model. The degree to which either the hostile or helpless position in this dyadic organization is identified with the self may depend on situational, temperamental, and cultural factors, as well as aspects of the individual's particular relationship history, and we would expect that a single individual could display either or both of these relational stances at different times or in different situations or relationships.

In support of the view that the two behaviorally distinct stances share important underlying commonalities, a variety of evidence indicates that D/secure and D/insecure infants sustain a similar degree of risk over time. First, in infancy, both subgroups of D infants exhibited clear indicators of conflict, apprehension, or dysphoria in relation to the caregiver at reunion. Second, both subgroups of disorganized infants were at risk for displaying highly aggressive behavior toward peers by ages 5 and 7 (Lyons-Ruth et al., 1993; Lyons-Ruth, Easterbrooks, & Cibelli, 1997; see also Shaw et al., 1996; Goldberg et al., 1995). Third, no subgroup differences were noted by Main et al. (1985) in the prediction from infant disorganization to controlling patterns of attachment behavior at age 6 in a sample in which the D/secure behavior pattern was the most prevalent form of disorganization. Fourth, Solomon, George, and De Jong (1995) have related the emergence by age 6 of both controlling–caregiving and controlling–punitive attachment strategies to increased externalizing symptoms, as well as to maternal self-representations as helpless in relation to the child. The relation between controlling attachment strategies and externalizing behavior has been replicated in several other cross-sectional studies (Moss et al., 1996, 1998; Speltz et al., 1990; Greenberg et al., 1991).

Even if a common hostile–helpless dyadic model underlies both fearful and threatening parental behavior, however, the parental behaviors exhibited in the presence of observers in the two subgroups are organized quite differently. Fearful or threatening parental behaviors also engender different forms of disorganized infant attachment behaviors, differences captured by the D/secure or D/insecure secondary classifications. These corresponding differences in the organization of infant behavior suggest that the differences in observed parental behavior are consistent with unobserved, day-to-day differences at home, differences sufficient to generate distinct patterns of infant attachment behavior over time. The corresponding differences in infant behavior weigh against the hypothesis that mothers in the fearful group simply inhibit aggressive behaviors when observed.

More work is clearly needed to examine both the maternal behavior patterns and the associated theoretical hypotheses emerging from this work. However, the accumulated evidence indicates that we need to continue to understand the developmental pathways associated with both helpless and hostile forms of disorganization. Further work is needed to explore the experiential, temperamental, and contextual factors that interact with disorganized attachment patterns to produce a differential likelihood of activating helpless or hostile behavior in intimate attachment relationships.

NOTE

1. Although the small numbers do not allow statistical comparisons, it is notable that mothers of D/ambivalent infants displayed behavior patterns in between those of D/secure mothers and D/avoidant mothers. Only 25% of D/ambivalent mothers had a high frightening score, while 50% were predominantly frightened. These frightened mothers differed from D/secure mothers in that they were more likely to display *high* levels of frightened behavior and were more likely to display concomitant dissociative behaviors than were D/secure mothers. However, they were less likely to display high frightening scores than mothers of D/avoidant infants.

REFERENCES

Ainsworth, M. D. S., Blehar, M., Waters, E., & Wall, S. (1978). *Patterns of attachment*. Hillsdale, NJ: Erlbaum.

Ainsworth, M. D. S., & Eichberg, C. (1991). Effects on infant–mother attachment of mother's unresolved loss of an attachment figure or other traumatic experience. In C. Parkes, J. Stevenson-Hinde, & P. Marris (Eds.), *Attachment across the life cycle* (pp. 160–186). New York: Routledge.

Atwood, G. (1995). *Adult attachment disorganization: A new classification and scoring scheme for the Adult Attachment Interview*. Unpublished doctoral dissertation, Harvard University, Cambridge, MA.

Baldwin, A. L., Cole, R. E., Baldwin, C. P., Fisher, L., Harder, D. W., & Kokes, R. F. (1982). The role of family interaction in mediating the effect of parental pathology upon the school functioning of the child. In A. L. Baldwin, R. E. Cole, & C. P. Baldwin (Eds.), Parental pathology, family interaction, and the competence of the child in school. *Monographs of the Society for Research in Child Development, 47*(5, Serial No. 197), 72–80.

Bowlby, J. (1969/1982). *Attachment and loss: Vol. 1. Attachment*. New York: Basic Books.

Bowlby, J. (1973). *Attachment and loss: Vol. 2. Separation*. New York: Basic Books.

Bowlby, J. (1980). *Attachment and loss: Vol. 3. Loss.* New York: Basic Books.

Cadoret, R. J., Winokur, G., Langbehn, D., Troughton, E., Yates, W. R., & Stewart, M. A. (1996). Depression spectrum disease: I. The role of gene–environment interaction. *American Journal of Psychiatry, 13,* 892–899.

Carlson, V., Cicchetti, D., Barnett, D., & Braunwald, K. (1989). Disorganized/disoriented attachment relationships in maltreated infants. *Developmental Psychology, 25,* 525–531.

Cassidy, J., & Berlin, L. (1994). The insecure/ambivalent pattern of attachment: Theory and research. *Child Development, 65,* 971–991.

Cassidy, J., & Kobak, R. (1988). Avoidance and its relation to other defensive processes. In J. Belsky & T. Nezworski (Eds.), *Clinical implications of attachment* (pp. 300–323). Hillsdale, NJ: Erlbaum.

Cassidy, J., & Marvin, R. S. (1987/1990/1991/1992). *Attachment organization in preschool children: Coding guidelines.* Unpublished coding manual, MacArthur Working Group on Attachment, Seattle, WA.

Clarke, A. S. (1993). Social rearing effects on HPA axis activity over early development and in response to stress in young rhesus monkeys. *Developmental Psychobiology, 26,* 433–447.

Crittenden, P. M. (1985). Maltreated infants: Vulnerability and resilience. *Journal of Child Psychology and Psychiatry and Allied Disciplines, 26,* 85–96.

Egeland, B., Jacobvitz, D., & Sroufe, L. A. (1988). Breaking the cycle of abuse. *Child Development, 59,* 1080–1088.

Egeland, B., & Sroufe, L. A. (1981). Attachment and early maltreatment. *Child Development, 52,* 44–52.

Fraiberg, S., Adelson, E., & Shapiro, V. (1975). Ghosts in the nursery. *Journal of the American Academy of Child Psychiatry, 14,* 387–421.

Freud, S. (1957). Mourning and melancholia. In J. Strachey (Ed. and Trans.), *The standard edition of the complete psychological works of Sigmund Freud* (Vol. 14, pp. 237–260). London: Hogarth Press. (Original work published 1917)

Gaensbauer, T. J., & Harmon, R. J. (1982). Attachment behavior in abused/neglected and premature infants: Implications for the concept of attachment. In R. N. Emde & R. J. Harmon (Eds.), *The attachment and affiliative systems* (pp. 245–279). New York: Plenum.

George, C., Kaplan, N., & Main, M. (1984/1985/1996). *Adult Attachment Interview.* Unpublished manuscript, University of California, Berkeley.

George, C., & Solomon, J. (1996). Representational models of relationships: Links between caregiving and attachment. *Infant Mental Health Journal, 17,* 198–216.

George, C., & Solomon, J. (1998, July). *Attachment disorganization at age six: Differences in doll play between punitive and caregiving children.* Paper presented at the meeting of the International Society for the Study of Behavioural Development, Bern, Switzerland.

George, C., & Solomon, J. (1999). Attachment and caregiving: The caregiving behavior system. In J. Cassidy & P. R. Shaver (Eds.), *Handbook of attachment: Theory, research, and clinical applications* (pp. 649–670). New York: Guilford Press.

Goldberg, S., Gotowiec, A., & Simmons, R. J. (1995). Infant–mother attachment and behavior problems in healthy and chronically ill preschoolers. *Development and Psychopathology, 7,* 267–282.

Greenberg, M. T., Speltz, M. L., DeKlyen, M., & Endriga, M. C. (1991). Attachment security in preschoolers with and without externalizing behavior problems: A replication. *Development and Psychopathology, 3,* 413–430.

Hann, D. M., Castino, R. J., Jarosinski, J., & Britton, H. (1991, April). *Relating mother–toddler negotiation patterns to infant attachment and maternal depression with an adolescent mother sample.* Paper presented at the biennial meeting of the Society for Research in Child Development, Seattle, WA.

Hertsgaard, L. Gunnar, M., Erickson, M. F., & Nachmias, M. (1995). Adrenocortical response to the Strange Situation in infants with disorganized/disoriented attachment relationships. *Child Development, 66,* 1100–1106.

Jacobsen, T., & Miller, L. (1998). Compulsive compliance in a young maltreated child. *Journal of the American Academy of Child and Adolescent Psychiatry, 37,* 462–463.

Jacobvitz, D., Hazen, N., & Riggs, S. (1997, April). *Disorganized mental processes in mothers, frightening/frightened caregiving, and disoriented/disorganized behavior in infancy.* Paper presented at the biennial meeting of the Society for Research in Child Development, Washington, DC.

Kraemer, G. W., & Clarke, A. S. (1996). Social attachment, brain function, and aggression. *Annals of the New York Academy of Sciences, 794,* 121–135.

Lyons-Ruth, K., Alpern, L., & Repacholi, B. (1993). Disorganized infant attachment classification and maternal psychosocial problems as predictors of hostile–aggressive behavior in the preschool classroom. *Child Development, 64,* 572–585.

Lyons-Ruth, K., & Atwood, G. (in press). Identification with a hostile or helpless attachment figure: Additional correlates of infant disorganization in the Adult Attachment Interview. In L. Atkinson (Ed.), *Attachment and psychopathology* (Vol. 2). Cambridge, UK: Cambridge University Press.

Lyons-Ruth, K., & Block, D. (1996). The disturbed caregiving system: Relations among childhood trauma, maternal caregiving, and infant affect and attachment. *Infant Mental Health Journal, 17,* 257–275.

Lyons-Ruth, K., Bronfman, E. & Parsons, E. (in press). Maternal disrupted affective communication, maternal frightened or frightening behavior, and disorganized infant attachment strategies. In J. Vondra & D. Barnett (Eds.), Atypical patterns of infant attachment: Theory, research and current directions. *Monographs of the Society for Research in Child Development, 64*(3, Serial No. 258).

Lyons-Ruth, K., Easterbrooks, A., & Cibelli, C. (1997). Infant attachment strategies, infant mental lag, and maternal depressive symptoms: Predictors of internalizing and externalizing problems at age 7. *Developmental Psychology, 33,* 681–692.

Lyons-Ruth, K., Kaufman, M., Masters, N., & Wu, J. (1991). Issues in the identification and long-term management of Munchausen by proxy syndrome within a clinical infant service. *Infant Mental Health Journal, 12,* 309–320.

Lyons-Ruth, K., Repacholi, B., McLeod, S., & Silva, E. (1991). Disorganized attachment behavior in infancy: Short-term stability, maternal and infant correlates, and risk-related subtypes. *Development and Psychopathology, 3,* 377–396.

Main, M. (1990). Cross-cultural studies of attachment organization: Recent studies, changing methodologies and the concept of conditional strategies. *Human Development, 33,* 48–61.

Main, M., & Cassidy, J. (1988). Categories of response to reunion with the parent at age 6: Predictable from infant attachment classifications and stable over a 1-month period. *Developmental Psychology, 24*(3), 415–426.

Main, M., & Goldwyn, R. (1985/1991/1994/1998). *Adult attachment scoring and classification systems.* Unpublished classification manual, University of California, Berkeley.

Main, M., & Hesse, E. (1990). Parents' unresolved traumatic experiences are related to infant disorganized attachment status: Is frightened and/or frightening parental behavior the linking mechanism? In M. Greenberg, D. Cicchetti, & E. M. Cummings (Eds.), *Attachment in the preschool years: Theory, research and intervention* (pp. 161–184). Chicago: University of Chicago Press.

Main, M., & Hesse, E. (1992). *Frightening, frightened, dissociated, or disorganized behavior on the part of the parent: A coding system for parent–infant interactions* (4th ed.). Unpublished manuscript, University of California, Berkeley.

Main, M., & Hesse, E. (1995). *Frightening, frightened, dissociated, or disorganized behavior on the part of the parent: A coding system for parent–infant interactions* (5th ed.). Unpublished manuscript, University of California, Berkeley.

Main, M., Kaplan, N., & Cassidy, J. (1985). Security in infancy, childhood and adulthood: A move to the level of representation. In I. Bretherton & E. Waters (Eds.), Growing points of attachment theory and research. *Monographs of the Society for Research in Child Development, 50*(1-2, Serial No. 209), 66–104.

Main, M., & Solomon, J. (1990). Procedures for identifying infants as disorganized/disoriented during the Ainsworth Strange Situation. In M. Greenberg, D. Cicchetti, & E. M. Cummings (Eds.), *Attachment in the preschool years: Theory, research and intervention* (pp. 121–160). Chicago: University of Chicago Press.

Main, M., Tomasini, L., & Tolan, W. (1979). Differences among mothers of infants judged to differ in security of attachment. *Developmental Psychology, 15,* 472–473.

Moss, E., Parent, S., Gosselin, C., Rousseau, D., & St-Laurent, D. (1996). Attachment and teacher-reported behavior problems during the preschool and early school-age period. *Development and Psychopathology, 8,* 511–526.

Moss, E., Rousseau, D., Parent, S., St-Laurent, D., & Saintonge, J. (1998). Correlates of attachment at school age: Maternal reported stress, mother–child interaction, and behavior problems. *Child Development, 69,* 1390–1405.

Nemeroff, C. (1996). The corticotropin-releasing factor (CRF) hypothesis of depression: New findings and new directions. *Molecular Psychiatry, 1,* 336–342.

Ogawa, J. R., Sroufe, L. A., Weinfield, N. S., Carlson, E. A., & Egeland, B. (1997). Development and the fragmented self: Longitudinal study of dissociative symptomatology in a nonclinical sample. *Development and Psychopathology, 9,* 855–879.

Radke-Yarrow, M., Cummings, E. M., Kuczynski, L., & Chapman, M. (1985). Patterns of attachment in two- and three-year-olds in normal families and families with parental depression. *Child Development, 56,* 884–893.

Robertson, J., & Robertson, J. (1969). *John, aged 17 months* [film]. London: Tavistock Institute of Human Relations.

Schuengel, C., van IJzendoorn, M., Bakermans-Kranenburg, M., & Blom, M. (1997, April). *Frightening, frightened and/or dissociated behavior, unresolved loss and infant disorganization.* Paper presented at the biennial meeting of the Society for Research in Child Development, Washington, DC.

Schuengel, C., Bakermans-Kranenburg, M., & van IJzendoorn, M. (1999). Frightening maternal behavior linking unresolved loss and disorganized infant attachment. *Journal of Consulting and Clinical Psychology, 67,* 54–63.

Shaw, D. S., Owens, E. B., Vondra, J. I., Keenan, K., & Winslow, E. B. (1996). Early risk factors and pathways in the development of early disruptive behavior problems. *Development and Psychopathology, 8,* 679–699.

Solomon, J., George, C., & De Jong, A. (1995). Children classified as controlling at age six: Evidence of disorganized representational strategies and aggression at home and at school. *Development and Psychopathology, 7,* 447–463.

Spangler, G., & Grossmann, K. E. (1993). Biobehavioral organization in securely and insecurely attached infants. *Child Development, 64,* 1439–1450.

Speltz, M. L., Greenberg, M. T., & DeKlyen, M. (1990). Attachment in preschoolers with disruptive behavior: A comparison of clinic–referred and nonproblem children. *Development and Psychopathology, 2,* 31–46.

Sroufe, L. A., Jacobvitz, D., Mangelsdorf, S., DeAngelo, E., & Ward, M. J. (1985). Generational boundary dissolution between mothers and their preschool children: A relational systems approach. *Child Development, 56,* 317–325.

Stevenson-Hinde, J., & Shouldice, A. (1995). Maternal interactions and self-reports related to attachment classification at 4. 5 years. *Child Development, 66,* 583–596.

Strage, A., & Main, M. (1985, April). *Attachment and parent–child discourse patterns.* Paper presented at the biennial meeting of the Society for Research in Child Development, Toronto, Ontario, Canada.

Terr, L. C. (1991). Childhood traumas: An outline and overview. *American Journal of Psychiatry, 148*(1), 10–20.

van IJzendoorn, M. H. (1995). Adult attachment representations, parental responsiveness, and infant attachment: A meta-analysis on the predictive validity of the Adult Attachment Interview. *Psychological Bulletin, 117,* 387–403.

van IJzendoorn, M. H., Schuengel, C., & Bakermans-Kranenburg, M. K. (1999). Disorganized attachment in early childhood: Meta-analysis of precursors, concomitants and sequelae. *Development and Psychopathology, 11,* 225–249.

Wartner, U. G., Grossmann, K., Fremmer-Bombik, E., & Suess, G. (1994). Attachment patterns at age six in South Germany: Predictability from infancy and implications for preschool behavior. *Child Development, 65,* 1014–1027.

Zahn-Waxler, C., & Kochanska, G. (1990). The origins of guilt. In R. Thompson (Ed.), *Nebraska Symposium on Motivation: Vol. 36. Socioemotional development* (pp. 183–258). Lincoln: University of Nebraska Press.

CHAPTER 3

Unresolved Loss and Infant Disorganization
Links to Frightening Maternal Behavior

CARLO SCHUENGEL
MARIAN J. BAKERMANS-KRANENBURG
MARINUS H. VAN IJZENDOORN
MARJOLIJN BLOM

One important contribution of John Bowlby's (1969/1982) theory of attachment has been the insight that all children form an attachment to their caregiver(s), even when the caregiving they receive is severely compromised. Like other primates, human infants are drawn to familiar adults in the face of real or perceived danger (Bowlby, 1969/1982). Infants who have been abused by a caregiver, however, find themselves in an irresolvable paradox (Main & Hesse, 1990). The person who should be their safe haven is at the same time frightening. This experience is likely to have a profound impact on the attachment relationship that is developing. Studies of abused infants have found that many exhibit anomalous forms of attachment behavior toward their parents (Carlson, Cicchetti, Barnett, & Braunwald, 1989; Crittenden, 1985; Egeland & Sroufe, 1981; Lyons-Ruth, Connell, Zohl, & Stahl, 1987). On the basis of these observations, Main and Solomon (1986) proposed a new attachment category: disorganized attachment.

A considerable number of infants of nonabusive parents have been found to have disorganized attachment as well. Perhaps without being fully aware, some parents may be a source of fear to their infants. This may explain another observation made by Main and Hesse (1990), that when parents show evidence of mental disorganization and disorientation when talking about a traumatic experience, for example, loss of a loved one, their infants are likely to fall into the disorganized category. On this basis, Main, DeMoss, and Hesse (1991) identified a new adult attachment category: unresolved regarding loss. In this chapter, we further examine how unresolved loss and disorganized attachment are linked to frightening parental behavior.

Since the publication of Ainsworth's work on 26 middle-class mother–infant dyads in Baltimore (Ainsworth, Blehar, Waters, & Wall, 1978), individual differences in the attachment relationships of babies and their caregivers have been studied with the use of a laboratory procedure, the strange situation. Babies are sensitive to natural clues to danger (Bowlby, 1985), some of which are provided by the strange situation. The procedure is so designed that the attachment behavioral system (Bowlby, 1969/1982) of the infant is increasingly activated as the procedure progresses. The setting is comfortable but unfamiliar; mother and baby are soon joined by a stranger, after which the parent twice leaves the infant for 3 minutes.

Ainsworth and her colleagues (1978) identified three groups of infants on the basis of their response to this procedure. The secure, avoidant, and ambivalent groups indicate different qualities of the attachment relationship. Main (1990) views the behavior of the infants in these groups as organized around different strategies for dealing with the fear produced by being left alone vis-à-vis their expectations of their parent.

A fourth group was later discovered when an increasing number of reports indicated that a sizable number of infants failed to fit one of the three organized patterns. Furthermore, forced classifications of these infants into a best-fitting alternative produced counterintuitive results. Main and Solomon (1986) found that this group of infants showed a (momentary) absence of organization of attachment behavior. Some of these children showed incompatible attachment strategies in response to the return of their parent, others showed conflict behaviors (Main & Weston, 1981), others seemed to lose their orientation toward their parent and the environment altogether, and still others displayed fear of their parent. Main and Solomon proposed a fourth, insecure, attachment category: disorganized/disoriented attachment (Group D).[1]

Although disorganization was often observed in maltreatment samples, disorganized attachment was also found in low-risk samples as well. In these samples, it was associated with parental unresolved loss as identified on the basis of response to the Adult Attachment Interview (AAI; George, Kaplan, & Main, 1984/1985/1996), an hour-long, semistructured interview focusing on attachment-related issues in childhood and adulthood, including experiences of loss by the death of someone important, for instance, an attachment figure (Ainsworth & Eichberg, 1991; Main & Hesse, 1990). Unresolved loss is identified on the basis of markers of mental disorganization or disorientation surrounding the loss. This is consistent with Bowlby's (1980) conceptualization of loss of a loved one as a "disorganizing" experience; he saw mourning as the process of reorganizing one's thoughts, feelings, and actions in the face of the permanent absence of the loved person. In 1995, van IJzendoorn reported a meta-analysis on nine studies using the AAI as well as the strange situation, in which unresolved traumatic experiences (such as loss) had an effect size of $r = .31$ on disorganized infant attachment.

Main and Hesse (1990) proposed that frightening parental behavior (threatening, frightened, or dissociated) forms the causal link between unresolved trauma and infant disorganization. Frightening behavior might be the result of parents being unable to control frightening memories or emotions associated with the loss. These memories or emotions might in turn be triggered by objects in the environment or by the actions and demands of their infant. Main and Hesse reasoned that frightening behaviors (such as looming, exaggerated startle, or freezing) may have an effect on infants that is similar to the aggressive and invasive behaviors of abusive parents. Infants who have these frightful experiences find themselves in a paradoxical situation. Fear activates the attachment behavioral system, and this system impels infants to seek out a safe haven. But what should be safe, the parent, is also the source of danger. Repeated experiences of this kind would result in disorganization of the attachment behavioral system. According to Main and Hesse, this happens irrespective of other dimensions of maternal behavior, for example, sensitivity. That way, frightening behavior accounts for otherwise apparently secure babies being classified as disorganized. This is also consistent with the fact that adults can be classified as unresolved regarding loss, while at the same time being classified as secure regarding their attachment representation. Figure 3.1 outlines the basic features of Main and Hesse's model.

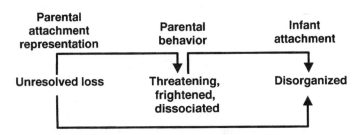

FIGURE 3.1. The theory of Main and Hesse (1990) linking unresolved loss and infant disorganization.

Before Main and Hesse's theory can be tested, several questions have to be answered. Can frightening behavior be observed under naturalistic conditions (Spangler, Fremmer-Bombik, & Grossmann, 1996)? And which population should we study? To test the role of unresolved loss in producing frightening behavior, a low-risk, middle-class population seems the best suited to reduce alternative explanations. However, social expectations might be confounding. The current pilot study focuses on frightening behavior as observed in the homes of 11 low-risk mothers. Furthermore, we investigated the links with unresolved loss, and with infant attachment.

METHOD

Participants

With the use of town hall records, we invited participants by mail to take part in a study on maternal life events and the role of these events in the development of the bond with their infants. The letter was unspecific as to which events we would focus on. Of the 157 mothers who were contacted 78 (50%) agreed to participate. We selected participants for the observational part of the study on the basis of their response to the Berkeley–Leiden Adult Attachment Questionnaire—Unresolved scale (BLAAQ-U; Main, van IJzendoorn, & Hesse, 1993), a questionnaire designed to discriminate participants likely to be classified as unresolved with regard to trauma. The BLAAQ-U results in scores on a scale for unresolved state of mind and for unusual beliefs associated with unresolved trauma. The BLAAQ-U has proven to have predictive validity and reliability (Main et al., 1993; Alkalay & Sagi, 1997). Out of the 78, we selected 7 mothers, on the basis of high scores on the BLAAQ-U, and 5 mothers, on the basis of low scores. (We favored high-scoring participants slightly to minimize the risk of having too low a number of unresolved participants in our pilot sample.) One low-scoring mother did not end up participating in the strange situation procedure and this dyad was excluded. The mean age of the final 11 mothers was 30 years (range 25 to 34). The mothers each had a minimum of 12 years of education.

Observation Procedures and Instruments

Frightening Maternal Behavior

We observed the home behavior of the mothers when their infants were 10 or 11 months old. The mothers were visited by Schuengel or a research assistant twice, once in the morning and once in the afternoon, on separate days. Appointments were made such that other household members (e.g., older children) would be absent during the home visits. Mothers were instructed to follow their normal routine as if they were alone with their child. The observer followed the dyad around with a camcorder and continuously recorded their behavior for 2 hours each visit—less if the infant had to be put to bed.

Coding proceeded in two stages. First, a selection of behavioral events was made by screening the videotapes for behaviors and interactions that could be frightening. In 10 cases, the tape was independently screened by two screeners (Schuengel and Blom). In one case, one observer completed the screening. As the coding progressed, some tapes had to be rescreened due to increased experience with frightening behavior, and due to changes in the coding system. The final coding of the screened tape fragments was done by consensus (among Main, Hesse, and the authors). First, coders decided on the type of frightening behavior. Second, the severity of the behavior was rated on a scale of 1 to 9. If a single behavior was rated higher than 5, the mother was considered "frightening." When several less intense behaviors seemed to form a pattern, this also resulted in a classification as frightening. When the highest event score was 5, the frightening behaviors had to be considered as a whole for a forced classification. Reliability between two coders was subsequently established on 16 cases ($r_s =$ .83). Coders were blind to AAI and strange situation procedure classifications.

The Main and Hesse (1992) coding system identifies three types of frightening behavior. The most obviously frightening one is *threatening behavior*. An example is "looming," a sudden movement into the area immediately surrounding the infant's face and eyes. Another example is vocally, verbally, or by movement or posture, attacking the baby. However, a parent acting *frightened* might be frightening to an infant as well. This is the case when the parental expression of fear is incomprehensible to the infant, or if the infant might get the idea it is him- or herself who frightens the mother. An example is exaggerated startling if the baby falls (without the mother appearing to cheer the baby up or to be playful). A pattern of behavior that conveys fearfulness is persistent and repeated backing away from the infant whenever he or she approaches. Another, less obvious type of frightening behavior is the category of *dissociated* behaviors, which includes "indications that a parent may have entered a somewhat dissociated state" (Main & Hesse, 1992; p. 10). An example showing that such behavior may frighten infants is a sudden drop in pitch in the parent's voice, as when a female voice suddenly takes on the quality of a male voice, again, without obvious playful or disciplinary intent. Another example is the mother assuming a trance-like posture or expression.

For exploratory purposes, two additional types of behavior were recorded. These behaviors might also be relevant to infants' disorganized attachment and parental unresolved trauma, but it is less clear whether these should also be regarded as frightening. One type includes behaviors that may indicate the activation of behavioral systems that conflict with expressions of attachment (infant) or caregiving (mother). This type of behavior includes treating the child as an attachment figure, or as an object of deference, as well as treating the child as a sexual/spousal partner. The other type includes dissociated behaviors that might not affect the child directly. This class includes rare behaviors such as treating inanimate objects as animate and acting as though the parent were a child.

Adult Attachment Interview

We conducted the AAI (George et al., 1984/1984/1996) with the mothers when the infants were about 12 months old. The AAI is a semistructured interview about the adults' childhood experiences with their own parents, about the influence of these experiences, and about their current relationship with their parents. Participants are also asked about attachment-related experiences of loss or other trauma and about their own children. A coding system is applied to the verbatim transcripts of participants' responses to arrive at an assessment of the state of mind with regard to their experiences (Main & Goldwyn, 1985/1991/1994). Bakermans-Kranenburg and van IJzendoorn (1993) report satisfactory reliability and discriminant validity for the instrument (see also Sagi et al., 1994; Crowell et al., 1996). van IJzendoorn's (1995) meta-analysis shows that the AAI classifications of parents have predictive validity with respect to the quality of the attachment relationship with their infants. For the present study, only the parts of the AAI that referred to losses and traumatic experiences were transcribed. Personal information that could identify the participant to the coder was deleted from the transcript. Marian Bakermans-Kranenburg coded the fragments for unresolved loss and for unresolved trauma. Having been trained by Mary Main and Erik Hesse, she has obtained good interrater reliability.

The category, unresolved state of mind with respect to loss experiences (Main et al., 1991), differs from other categories that have been considered indicative of unresolved or pathological mourning in clinical contexts (see Stroebe, Stroebe, & Hansson, 1993, for a review). Incomplete mourning, failure to mourn, or emotionality during the discussion of loss is not coded as unresolved loss.

Participants can be classified as unresolved only on the basis of apparent mental disorganization or disorientation during the discussion of a loss. This can be manifest in (1) lapses in the monitoring of reasoning (i.e., a discussion about the loss contains references to actions of the deceased in the present); (2) lapses in the monitoring of discourse (i.e., the discussion of the loss takes a direction that is not appropriate for the immediate discourse context, such as unusual attention to detail in their descriptions of the event or their immediate reaction to it); or (3) lapses in the monitoring of behavior, as in reports of extreme behavioral reactions to the loss (e.g., suicide or nervous breakdown in the absence of convincing evidence that the participant has now regained mental and behavioral control). The Main et al. (1991) coding system requires that each instance of these lapses is rated on a 9-point scale. Instances are then combined in a final score on the same 9-point scale, which forms the basis of the classification. Scores higher than 5 automatically lead to unresolved classification, and with a score of 5, the decision is left to the judgment of the coder.

Strange Situation

The strange situation procedure (Ainsworth & Wittig, 1969) was administered when the infants were around 14 months old. This procedure involves a structured series of episodes in which the infant is exposed to mildly stressful events, including the entrance of an unfamiliar adult and two separations from the parent, followed by reunions. We used the traditional Group A (avoidant), Group B (secure), and Group C (ambivalent) classification system (Ainsworth et al., 1978) and the directions of Main and Solomon (1990) for Group D (disorganized/disoriented) attachment. Infants in the secure group can respond to the separation from their parent with distress, but they actively seek contact on her return and are relatively easily consoled. Infants in the avoidant group typically do not show distress and avoid the proximity of their parent on reunion. Infants in the ambivalent group generally are very distressed by separation and on reunion show contact seeking as well as resistance to the parent. These infants are very difficult to console. Main and Solomon's system includes a 9-point rating scale for disorganized behavior. A score higher than 5 leads to the classification as disorganized. When the behavior qualifies for a classification as disorganized, a best-fitting traditional classification is also assigned. In rare cases, infants can be classified CC (cannot classify) when the pattern of infant behavior is inconsonant with one of the traditional and disorganized categories (Main & Solomon, 1990). In these cases, a best-fitting secondary classification is assigned. Coders were blind to all other information about the dyads. Intercoder reliabilities were adequate for all three coders (Schuengel, Bakermans-Kranenburg, & van IJzendoorn), with percentage agreement on disorganized versus not disorganized ranging from 83 to 96. All were trained by Mary Main and Erik Hesse.

CASE DESCRIPTIONS

The case descriptions are organized in four sets. First, we describe the cases in which there was concordance in the classification of maternal state of mind regarding trauma, maternal behavior at home, and infant strange situation behavior. These concordant cases are grouped by maternal AAI classification: unresolved loss and no unresolved loss. Second, we discuss the cases in which there was discordance. The final case description concerns a mother who had recently experienced a loss of a loved one when we observed her home behavior. Data on the dyads in our sample are summarized in Table 3.1.

Concordance in Mothers with Unresolved Loss

Mrs. H and Nina

Mrs. H was 30 years old when she had Nina, her second child. She had lost her maternal grandmother at age 27. She had also experienced physical abuse by her father. She reported still feeling fearful sometimes of her father hitting her when she did something wrong; however, it was not clear whether this constituted unrealistic fear associated with unresolved trauma. An unresolved state of mind was apparent regarding the loss of her grandmother, when Mrs. H revealed she could sometimes feel her grandmother's presence.

At first, maternal behavior during both home visits appeared only overstimulating, but not frightening. However, Mrs. H engaged in severe tickling, to the point that Nina cried helplessly as she unsuccessfully tried to ward off her mother. Furthermore, Mrs. H would occasionally move her face close to Nina's and show a frightening grin with bared teeth. This type of aggressive looming behavior is considered frightening.

There was also some hint of dissociated behavior. Mrs. H had an eerie facial expression when she crawled catlike toward Nina and mauled her. Within a few seconds, her expression became angry and unhappy, and then changed into a smile. In itself, this would not be enough to count as definitely frightening, even though the rapid changes of affective tone suggest unusual shifts in Mrs. H's emotional and behavioral state.

Four months later, Nina could be observed to display disorganized attachment behavior, as on second reunion, she inexplicably lay flat on the floor, without looking at her mother. She then moved toward her mother, but just before reaching her, she again lay flat on the floor. Besides disorganized, she was classified as secure.

Mrs. C and Dave

Mrs. C was 28 years old when she had her first child, Dave. At 27 years of age, she had lost her best friend, and this had prompted her to want to

TABLE 3.1. Summary Data

Infant's name	Mother's name	Unresolved loss (yes/no)	Frightening behavior (yes/no)	Threatening, frightened, or dissociated behavior	Primary infant attachment classification	Secondary infant attachment classification
			Concordance in mothers with unresolved loss			
Nina	Mrs. H	Yes	Yes	Threatening	Disorganized	Secure
Dave	Mrs. C	Yes	Yes	Threatening	Disorganized	Avoidant
Johanna	Mrs. Y	Yes	Yes	Threatening	Secure	Disorganized
Donna	Mrs. S	Yes	Yes	Frightened	Disorganized	Secure
			Concordance in mothers without unresolved loss			
Robby	Mrs. G	No	No	Threatening	Secure	—
Mandy	Mrs. O	No	No	Threatening	Avoidant	—
			Discordance in a mother with unresolved loss			
Violet	Mrs. D	Yes	Yes	Threatening	Secure	—
			Discordance in mothers without unresolved loss			
Vonne	Mrs. N	No	Yes	Threatening	Secure[a]	—
Deborah	Mrs. R	No	Yes	Frightened	Secure[a]	—
Jolene	Mrs. P	No	Yes	Threatening	Secure	—
			Recent loss			
Ariadne	Mrs. F	No	No	—	Disorganized	Secure

Note. All mothers had experienced loss.
[a]Displayed disorganized attachment behavior at home, sufficient for classification as disorganized.

have a child. Her discourse about the loss and the subsequent birth of Dave showed lapses in the monitoring of reasoning. She stated that Dave was born within 1 day of the first anniversary of her friend's death. In another sentence, she implicated (in a slip of the tongue) that this friend was Dave's father. This indicated an unresolved state of mind regarding this loss. An important incident occurred when Dave was 8 months old. Mrs. C found him lifeless in his crib. He was saved, but a monitoring device was placed in his bedroom to alert his parents if he should stop breathing. At the time of the first home visit, Dave was 10 months old. Both parents were present and talked to the cameraperson. They were no longer worried that Dave would die in his crib, and they had shut the monitor off, because it had been going off frequently without any reason.

Mrs. C displayed threatening behavior. While she was sitting on a chair with Dave lying on his back on the floor below, she clawed repeatedly toward Dave's face and pushed his nose. This became more frightening because Dave's reactions of fear and distress did not stop her from going on with this disagreeable and fear-provoking behavior. She was also observed to deliberately startle Dave with her voice and with her gestures.

When he was 14 months old, Dave displayed a mixed and confused sequence of avoidance, proximity seeking, and distress during the second reunion of the strange situation. Apart from being deemed disorganized, he was classified as avoidant.

Mrs. Y and Johanna

Mrs. Y was the youngest mother in our sample, having given birth to Johanna when she was 25 years old. At about age 14 or 15, she had lost someone who was very dear to her, the mother of her high school friend. She went into unusual detail when asked about her reactions to the loss, indicating a lapse in the monitoring of discourse. For example, she described how, when she waited for the school headmaster to tell her the news, "through the crack in the door we saw someone walk or something."

At the 10-month home visits, Mrs. Y appeared extremely focused on behavior of her baby that was potentially hurtful or dangerous. However, in addition to making warning noises, she occasionally became scary by using a very low voice and making odd, "spooky" sounds. The pattern of warning and being simultaneously "dangerous" was deemed frightening, although no single instance would have been sufficient to put her in the frightening category.

When she was 14 months old, Johanna showed simultaneous avoidance and proximity seeking during the strange situation, but it was not quite sufficient for definite placement in the disorganized category. Disorganized was her secondary classification, however, whereas the primary classification was secure.

Mrs. S and Donna

Mrs. S had her second child, Donna, when she was 31. She had lost her mother when she was 22. An unresolved state of mind was indicated by her extreme behavioral reaction. She reported that some time afterward, she developed psychological and physiological symptoms, and underwent hypnotherapy to resolve the loss. Although she stated that the therapy had been successful, in later, related discussion, it became apparent that the loss continued to influence her behavior. She reported she was too afraid to take her elder son to the beach, for fear she might lose him.

On two occasions during the 10-month home observation, Mrs. S displayed exaggerated startling when Donna fell on her bottom. Both times, she followed this by pulling back from the baby. The first time she put out her arm as if she was under attack, and the second time, her face expressed startle and fear—to the observers, Donna's fall did not seem very sudden or serious. This type of frightened behavior qualified for the frightening category.

In the strange situation, Donna displayed a sequential contradictory behavior pattern of calling out and crying during separation, but avoiding her mother on reunion. The primary classification was disorganized; the secondary classification was secure.

Concordance in Mothers without Unresolved Loss

Mrs. G and Robby

Mrs. G had Robby at age 31. He was her first child. The only loss she experienced was of the mother of her sister-in-law, but she did not discuss this in the AAI. This failure to discuss a loss was not considered indicative of unresolved loss, because she might have regarded this loss as unimportant.

During the home visit, when Robby was 10 months old, we saw that the mother frequently engaged in rough play in which she growled at Robby and chased him. This was, however, accompanied by warm metasignaling. Mrs. G appeared to discipline Robby somewhat harshly and this also could have made Robby somewhat afraid, although disciplining provides a context that makes such behavior comprehensible. We judged her behavior to be moderately to slightly threatening, but not enough for placement in the category.

In the strange situation, Robby exhibited a very secure pattern of attachment behavior and no signs of disorganization.

Mrs. O and Mandy

Mrs. O had her first child, Mandy, when she was 28. Mrs. O had experienced a difficult upbringing in which she was physically abused by her father. She had been in therapy and had undergone hypnotic regression. She lost a good friend when she was 18. However, Mrs. O was not classified as unresolved for either the abuse or the loss. In fact, she dismissed any negative effects regarding her abuse experiences and stated that she regarded the influence on her as entirely positive. Although perhaps clinically relevant, for our purposes, this dismissive attitude toward a trauma is not considered indicative of an unresolved state of mind.

During the home observations, we saw Mrs. O startling Mandy and provoking fear in her in the context of rough, overstimulating play. We rated the behavior as moderate but not enough for classification as frightening, because of the clear signals toward Mandy that it was some sort of play. We also saw Mrs. O lapse into absorption during her interaction with Mandy, staring and not noticing her baby, but these brief moments only qualified for a low rating of dissociated behavior.

The strange situation behavior of Mandy was somewhat atypical, as she displayed proximity seeking on the first reunion but failed to do so on the second, passing her mother instead by the door. This sequence, although unusual is not inexplicable or contradictory enough to be considered disorganized. Instead, the overall best-fitting classification was avoidant.

Discordance in a Mother with Unresolved Loss

Mrs. D and Violet

Violet was Mrs. D's third child, born when Mrs. D was 30. Mrs. D's mother had died when Mrs. D was 20, and Mrs. D displayed an unresolved state of mind regarding that loss. The circumstances surrounding the loss were traumatic. Mrs. D discovered her mother after she had committed suicide, and for this reason she was still angry with her. This anger led to lapses in the monitoring of discourse and (implicitly) of reasoning, because she started addressing her mother ("How could you ever have done that!"). Other lapses included dysfluency, as she was repeatedly unable to name the cause of death (e.g., "And I still am angry with her, because she . . . because she, yes, . . . ").

Rage appeared to play a role in her behavior toward Violet as well. She was observed to engage in an angry fit that resulted in uncontrolled battering of the toy Violet was holding, taking Violet by the shoulders and shaking her, and emitting an uncontrolled angry scream. This only took about 10 seconds, but this incident nevertheless placed her in the frightening category.

Mrs. D also displayed timid/deferential behavior toward Violet. Several times, in reaction to Violet's noncompliance, she retracted her hands and folded them before her chest with her shoulders lowered and her gaze downward. Her facial expression did not display dramatic license; instead, she honestly apologized to Violet. As noted before, this type of behavior is not considered in the classification of frightening behavior, but it is recorded and coded on a similar scale. We rated her timidity/deference as moderate to low.

When she was 14 months old, Violet displayed "underwater" movements in response to the second reunion in the strange situation. She lifted her arms in a slow, smooth gesture, and continued moving slowly after she was picked up. On the tape, it looked as if the videotape was being played in slow motion. This type of behavior can be ambiguous, however, and it would have to be very distinct to lead to disorganized classification, which was not the case here. The baby was classified as secure.

Discordance in Mothers without Unresolved Loss

Mrs. N and Vonne

For Mrs. N, Vonne was her second daughter, whom she had at age 31. When Mrs. N discussed the loss of her best friend when she was 18, she seemed somewhat unsettled, but there were not enough signs to consider her unresolved.

The home behavior of Mrs. N was at times simply overstimulating, but the aggression that went with it made it definitely threatening as well. She tossed Vonne around, accompanied by baring her teeth and making growling noises. In the context of feeding, she also showed aggression and looming behavior toward Vonne.

At 10 months of age, Vonne was observed to display disorganized behavior during the home visits.[2] There were some signs of disorganization when Mrs. N engaged in overstimulating behavior. Vonne swept at Mrs. N's face in a way that looked casual, but in fact, it was aimed at Mrs. N's eye. This is usually regarded as a strong marker of disorganization, although the fact that Vonne was not in a good mood at the same time made it less severe. Vonne also exhibited stereotypical movements while she was held by the parent (but these were not marked and Vonne was distressed, so this was also not a strong marker), a confused cry–laugh that sounded fearful (a definite sign of disorganization), and other stereotypical movements while not distressed. Together, these behaviors would have led to a classification as disorganized when shown in the context of the strange situation.

At 14 months of age, Vonne showed little disorganized behavior within the strange situation, and her classification was secure. It was noted, however, that her behavior deteriorated from the first to the second reunion, showing active resistance on second reunion, but no resistance on the first.

Mrs. R and Deborah

Mrs. R had Deborah, her fourth child, at the age of 34. The losses of both her grandparents (during adolescence and adulthood) were not classified as unresolved.

During both home visits, the cameraperson noted that Mrs. R was very shy. She repeatedly asked the cameraperson permission to do her household chores or to take care for her infant, and she had to be reinstructed a couple of times to go about her normal business. This meant we had to be careful not to mistake her camera-shy behavior for frightened or timid/deferential behavior. These behaviors occurred, however, following actions of the infant, and the behaviors were specifically directed at the infant. In fact, we deemed her behavior frightened because of the consistent backing away from the infant and displays of caution toward the infant. Mrs. R also showed minor forms of threatening, dissociated, and timid/deferential behavior. Apart from these behaviors and reactions, she interacted little with the infant, only to discipline her or take care of diapers, clothing, or to administer drinks.

Oddly enough, although apparently frightened by her infant, Mrs. R treated her in a cold and harsh manner, perhaps as a way to control her fearfulness. Similar to Vonne, Deborah reacted with disorganized behavior. On one occasion, she heard her mother approach and displayed an asymmetrical facial expression by pulling one corner of her mouth down. She also engaged in mistimed movements: an inexplicable bout of activity, jerking her head and chest back and forth. When Mrs. R stood before her, ready to pick her up, Deborah looked up with a fearful facial expression: Her eyes bulged, her mouth was open and her shoulders were tense.

But in the strange situation procedure 4 months later, Deborah did not show disorganized behavior, and she was actually classified as secure. There was unusual behavior at the second reunion, however. Deborah cried and signaled weakly to be picked up. After being picked up, she stopped crying, and Mrs. R kneeled and held the infant in an awkward position. Because Deborah was put in this position by her mother, it cannot be coded as disorganized behavior. But it is odd for a secure infant to stay immobile when in an uncomfortable position on her mother's lap. Normally, secure babies sink in comfortably. This infant sat passively but uncomfortably and sucked her thumb.

Mrs. P and Jolene

Mrs. P had her first child, Jolene, when she was 30. She had lost two grandparents when she was 5 and 6 years old, but she was not unresolved.

In the home, when the baby was 10 months old, Mrs. P struck the observers as being harsh and aggressive toward Jolene. She frequently stood watching Jolene or commanded her in a way that reminded the observers of an (old-fashioned) prison guard. She also frequently displayed an ominous facial expression, and at two instances, we observed brief moments of her threatening Jolene by sticking her chin out, eyes bulging, and moving her face close to Jolene's. It was not accompanied by metasignaling that this was play. We judged Mrs. P as moderately threatening toward Jolene.

In the strange situation procedure, Jolene did not show signs of disorganization, and she was classified as securely attached.

Recent Loss

Mrs. F and Ariadne

Ariadne was Mrs. F's first child, born when she was 32. Nine months after Ariadne was born, Mrs. F's mother died. At the AAI, 3 months later, she did not show any signs of unresolved loss.

When Ariadne was 10 months old, the mother–infant interaction was very pleasant, and there was no sign of frightening behavior. The parent also did not strike us as being depressed or inhibited in her interaction with Ariadne.

Ariadne had a secondary secure classification on the basis of her strange situation behavior, but, quite unexpectedly, her primary classification was disorganized. Her disorganized behavior was moderate to definite in the first-reunion episode: She fell prone in a depressed posture, and lay still for some time.

DISCUSSION

On the basis of the descriptions of 11 dyads, we can examine the evidence for Main and Hesse's (1990) theory that frightening behavior is the causal link between unresolved loss and infant disorganization/disorientation. All 5 unresolved mothers displayed frightening behavior, and 4 of these 5 infants were classified as disorganized (primary or secondary). There were no children classified as disorganized in the group of children whose mothers who were not unresolved nor frightening. Up to this point, our observations were consistent with the theory. However, frightening behavior was also found in 3 mothers without unresolved loss, and their infants were not disorganized. Although these mothers had no unresolved loss, we would still have predicted that their frightening behavior would have led to attachment disorganization. However, this was not the case.

Several interpretations are possible. One possibility is that frightening behavior has nothing to do with disorganization at all, and that some other unknown factor determined attachment behavior. However, such a factor has to account for the association between unresolved loss and infant disorganization also. Perhaps shared genetic factors such as temperament predispose adults to react with mental disorganization or disorientation to traumatic experiences, and predispose infants to develop disorganized attachment. Another possibility is that unresolved loss disrupts caregiving, in multiple ways, and frightening behavior might just be one aspect of disrupted caregiving leading to infant disorganization. In future tests of Main and Hesse's theory, other aspects of maternal behavior should be measured also in order to test this possibility. In a sample of 85 dyads, Schuengel, Bakermans-Kranenburg, and van IJzendoorn (1999) tested whether other aspects of maternal behavior (sensitivity) or mental status (depression) explained the correspondence between unresolved loss and infant disorganization. This was not the case.

Another interpretation of the lack of correspondence between frightening behavior and disorganization could be methodological. We found two infants that showed disorganized attachment behavior in the home but were not disorganized during the strange situation. It was an informal observation, and it must be viewed with caution, because these infants were about 10 to 11 months old. The finding does, however, warrant further investigation of the ways in which disorganization can be reliably and validly assessed. For example, evidence on the stability of the disorganized classification is mixed (van IJzendoorn, Schuengel, & Bakermans-Kranenburg, 1999). Classification of disorganized attachment might be less robust than classification into the traditional attachment groups. In contrast to the classification of avoidant and secure attachment, the classification of disorganized attachment is entirely dependent upon positive evidence. The coding system does not identify behaviors that are negative indicators of disorganization, showing organization. In fact, it is possible that on the basis of just a single behavior, perhaps lasting a few seconds, an otherwise "organized" baby might be classified as disorganized. Furthermore, the predictive validity of disorganized attachment behavior in the lab with respect to attachment behavior in the home has never been studied, but, as indicated by our observations, it should be a topic of investigation.

However, apart from reliability or validity issues, the possibility of real change also must not be discounted. Perhaps Deborah and Vonne learned to construct an organized strategy in the 4 months between home observation and strange situation. This does not imply that disorganization is "just a phase." A sizable proportion of infants is still disorganized at 14 months, and disorganization corresponds to unresolved loss experiences of the attachment figure. However, one could speculate that some forms of frightening parental behavior might lead to disorganization in a 10-month-old child, but not in a 14-month-old child.

Then, there is the possibility that frightening behavior is important in the transmission of the effects of unresolved loss, but that the causal model is incomplete. In fact, this is what our limited data suggest. One way to look at the various concordances and discordances is that frightening behavior predicts disorganization when mothers are unresolved, but does not predict disorganization when mothers are not unresolved (see Table 3.1). We now reexamine the theoretical basis of the current model, with a particular focus on possible moderating factors.

Unresolved Loss and Dissociation

To recapitulate, on the basis of discussions about loss and traumatic experiences in the AAI, an adult is classified as having unresolved loss when he or she displays lapses in the monitoring of reasoning, discourse, or behavior (Main & Goldwyn, 1985/1991/1994). An example of a lapse in the monitoring of reasoning can be found in Mrs. H, who still seems to believe her grandparent is still around, even though Mrs. H also knows she is dead. An example of a lapse in the monitoring of discourse can be found in Mrs. Y, who lost herself in detailed description and visual images when asked about her reactions to her loss. Main and Morgan (1996) argue that dissociation may underlie these lapses. This is consistent with the hypothesized (but unproven) link between traumatic experiences and dissociation (Hacking, 1995). Lapses similar to those described in the coding system for the AAI seem to be observable in dissociative disorder patients when they discuss traumatic experiences (e.g., intrusion of visual–sensory images; van der Kolk & Fisler, 1995).

Dissociation can be seen as a defense mechanism for handling the overwhelming emotions that accompany traumatic experiences—especially emotions of fear (Putnam, 1991). During a traumatic experience, it is believed that the person processes his or her perceptions and reactions in separate mental "compartments." Because the memories about the event are stored separately, the working through of the traumatic experience can be hampered (Classen, Koopman, & Spiegel, 1993; Spiegel, 1991). For the dissociatively disorded patient, this results in a disruption of the usually integrated functions of consciousness, memory, identity, and perception of the environment (see DSM-IV, American Psychiatric Association, 1994). van der Kolk and Fisler (1995), following the French psychiatrist Janet, have argued on the basis of interviews with traumatized individuals, that dissociation during traumatic experience produces traumatic memories that consist of images, sensations, affective, and behavioral states that are only partially, or not at all, integrated into a narrative. Under special circumstances, these unintegrated memories can be unconsciously evoked. When dissociated memory content temporarily becomes conscious or semiconscious, the person's behavior is likely to change. To bystanders, the resulting behavior can be inexplicable and frightening to experience.

Lapses in monitoring associated with unresolved status in the AAI suggest that memories about traumatic events are being processed in a somewhat altered state, that is, in a different cognitive "register" (Main &

Morgan, 1996). This may lead to multiple representational models. However, in normative samples, participants classified as unresolved are generally functioning well; if unresolved loss and dissociated disorder (massive breakdown of integrative functions of the mind) are on the same continuum, then they are at opposite ends.

In any case, the phenomenon of dissociation highlights the particularly erratic character of the continuing emotional and behavioral reactions of the traumatized individual. Dissociation therefore provides a useful framework in which to understand the behavior of traumatized individuals. But, as noted by Bowlby (1980), the broader principle of the "defensive exclusion of unwelcome information" may underlie this particular phenomenon, as well as other phenomena such as repression, denial, and splitting. It is still unclear whether dissociation fully explains unresolved loss, or that other forms of defensive exclusion are relevant also. George and Solomon (in press) adopt the broader starting point and discuss how defensive exclusion of trauma-related information as a process might have an impact on the caregiving system. It could be that the current focus on dissociation as the reaction to trauma is too narrow, and that it would be worthwhile to return to Bowlby's (1980) earlier thinking about defensive exclusion and the ways it might lead to multiple representational models (see Solomon & George, Chapter 1, this volume).

Given that unresolved loss is a manifestation of the existence of multiple representational models (Main & Hesse, 1990; George & Solomon, in press), the questions arise: How are altered states that are connected with multiple models provoked under natural circumstances, while during the AAI these might be provoked by the interview questions? And, crucial for our purposes, do these altered states influence behavior in a way that is noticeable to infants; are these responsible for the behaviors we classify as frightening? These questions are as yet without answer.

It has been noted for people with trauma histories that any affective state related to their traumatic experiences may trigger their recalling or even reexperiencing of the original event. These triggering affective states can be daily emotions, such as fear, longing, and intimacy (van der Kolk & Fisler, 1995) that any parent of young children may experience. A parent who shifts into a traumatized state might be quite scary for an infant. To begin with, the shifting of states could, in itself, be frightening for infants to witness, when the parent, for example, enters a trance-like state. In addition, changes in the level of arousal of the parent could occur, which could lead to intense and aggressive, overstimulating behavior, as we saw in some of the mothers in our sample. Alternatively, perceptions by the parent of objects within the environment (Liotti, 1992) or actions of the infant could be distorted due to a traumatic state of mind. Relatively harmless actions by the infant, for example, could provoke anger or fear in the parent if they resonate with the parent's experience of loss (Bowlby, 1988). Bowlby noted, furthermore, that these reactions of fear could become disconnected from their source; thus, the parent may be angry or fearful in the absence of triggering objects or events.

In summary, frightening behavior originating from traumatic experiences can be the result of various mechanisms. In addition, it seems that these mechanisms are likely to be activated during daily interactions with infants. We identified several mechanisms that suggest that the resulting behavior will not only be scary but also inconsistent with the context, with preceding infant behavior, and with preceding parental behavior. We propose that this inconsistency might be the dimension that modifies the impact of frightening behaviors on infants.

The Inconsistency Hypothesis

Bowlby (1985) described the alertness of infants to clues to danger within the environment. As we say at the beginning of this chapter, the natural reaction of infants to these clues is to seek a safe haven, normally, the attachment figure. However, when the attachment figure is simultaneously the source of perceived danger, infants are placed in a paradoxical situation and will be unable to find a solution for their fear. It is presumed that this makes it impossible for infants to develop a coherent and organized strategy for dealing with fear and distress in the presence of their attachment figure. These infants display disorganized attachment behavior within the strange situation (Main & Hesse, 1990). However, when infants are able to ignore the frightening behavior of their parent, they will not necessarily become disorganized. This would involve a strategy similar to the one avoidantly attached infants seem to use within stressful situations (Main, 1990) as they ignore the presence or absence of their parent and suppress their emotions of distress. Main notes that the strategy of these infants is primarily based on a mental act: the turning away of their attention from the whereabouts of the attachment figure. Avoidantly attached infants ignore that their parent may be rejecting. Infants who ignore that their parent is sometimes scary may be able to fall back on their underlying secure, avoidant, or ambivalent attachment strategy; they do not reach the state of disorganization. This might only be possible under two conditions: (1) parental behavior is only slightly frightening; or (2) slightly or moderately frightening behavior occurs in a consistent pattern. We do not expect that infants can adapt to highly frightening behavior, even if it is displayed in a consistent way.

In our study, mothers with moderately to highly frightening behavior were classified as frightening. In some cases, consistency lowered the score; in others, consistency elevated the score. On the one hand, for example, the somewhat harsh behavior of the mother of Robby was rated low, because this behavior was consistently connected with disciplining. Also, instances of overstimulating, attacking, and chasing were mitigated when the mothers used metasignaling that this was all part of play, which could also be a consistent pattern. On the other hand, the spooky warning sounds of Mrs. Y only received a rating sufficient for placement in the frightening category, just *because* this was a fairly consistent pattern of behavior. Of many other maternal behaviors, it was not possible to evaluate whether the frightening behaviors were part of a consistent pattern.

It is interesting to note that two of the three children whose mothers were frightening in the absence of unresolved loss, Vonne and Deborah, showed a secure attachment pattern but also showed anomalous behavior patterns. These infants had shown disorganized behavior in the home. It might be that in the 4 months between the home observations and the strange situation, these infants completed the more challenging work of developing an organized strategy in response to a mother whose frightening behavior was moderate but consistent. This may explain their secure but relatively atypical behavior compared to children who had organized their attachment strategy more early on.

A developmental shift from disorganization to nondisorganization might only be possible when frightening maternal behavior is relatively mild. Under that condition, infants may after some time be able to use an organized shift of attention away from the fact that their mother is a source of fear. But the situation of these infants may also be considered in a different way, as a balance between fear of the mother and fear of the situation. When the fear provoked by the situation overrides the fear for the parent, the attention of the infant may be shifted from the fact that she, too, is a source of danger. Then, we would predict that these children do show disorganized behavior in circumstances that are stressful enough to activate the attachment behavioral system to some extent (e.g., within the home), but not necessarily under the greater stress of the strange situation. Continuous scores for disorganization in the strange situation might adequately reflect the fact that some infants might have some difficulty organizing a response, but ultimately succeed in doing so.

Thus, a new model might take inconsistency of frightening behavior into account. At the same time, the model should reflect that inconsistency will only be important if frightening behavior is moderate. It will be relatively unimportant if frightening behavior is either very low or very high. Probably its influence will only be detectable in low-risk samples, and in the absence of multiple, severe trauma to parent and to child.

The addition of the inconsistency dimension will necessitate even more extensive observation than already is required to observe frightening behavior. Perhaps the problem can be approached by using a more strictly event-based scoring method and applying techniques for sequential analysis. Or perhaps the contexts in which frightening behaviors occur should be recorded: If a particular behavior occurs across several contexts (i.e., is not tied to a particular context), this may be an indicator of inconsistency. It could also be fruitful to interview parents afterward about possible conscious motives for their behavior, although it will depend on the context whether this would be ethically acceptable.

Notwithstanding the practical difficulties, inconsistency can be one of the identifying features of frightening behavior that is responsible for second-generation effects of unresolved trauma, distinguishing from frightening behavior that is linked to other processes (e.g., depression, personality, beliefs about child rearing). This is suggested by our case examples. Frightening behavior by not unresolved mothers did not predict disorganization, whereas frightening behavior by unresolved mothers did predict disorganization.

CONCLUSIONS

Our study shows that in a normal sample within a naturalistic setting, one can observe frightening parental behavior. One can even observe disorganized infant behavior. Using the same observational strategy, Schuengel et al. (1999) did establish in a sample of 85 dyads that frightening behavior indeed predicted disorganized attachment. Frightening behavior was predicted by the interaction between unresolved loss and maternal attachment security. Our case-level approach did, however, yield some important additional hypotheses when we examined mismatches between parental behavior and infant attachment. Frightening behavior seems to be an important new category of parental behavior that has the potential of elucidating second-generation effects of traumatic experiences. However, not only the severity of the behavior but also the patterning might be important. On the basis of theory as well as case material, the consistency of patterns of frightening behavior should be further investigated.

ACKNOWLEDGMENTS

We are indebted to Mary Main and Erik Hesse of the University of California at Berkeley for their participation in the coding of parental home behavior. We wish to thank Tirtsa Joels of Haifa University for her assistance in the classification of the strange situations. This study was supported by a Pioneer award from the Netherlands Organization for Scientific Research (NWO, Grant No. PGS 59-256) to Marinus H. van IJzendoorn.

NOTES

1. The same difficulties in classifying these infants were noticed by Crittenden (1985), Lyons-Ruth et al. (1987), and Carlson et al. (1989).

2. We had not predicted disorganized behavior in the home when we conducted the study. We are, to our knowledge, the first to report disorganized attachment behavior outside the laboratory situation. In future research, this behavior has to be excluded by a screener in order to keep coders of frightening maternal behavior unaware of the attachment status of the baby.

REFERENCES

Ainsworth, M. D. S., Blehar, M. C., Waters, E., & Wall, S. (1978). *Patterns of attachment.* Hillsdale, NJ: Erlbaum.

Ainsworth, M. D. S., & Eichberg, C. (1991). Effects on infant–mother attachment of mother's unresolved loss of an attachment figure, or other traumatic experience. In C. M. Parkes, J. Stevenson-Hinde, & P. Marris (Eds.), *Attachment across the life cycle* (pp. 160–183). London: Routledge Tavistock.

Ainsworth, M. D. S., & Wittig, B. A. (1969). Attachment and exploratory behavior of one year olds in a strange situation. In B. M. Foss (Ed.), *Determinants of infant behavior* (pp. 113–136). London: Methuen.

Alkalay, S., & Sagi, A. (1997, April). *Identifying unresolved states of mind among holocaust survivors in Israel.* Poster presented at the biennial meeting of the Society for Research in Child Development, Washington, DC.

American Psychiatric Association. (1994). *Diagnostic and statistical manual of mental disorders* (4th ed.). Washington, DC: Author.

Bakermans-Kranenburg, M. J., & van IJzendoorn, M. H. (1993). A psychometric study of the Adult Attachment Interview: Reliability and discriminant validity. *Developmental Psychology, 29,* 870–880.

Bowlby, J. (1969/1982). *Attachment and loss: Vol. 1. Attachment* (2nd ed.). London: Penguin.

Bowlby, J. (1973). *Attachment and loss: Vol. 2. Separation.* London: Penguin.

Bowlby, J. (1980). *Attachment and loss: Vol. 3. Loss.* London: Penguin.

Bowlby, J. (1988). *A secure base: Clinical applications of attachment theory.* London: Routledge.

Carlson, V., Cicchetti, D., Barnett, D., & Braunwald, K. (1989). Disorganized/disoriented attachment relationships in maltreated infants. *Developmental Psychology, 25,* 525–531.

Classen, C., Koopman, C., & Spiegel, D. (1993). Trauma and dissociation. *Bulletin of the Menninger Clinic, 57,* 178–194.

Crittenden, P. M. (1985). Maltreated infants: Vulnerability and resilience. *Journal of Child Psychology and Psychiatry and Allied Disciplines, 26,* 85–96.

Crowell, J. A., Waters, E., Treboux, D., O'Connor, E., Colon-Downs, C., Feider, O., Golby, B., & Posada, G. (1996). Discriminant validity of the Adult Attachment Interview. *Child Development, 67,* 2584–2599.

Egeland, B., & Sroufe, L. A. (1981). Attachment and maltreatment. *Child Development, 52,* 44–52.

George, C., Kaplan, N., & Main, M. (1984/1985/1996). *Adult attachment interview.* Unpublished manuscript, University of California, Berkeley.

George, C., & Solomon, J. (in press). The development of caregiving: A comparison of attachment and psychoanalytic approaches to mothering. In D. Diamond, S. Blatt, & D. Silver (Eds.), Psychoanalytic Theory and Attachment Research: I. Theoretical Considerations. *Psychoanalytic Inquiry, 19* [Special issue].

Hacking, I. (1995). *Rewriting the soul: Multiple personality and the sciences of memory.* Princeton, NJ: Princeton University Press.

Liotti, G. (1992). Disorganized/disoriented attachment in the etiology of the dissociative disorders. *Dissociation, 5,* 196–204.

Lyons-Ruth, K., Connell, D. B., Zoll, D., & Stahl, J. (1987). Infants at social risk: Relations among infant maltreatment, maternal behavior, and infant attachment behavior. *Developmental Psychology, 23,* 223–232.

Main, M. (1990). Cross-cultural studies of attachment organization: Recent studies, changing methodologies, and the concept of conditional strategies. *Human Development, 33,* 48–61.

Main, M., DeMoss, A., & Hesse, E. (1991). Unresolved/disorganized/disoriented state of mind with respect to experiences of loss. In M. Main & R. Goldwyn (Eds.), *Adult attachment scoring and classification systems* (pp. 103–133). Unpublished classification manual, University of California at Berkeley.

Main, M., & Goldwyn, R. (1985/1991/1994). *Adult attachment scoring and classification systems.* Unpublished classification manual, University of California at Berkeley.

Main, M., & Hesse, E. (1990). Parents' unresolved traumatic experiences are related to infant disorganized attachment status: Is frightened and/or frightening parental behavior the linking mechanism? In M. T. Greenberg, D. Cicchetti, & E. M. Cummings (Eds.), *Attachment in the preschool years: Theory, research, and intervention* (pp. 161–182). Chicago & London: University of Chicago Press.

Main, M., & Hesse, E. (1992). *Frightening, frightened, timid, dissociated or disorganized behavior on the part of the parent: A coding system for use with videotaped parent–infant interactions in the home or laboratory setting.* Unpublished scoring manual, University of California at Berkeley.

Main, M., & Morgan, H. (1996). Disorganization and disorientation in infant Strange Situation behavior: Phenotypic resemblance to dissociative states? In L. Michelson & W. Ray (Eds.), *Handbook of dissociation: Theoretical, empirical and clinical perspectives* (pp. 107–138). New York: Plenum.

Main, M., & Solomon, J. (1986). Discovery of an insecure–disorganized/disoriented attachment pattern. In T. B. Brazelton & M. W. Yogman (Eds.), *Affective development in infancy* (pp. 95–124). Norwood, NJ: Ablex.

Main, M., & Solomon, J. (1990). Procedures for identifying infants as disorganized/disoriented during the Ainsworth Strange Situation. In M. T. Greenberg, D. Cicchetti, & E. M. Cummings (Eds.), *Attachment in the preschool years: Theory, research, and intervention* (pp. 121–160). Chicago: University of Chicago Press.

Main, M., van IJzendoorn, M. H., & Hesse, E. (1993, March). *Adolescent attachment organization: Findings from the BLAAQ self-report inventory, and relations to absorption and dissociation.* Paper presented at the biennial meeting of the Society for Research in Child Development, New Orleans, LA.

Main, M., & Weston, D. R. (1981). The quality of the toddler's relationship to mother and to father: Related to conflict behavior and the readiness to establish new relationships. *Child Development, 52,* 932–940.

Putnam, F. W. (1991). Dissociative phenomena. In A. Tasman & S. M. Goldfinger (Eds.), *American Psychiatric Press review of psychiatry* (Vol. 10, pp. 145–160). Washington, DC: American Psychiatric Press.

Sagi, A., van IJzendoorn, M. H., Scharf, M., Koren-Karie, N., Joels, T., & Mayseless, O. (1994). Stability and discriminant validity of the Adult Attachment Interview: A psychometric study in young Israeli adults. *Developmental Psychology, 30,* 771–777.

Schuengel, C., Bakermans-Kranenburg, M. J., & van IJzendoorn, M. H. (1999). Frightening maternal behavior linking unresolved loss and disorganized infant attachment. *Journal of Consulting and Clinical Psychology, 67,* 54–63.

Spangler, G., Fremmer-Bombik, E., & Grossmann, K. (1996). Social and individual determinants of infant attachment security and disorganization. *Infant Mental Health Journal, 17,* 127–139.

Spiegel, D. (1991). Dissociation and trauma. In A. Tasman & S. M. Goldfinger (Eds.), *American Psychiatric Press review of psychiatry* (Vol. 10, pp. 261–266). Washington, DC: American Psychiatric Press.

Stroebe, M. S., Stroebe, W., & Hansson, R. O. (Eds.). (1993). *Handbook of bereavement: Theory, research, and intervention.* Cambridge, UK: Cambridge University Press.

van der Kolk, B. A., & Fisler, R. (1995). Dissociation and the fragmentary nature of traumatic memories: Overview and exploratory study. *Journal of Traumatic Stress, 8,* 505–525.

van IJzendoorn, M. H. (1995). Adult attachment representations, parental responsiveness, and infant attachment: A meta-analysis on the predictive validity of the Adult Attachment Interview. *Psychological Bulletin, 117,* 387–403.

van IJzendoorn, M. H., & Bakermans-Kranenburg, M. J. (1996). Attachment representations in mothers, fathers, adolescents and clinical groups: A meta-analytic search for normative data. *Journal of Consulting and Clinical Psychology, 64,* 8–21.

van IJzendoorn, M. H., Schuengel, C., & Bakermans-Kranenburg, M. J. (1999). Disorganized attachment in early childhood: Meta-analysis of precursors, concomitants, and sequelae. *Development and Psychopathology, 11,* 225–249.

CHAPTER 4

Individual and Physiological Correlates of Attachment Disorganization in Infancy

GOTTFRIED SPANGLER
KARIN GROSSMANN

Attachment formation is a developmental task that must be successfully resolved first in infancy and then continually throughout childhood, as it remains critical to a child's adaptation (Bowlby, 1969/1982; Cicchetti, Cummings, Greenberg, & Marvin, 1990). From the very start, attachment formation requires organization, coordination, and integration of perceptions, emotions, and behaviors as the infant adapts to his or her caregiving environment (Ainsworth, 1973). The process of attachment formation is interactive, depending on the one hand, on species-specific adaptations and the individual social responsiveness to the infant. On the other hand, it depends also on the individual readiness of the caretaker to minister to the infant's needs. By the end of the first year, individual differences in attachment patterns during infancy can be assessed using Ainsworth's strange situation (Ainsworth, Blehar, Waters, & Wall, 1978), yielding the traditional classification of an infant as securely attached (B), insecure–avoidantly attached (A), or as insecure–ambivalently attached (C). These categories were derived from well-defined, specific behavioral strategies of infants in dealing with reunion with the attachment figure following separation, under the assumption that even short separations lead to an activation of the attachment behavioral system. The predictive power of these patterns of infant–mother attachment for the development of social–emotional competence of the child has been demonstrated repeatedly (e.g.,

Main, Kaplan, & Cassidy, 1985; Matas, Arend, & Sroufe, 1978; Suess, Grossmann, & Sroufe, 1992).

Investigators of infant attachment behavior have often noticed, although not always published, that the three traditional attachment classifications do not adequately capture the observed variations in infant behavioral strategies after reunion with the attachment figure. Analyses of the behaviors of such infants by Main and Solomon (1986) or Crittenden (1985) resulted in the description of an additional set of behaviors seen as a new behavioral dimension conceptualized as disorganization/disorientation (D) by Main and Solomon (1990). Some of the nonclassifiable infants seemed unable to build up a coherent behavioral strategy upon reunion in coping with the emotional challenge caused by the separation from the mother. Their behaviors were marked by a temporal disorder, by functional contradictions such as proximity seeking with avoiding gaze, incompleteness or interruptions of movements, breaks, stereotypies, confusion, and apprehension. Main and Solomon report as their central discovery the striking *absence* of a common reunion behavioral pattern (1990, p. 97; emphasis in original). The newly observed behaviors of these infants seemed to lack a readily observable goal, intention, or explanation. Main and Solomon advised investigators to code for disorganized/disoriented behaviors separately, in addition to the traditional secure and insecure patterns of attachment. Thus, the quality of infant–parent attachment can be described with respect to two conceptually different behavioral dimensions, the security of the attachment relationship, as well as the coherence or organization of a specific attachment pattern.

Studies reporting on disorganized attachment status of infants often focused on mothering disorders in high-risk populations (Carlson, Cicchetti, Barnett, & Braunwald, 1989; Crittenden, 1988; Lyons-Ruth & Block, 1996). In a sample of maltreated infants, Carlson and colleagues (1989) found a preponderance of infants with disorganized attachment status (82%). Other studies showed a greater percentage of disorganization among infants known to have been abused or neglected (Lyons-Ruth, Repacholi, McLeod, & Silva, 1991). Still other studies reported an association between attachment disorganization in infants and a caregiving environment characterized by inconsistent care, such as that arising from maternal depression (Radke-Yarrow, Cummings, Kuczynski, & Chapman, 1985). Main and Hesse suggested that in an otherwise adequate caregiving relationship, there may sometimes be elements of fear in the interactions arising from frightening or frightened behavior of the parent (Main & Hesse, 1990). Such parental behavior may have a disorganizing effect on the infant's attachment behavior. A parental factor that has been linked to disorganization in older children from a nonrisk population was a subjective feeling of helplessness in mothers (George & Solomon, 1996). Another parental variable found to be linked to disorganized infant attachment was an attachment representation as assessed in the Adult Attachment Interview considered unresolved–disorganized (van IJzendoorn, 1995). This category is given on the basis of lapses in the monitoring of reasoning or discourse occurring specifically during discussions of potentially traumatic events (Main & Goldwyn, 1985/1991/1994).

In all of these studies, none or very little information was provided about the infants' individuality independent of their interactions with the caretaker. Although temperament by itself rarely predicts quality of infant attachment (Seifer, Schiller, Sameroff, Resnick, & Riordan, 1996), it is noteworthy that a preponderance of attachment disorganization is found in high-risk populations. Research on determinants of child abuse (Starr, 1988) points to child as well as parental factors. Therefore, we consider it important for the dimension of infant attachment disorganization to explore the effect of child characteristics.

In this chapter, we provide accumulating evidence from our own longitudinal studies for such influences. First, we address the psychobiology of disorganization in its manifestations in infants' cardiac and adrenocortical responsiveness. These data point to an interpretation of disorganization status as indicating a dysfunctional behavioral style in dealing with the demands of the strange situation. Second, we propose that newborn behavioral organization and cross-parental stability suggest a strong individual component of infant disorganization. We show that individual differences in the neonatal period predict infant disorganization at 12 months, and that behavioral disorganization in infancy with one parent predicts disorganized/controlling behavior at 6 years with the other parent. Finally, on the basis of our longitudinal data, we conclude that disorganization can also be conceptualized as an individual construct rather than as a property of a relationship.

The data we present come from three different longitudinal samples: the Bielefeld Longitudinal Sample (e.g., Grossmann, Grossmann, Spangler, Suess, & Unzner, 1985), the Regensburg Longitudinal Sample I (e.g., Wartner, Grossmann, Fremmer-Bombik, & Suess, 1994), and the Regensburg Longitudinal Sample III (e.g., Spangler & Grossmann, 1993; Spangler, Schieche, Ilg, Maier, & Ackermann, 1994). A short characterization of the three samples, including assessment procedures and analyses, is depicted in Table 4.1.

PSYCHOBIOLOGY OF INFANT DISORGANIZATION

Disorganized Behaviors as an Alarm Response: Evidence from Cardiac Responsiveness

Main and Hesse (1990) have suggested that disorganization reflects on the part of an infant an intense alarm response that is elicited in a stressful situa-

TABLE 4.1. Description of the Longitudinal Samples Referred to in This Chapter

Sample	Bielefeld Longitudinal Sample (e.g., Grossmann et al., 1985)	Regensburg Longitudinal Sample III (e.g., Spangler & Grossmann, 1993)	Regensburg Longitudinal Sample I (e.g., Wartner et al. 1994)
Sample size	$N = 47$	$N = 41$	$N = 41–47$
Selection criterion	Nonrisk pregnancy and birth	Nonrisk pregnancy and birth	Nonrisk pregnancy and birth
Socioeconomic status	Lower to upper middle-class	Lower to upper middle-class	Lower to upper middle-class
Data assessments included	• NBAS at newborn age • Home observations during the first year • Strange situation at 12 months	• NBAS at newborn age • Behavioral observations during the first year • Strange situation at 12 months	• Strange situation with mother at 12 or 18 months • Clown session with father and mother at 12 or 18 months • 6-year reunion procedure with mother
Measures	• Newborn behavioral organization • Maternal sensitivity ratings during the first year • Attachment security and disorganization at 12 months	• Newborn behavioral organization • Maternal sensitivity during the first year • Attachment security and disorganization at 12 months • Heart-rate/cortisol measures in strange situation	• Disorganization in clown session • Attachment security and disorganization at 12 months • Attachment security and disorganization (controlling/unclassifiable) at 6 years
Analyses conducted		Psychobiological processes in disorganized infants	Cross-parental stability of disorganization
Combined analyses	Prediction of attachment security and disorganization from maternal sensitivity and newborn behavioral organization (e.g., Spangler, Fremmer-Bombik, & Grossmann, 1996)		

tion. In the presence of, or upon return of the mother, the infant seems to experience a strong conflict between approach (activated by separation) and withdrawal (presumably activated by fear of the parent) such that the activation of attachment behavior cannot be systematically controlled by an organized, goal-oriented behavioral strategy. The status of attachment disorganization during the strange situation, according to Main and Solomon (1990), is based on the identification of specific behavioral events grouped into seven categories: (1) sequential or (2) simultaneous display of contradictory attachment behavior patterns, for example, proximity seeking accompanied or immediately followed by avoidance; (3) undirected, incomplete, and interrupted movements and expressions, for example, upon becoming distressed, the infant moves away from the parent rather than to parent; (4) stereotypies, asymmetrical, and mistimed movements and anomalous postures; (5) freezing, stilling, and slowed movements and expressions; (6) direct indices of apprehension regarding parent, for example, jerking back from parent with fearful expression; and (7) direct indices of disorganization or disorientation; for example, clear indices of confusion in the first moment of reunion, fall while approaching parent. These behavioral criteria are scored on a 9-point scale ranging from "no such behaviors" (1) to "moderate indices of disorganization/disorientation" (5) to "definite qualification for disorganized attachment status" (9) (see Appendix).

The identification of behaviors indicative of disorganization is difficult because of the subtlety and variety of behaviors that cannot be characterized in terms of some kind of similarity. Most of them "do not . . . have even a superficial similarity" (Main & Solomon, 1990, p. 147). Some of these behaviors are so subtle and short in duration that they can only be observed with the help of repeated slow-motion video editing (p. 147). High scores on the disorganization scale can be due to a single event of a marked symptomatic behavior (which can be easily identified because of its intensity, but raises the issue of reliability because of its low frequency of occurrence), or due to an accumulation of various minor, disorganized behaviors.

Supporting evidence for interpreting disorganized behaviors as indications of alarm could be accomplished by using external criteria. Specifically, changes in cardiac activity have been used as indicators of the context evaluation of an individual. An increase in heart rate may be part of a defensive response (Graham & Clifton, 1966) or may be interpreted as an index of emotional and behavioral activation (Fowles, 1980). According to Ursin, Baade, and Levine (1978), heart rate may indicate a fast-acting and short-lasting activation to cope with aversive situations. If disorganized behaviors in infants were indicative of alarm and reflected the infant's evaluation of the situation as threatening, we would expect cardiac responses, in particular, a phasic heart-rate acceleration, immediately upon their occurrence. In contrast, if disorganized behaviors were of no emotional significance, no systematic variations in heart-rate responses would be expected. Furthermore, if the notion of alarm is correct, we would expect, especially during separation, a higher overall cardiac activation (tonic response) in disorganized infants as compared to nondisorganized ones. In summary, assessment of cardiac activity can provide useful information for the concept of disorganization in two ways. Phasic responses accompanying specific infant behaviors labeled disorganized may support the validity of those behaviors as indications of alarm. And, in addition, a tonic activation during separation may indicate an extreme emotional activation such as that assumed to be experienced by disorganized infants. Both types of cardiac activation, however, may also reflect a greater effort of disorganized subjects to produce an effective coping response (e.g., Lundberg & Frankenhaeuser, 1980).

In the Regensburg III longitudinal study, 41 infants were classified for their patterns of attachment to their mothers, including status of disorganization in the strange situation at 12 months (see Table 4.1). The infant's cardiac activity was simultaneously assessed during the strange situation. Three disposable electrocardiogram (EKG) electrodes were placed in a triangular pattern on the infant's chest. Then, interbeat intervals were continuously recorded by a portable heart-rate recorder and converted to heart rates (beats per minute) later. Quality of infant–mother attachment was determined by trained observers (see Spangler & Grossmann, 1993, for details). The interrater reliability for the traditional attachment categories (secure, avoidant, ambivalent) was 90%. Regarding disorganization, each occurrence of any kind of disorganized behavior was exactly marked on the time axis and assigned to one of the behavioral groups specified by Main and Solomon's (1990) system. Reliability of the observers for the disorganization (5 or above) of the infants was 82%. Subsequently, all disagreements were conferenced. For the present purpose, two types of analyses were conducted. First, mean heart-rate response scores for each episode of the strange situation were calculated for each infant. To control for individual differences in basic heart-rate level, change scores were used by subtracting the heart-rate scores per episode from the mean heart rate in the second episode of the strange situation. Second, exact time and type of each disorganized behavior as identified on the videotapes were taken from the written records. For each of these behavioral events, heart-rate change scores were calculated by subtracting the mean heart rate during the 3 seconds immediately before the behavioral event from the respective heart-rate scores after the onset of the specified behavior. We combined the seven behavioral groups of the Main and Solomon system into three conceptually consistent categories: (a) *contradictory behaviors* (Groups 1 and 2, regarding the simultaneous or sequential display of contradictory behavior patterns; (2) *behaviors lacking goal orientation* toward the attachment person (Groups 3, 4, and 5, concerning undirected movements, stereotypies, and slowed movements or stilling); and (3) *direct indices of disorganization and apprehension* (Groups 6 and 7; specifying clear behavioral symptoms of disorganization). For further analysis, the heart-rate responses for each of these three groups of disorganized behaviors were collapsed for each subject.

In this sample, 9 out of 41 infants (22 %) were classified as disorganized. The proportion of disorganized infants was comparable to previous findings (Main & Hesse, 1990; Ainsworth & Eichberg, 1991). The proportion of infants showing one of the three traditional attachment patterns was 56% (23), 15% (6), and 2.5% (1) for the secure, avoidant, and ambivalent pattern, respectively. More than half of the infants ($n = 23$, 56%) showed no or only minimal signs of disorganization (D-score < 2). Mild indices of disorganization (scores of 3 or 4) were observed in 9 infants (22%). Regarding the three categories of disorganized behavior, *contradictory behaviors* were observed in 10 infants (24%), *behaviors lacking goal orientation* were observed in 15 infants (37%), and *direct indices of disorganization* were observed in 6 infants (15%).

As described in Spangler and Grossmann (1993), results showed significant differences for overall cardiac activation during separation between infants according to their attachment pattern and status of disorganization. All infants exhibited an overall cardiac activation during the second separation (see Figure 4.1). However, high cardiac activation was most prominent in disorganized infants who showed a more intense cardiac responsiveness than infants classified either secure or avoidant in their

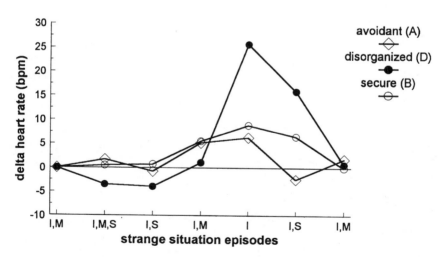

FIGURE 4.1. Changes in heart rate during the strange situation episodes for different attachment groups (M, mother, I, infant, S, stranger). Only one infant was classified insecure–ambivalent (C); thus, heart rates were not displayed for this class. From Spangler and Grossmann (1993). Copyright 1993 by University of Chicago Press. Reprinted by permission.

attachment. Extending the assumption of Main and Hesse (1990) that disorganized infants experience alarm in the presence of the mother, our findings provide evidence that disorganized infants also seem to experience more intense alarm during separation.

A specific analysis of the phasic heart-rate responses of the infants immediately after the occurrence of disorganized behaviors was performed. For each of the three major categories of disorganized behaviors, a separate multivariate analysis of variance (MANOVA) with one repeated-measures factor (1 to 6 seconds after the onset of the behavior) was conducted with heart-rate response as the dependent variable. Whereas we found no effect in heart-rate responsivity for the category *contradictory behaviors*, the heart-rate responses were significantly above zero after the onset of *behaviors lacking goal orientation*, $F(1,14) = 4.70$, $p < .05$, and after the onset of behaviors in the category *direct indices of disorganization*, $F(5,25) = 21.89$, $p < .001$ (Figure 4.2). Graham and Clifton (1966) interpreted heart-rate acceleration as a defensive response linked to negative emotions. In this view, our findings suggest that disorganized behaviors in the presence of the attachment figure that were followed by heart-rate acceleration may have been accompanied by a negative emotional response. This indicates at least a momentary lack of physiological relaxation after reunion with the attachment figure for the infants showing these types of behaviors. The finding that *contradictory behaviors* were not

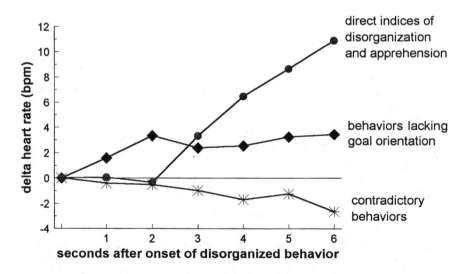

FIGURE 4.2. Heart rate responses following the onset of different categories of disorganized behavior.

associated with heart-rate accelerations may be due to one or several reasons. As *contradictory behaviors* may occur either simultaneously or sequen-
tially, cardiac responses may be masked by heart-rate changes due to different motor behaviors. Furthermore, because of the complexity of such
behaviors, the exact onset of the critical behavior (is it the first or the contradictory one?) is difficult to determine. Of course, it may also be possible
that no specific cardiac response is accompanying these kinds of disorganized behaviors.

In conclusion, attachment disorganization is reflected in increased
cardiac activity during the strange situation in two ways. First, heightened
tonic heart rate during separation suggest a more intense alarm during
separation in disorganized infants than in infants with an organized attachment pattern. Second, most infant behaviors defined as indicative of
attachment disorganization in the presence of the attachment figure are
accompanied by phasic heart-rate accelerations. They seem to have an
important emotional significance for the organism. They may signal a
physiological alarm reaction associated with negative emotions in the presence of the caregiver or, according to Lundberg and Frankenhaeuser
(1980), the heightened heart rates may indicate the greater effort of disorganized infants to organize their behavior.

Disorganization as a Nonfunctional Attachment Behavior Strategy: Evidence from Adrenocortical Activity

Ainsworth considered the secure attachment pattern to be the most adaptive behavioral pattern for dealing with separation stress in infancy, both
from a phylogenetic and an ontogenetic point of view (Ainsworth et al.,
1978); that is, a secure attachment behavioral pattern indicates a well-
balanced strategy of seeking consolation when distressed and using it effectively, but also relying on the attachment person as a secure base from
which to explore when not distressed. The insecure patterns have been
interpreted as less functional with respect to the attachment–exploration
balance, either because distress does not lead to appropriate behaviors for
consolation (avoidant pattern), or because the attachment behaviors are
not effective in alleviating the distress (ambivalent pattern) (Sroufe, 1979).
For example, the avoidant pattern is considered a defensive strategy ("displacement behavior"; Ainsworth et al., 1978) that helps to reduce observable emotional arousal. It cannot be considered effective, though, since it
does not reduce tonic physiological arousal (Ursin et al., 1978, p. 7). Nevertheless, both insecure attachment patterns (avoidant and ambivalent) are
seen as coherent, though less effective, behavioral strategies. Main and Solomon (1986) provided arguments to consider the status of disorganization
as a form of insecurity irrespective of the underlying attachment pattern,

because disorganized infants lack any coherent strategy in dealing with the demands of the strange situation. Still, one issue remains open. Is the disorganization status of an infant indicative of an overall disorganization of behavioral regulation or do the specific disorganized behaviors signify only a momentary emotional overreaction?

In order to test the adaptiveness of the status of disorganization, we again took a psychobiological approach by including adrenocortical processes. The adrenocortical system seems to be sensitive to stressful situations involving novelty, uncertainty, and/or negative emotions (Levine, 1983). From an arousal model perspective, one would expect heightened adrenocortical activity in the disorganized infants when assuming either an intense alarm in these subjects or a greater effort to organize their behaviors (Lundberg & Frankenhaeuser, 1980). Moreover, animal research (Levine, Wiener, Coe, Bayart, & Hayashi, 1987; von Holst, 1986), as well as studies of human newborns (e.g., Spangler & Scheubeck, 1993), have shown that adrenocortical activation is most prominent in subjects with no or inappropriate behavioral coping strategies. Thus, the adrenocortical system can provide useful information. The coping model offers several hypotheses regarding adrenocortical activation during the strange situation. From a narrow attachment perspective, cortisol increases could be expected in infants who do not show adequate stress-reducing behavioral strategies (avoidant and ambivalent patterns) and in disorganized infants who do not have any coherent strategy at all. No or only small increases in cortisol level would be expected for securely attached infants exhibiting an adequate behavioral coping strategy by seeking protection from their attachment figure. If, on the other hand, and in line with the coping model, the two traditional insecure patterns (avoidant and ambivalent) are considered coherent and even functionally adaptive for a given infant–mother pair (Hinde & Stevenson-Hinde, 1990), although at some psychological cost (Main, 1981), a low cortisol increase would also be expected in these groups. Under any assumption, however, heightened adrenocortical activity can be expected in disorganized infants whose behavior suggests an ineffective or noncoherent coping strategy.

Previously presented evidence (Spangler & Grossmann, 1993) confirms the notion that status of disorganization reflects an ineffective response to separation and/or reunion. Figure 4.3 (taken from Spangler & Grossmann, 1993, p. 1447) shows these findings. No increase in adrenocortical activity was found in the infants with a secure attachment pattern assessed 30 minutes after the strange situation procedure. However, significant increases in cortisol levels were found in infants with insecure attachment patterns, and, most prominently, in infants with disorganized attachment status. The latter finding has been replicated in a recent study by Hertsgaard, Gunnar, Erickson, and Nachmias (1995).

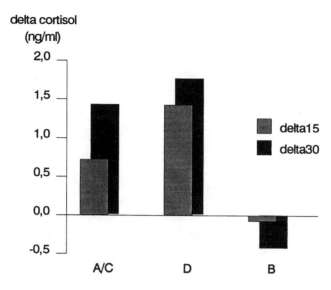

FIGURE 4.3. Cortisol change during the strange situation for secure (B), insecure–avoidant and insecure–ambivalent (A/C), and disorganized infants (D); post-assessment 15 minutes (delta 15) and 30 minutes (delta 30) after the strange situation. From Spangler and Grossmann (1993). Copyright 1993 by University of Chicago Press. Reprinted by permission.

Our research on the psychobiology of infant behaviors considered disorganized/disoriented provided evidence for the validity of the concept of infant disorganization of attachment behavioral strategies in the strange situation on a physiological level. Although the assessment of disorganization is based on a great variety of behaviors, including stereotypies, and clinical indicators of stress, including quite subtle behavioral elements, these behaviors seem to be symptomatic of poor psychophysiological organization of the infant. Disorganized infants, irrespective of their underlying attachment category, seem to experience more intense alarm and negative emotional arousal on a physiological level during the strange situation as compared to infants not classified as disorganized. Disorganized infants seem to have more difficulties or indicate more effort to organize an effective coping response.

Our findings allow two interpretations. First, infants with disorganized attachment status may be more easily or intensely alarmed by the strange situation, which is reflected in their cardiac responses, which peak when the infant is alone. Thus, it may be more difficult for them to organize effective coping strategies, which in turn leads to an adrenocortical activation. Second, according to Lundberg and Frankenhaeuser (1980), the infants' alarm response may be reflected in the increased adrenocortical activity, and the heightened cardiac activity may indicate their effort and difficulty in organizing an effective coping response. In short, we suggest that status of disorganization indicates a physiological state of alarm in an infant who has no appropriate behavioral response to deal with the challenge.

INFANT DISORGANIZATION AS AN INDIVIDUAL VERSUS RELATIONSHIP CONSTRUCT

Attachment security as defined by the three traditional attachment categories (A, B, C) is seen as a feature of the individual dyadic relationship. Main (1996) enumerated the evidence for the influence of the parent's contribution to infant attachment status. Her main points were as follows: (1) Quality of mother–infant interaction during the first year predicted quality of infant–mother attachment (Ainsworth et al., 1978; Grossmann et al., 1985); it should be noted, however, that the same correlation was not found for infant–father attachment (Volling & Belsky, 1992); (2) classifications of Adult Attachment Interviews obtained from expectant parents predicted subsequent classifications of their infants in the strange situation procedure (Steele, Steele, & Fonagy, 1996); and (3) attachment classifications to mother and to father were usually independent (van IJzendoorn & Bakermans-Kranenburg, 1996). This indicates that an infant can form qualitatively different attachments to different caregivers. Although Fox, Kimmerly, and Schafer (1991) reported evidence for a statistically significant but small proportion of common variance uncovered in a meta-analysis of 672 families, this finding cannot be used as an argument for attachment strategies as an individual disposition because the common variance could also be due to similarities in parent's interactive behaviors (see Grossmann & Grossmann, in press, for concordances between parental interactive behaviors.)

As with attachment security, Main and Solomon (1990) considered infant status of disorganization in the strange situation to be a feature of the specific dyadic relationship (i.e., to be independent across caregivers). They reported less than 10% concordance of infant attachment disorganization between mother and father in the strange situation. Additional evidence came from a study by Steele et al. (1996). None of the 8 infants classified as disorganized with mother was classified disorganized with father. All of these studies addressed infant status of disorganization in the strange situation, but none of the studies provided information about precursors of infant disorganization.

In the next section, we present data from two nonclinical samples concerning individual and social predictors of disorganization in the strange situation. We also provide data indicating common variance of disorganized behaviors in infants across the two parents in a situation different from the strange situation.

Individual and Social Predictors of Attachment Security and Disorganization

There is considerable empirical evidence concerning the social and individual antecedents of attachment security (the traditional attachment classification A, B, C). First, a secure pattern of attachment has been associated with higher maternal sensitivity during the first year than the insecure patterns (Ainsworth et al., 1978; Belsky, Rovine, & Taylor, 1984; Grossmann et al., 1985; for a review, see Goldsmith & Alansky, 1987). Maternal sensitivity also contributes to a substantial part of the transgenerational transmission of attachment patterns (e.g., Grossmann, Fremmer-Bombik, Rudolph, & Grossmann, 1988; for a review, see van IJzendoorn, 1995).

Second, associations between aspects of newborn behavior such as irritability, orientation to external stimuli, or regulation of internal state and later attachment classification have been documented. High newborn irritability has been significantly related not only to the ambivalent pattern (Miyake, Chen, & Campos, 1985; Egeland & Farber, 1984) but also to the avoidant pattern (Crockenberg, 1981; van den Boom, 1994). In the study of Grossmann et al. (1985), low newborn orientation has been associated with an avoidant pattern of infants to mother as well as to father.

In contrast, only recently, researchers have accumulated some knowledge about the origins of attachment disorganization. Findings from high-risk samples indicated an occurrence of a high rate of disorganization in maltreated infants (Carlson et al., 1989). Attachment disorganization was also more often observed in infants with family risk factors and in infants experiencing hostile–intrusive and low-involved mothering styles (Lyons-Ruth et al., 1991). Studies by Ainsworth and Eichberg (1991) and Main and Hesse (1990) reported a link between disorganization of infant attachment behavior and unresolved traumatic attachment experiences of the mother. Traumatized mothers are assumed to exhibit frightened or frightening behavior in specific situations, which then cause disorganization in infant attachment behavior (Main & Hesse, 1990). This relation was shown for mothers with an insecure attachment representation, although not for mothers with a secure representation (Schuengel, van IJzendoorn, Bakermans-Kranenburg, & Blom, 1997). But, as shown in a meta-analytic report, despite a significant prediction of infant disorganization by an attachment representation indicative of unresolved traumatic experiences, only 53% of disorganized infants actually had parents classified as having an unresolved attachment representation (van IJzendoorn, 1995). Thus, multiple pathways to disorganization seem to exist.

Predictability of Attachment Disorganization from Newborn Behavioral Organization

The newborn data of two of our studies allowed us to investigate the relative contribution of newborn behavioral organization as a potential precursor of later infant attachment disorganization. For this analysis, data from two longitudinal samples were combined: the Bielefeld Longitudinal Sample and the Regensburg Longitudinal Sample III (see Table 4.1). In both samples, newborn behavioral organization, maternal sensitivity during the first year, and infant attachment security as well as disorganization were assessed at 12 months, using comparable assessment schedules and the same methods for behavioral analyses. The results have been published recently by Spangler, Fremmer-Bombik, and Grossmann (1996).

Newborn behavioral organization was assessed twice during the first 6 days after birth by using the Brazelton Neonatal Behavioral Assessment Scale (NBAS, Brazelton, 1984). Two indices were composed: newborn's orientation to external stimuli (e.g., responsiveness to sounds and sights), and newborn's emotional regulation (e.g., peak of excitement, consolability). These indices comprise the newborn's ability to cope with induced arousal and external and internal stimuli. Maternal sensitivity was rated at three observation periods throughout the first year (2-3 months, 6 months, 9-10 months) using Ainsworth's scale for maternal sensitivity (Ainsworth, Bell, & Stayton, 1974). At 12 months, infants' attachment security (traditional attachment classification A, B, C) and status of disorganization were classified in the strange situation. Complete data sets were available for a total sample of 88 mother–infant pairs (see Spangler et al., 1996). In terms of the three traditional attachment patterns, 44 (50%) of the infants were classified securely attached (B), 31 (35%) insecure–avoidant (A), 7 (8%) insecure–ambivalent, and 6 (7%) were considered unclassifiable. Fifteen, or 17%, of the infants were classified as disorganized, 7 with an underlying secure pattern, 5 with an underlying avoidant or ambivalent pattern, and 3 of the 6 unclassifiable with respect to the underlying traditional classification.

A clear pattern of findings emerged (see Figure 4.4). As expected, security of attachment was predicted by maternal sensitivity. No significant differences with respect to newborn behavioral organization were found between securely and insecurely attached infants, however. In contrast, in these two nonclinical samples, infant attachment disorganization was not associated with maternal sensitivity. However, infant disorganization was predictable from newborn behavioral organization. Infants classified as

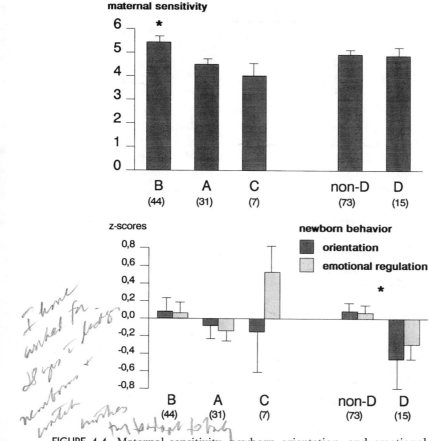

FIGURE 4.4. Maternal sensitivity, newborn orientation, and emotional regulation in securely attached (B), insecure–avoidantly attached (A), and insecure–ambivalently attached (C) infants, in disorganized (D) and nondisorganized (non-D) infants. Error bars indicate 1 *SE*. The asterisk indicates the significant statistical difference between D and non-D, *p* < .05. From Spangler, Fremmer-Bombik, and Grossmann (1996). Copyright 1996 by Michigan Association for Infant Mental Health, Inc. Reprinted by permission.

disorganized at 12 months in the strange situation, as compared to nondisorganized ones, exhibited lower orientation and somewhat lower emotional regulation already during the neonatal period. These findings clearly demonstrate that behavioral disorganization during the strange situation could indicate a more general deficit in behavioral regulation that can already be observed during the newborn period. Thus, individual characteristics of the infant contribute to disorganization of attachment behavior in the strange situation.

Infant Attachment Disorganization as Related to Behavioral Regulation during the First Year

Given the link between infant status of attachment disorganization, and newborn behavioral organization we next asked whether behavioral organization throughout the first year predicted infant disorganization at 12 months. We conducted further analyses within the Regensburg III longitudinal sample (see Table 4.1) with specific infant behaviors observed during the first year. At the ages of 3, 6, and 9 months, the 41 infants of this sample were videotaped in two different situations, a 15 minute free-play session with mother and a Bayley exam. These observations were video-recorded at home when infants were 3 months old and in the laboratory playroom at the ages of 6 and 9 months. Negative emotionality, defined as negative vocalization and motoric restlessness, were coded in order to determine the infant's ability to regulate his or her behavior in two challenging situations. Infants' negative vocalizations and motoric restlessness were rated for their intensity on two 6-point scales for each consecutive 30-second interval in the two situations. Negative vocalization included protest, fussing, or crying. Motoric restlessness included all undirected or spontaneous movements of the infants that were not coordinated with external events or organized in a goal-corrected manner to objects or persons, or accompanied by indications of positive emotions (e.g., bouncing) (see Spangler et al., 1994). Both the intensity and the variability of negative vocalization and motoric restlessness were calculated separately for each type of situation at each age point. Intensity was defined as the mean rating of all 30-second intervals per situation and was used as an index for emotional stress. Variability was defined as the mean square of differences of successive 30-second intervals and was used as an index for emotional lability. Thus, four measures were available for each situation at each age: intensity and variability of negative vocalization, and intensity and variability of motoric restlessness.

Systematic differences between infants with and without disorganization with respect to the four indices of behavioral regulation during the first year were examined with three-way MANOVAs with age (3, 6, 9 months) and situation (free play, Bayley exam) as repeated measure factors and disorganization (D, non-D) as an independent factor.[1] The MANOVA for intensity of negative vocalization revealed main effects for age $F(2,66) = 38.19$, $p < .001$; situation, $F(1,33) = 4.27$, $p < .05$; and disorganization, $F(1,33) = 9.86$, $p < .01$. There were no interaction effects. The intensity of negative vocalizations decreased with age and was always higher during the exam sessions as compared to free-play sessions (Figure 4.5). Most important for our argument in this chapter, disorganized infants as compared to nondisorganized ones exhibited more intense negative vocalizations throughout the first year and in both situations (i.e., in unstructured inter-action with the mother and in structured interaction with the examiner).

The three-way MANOVA for variability of negative vocalization revealed main effects for age, $F(2,66) = 24.64$, $p < .001$, and disorganiza-tion, $F(1,33) = 8.45$, $p < .01$. In addition, the interaction between age and disorganization, $F(2,66) = 5.9$, $p < .01$, approached significance, $F(2,66) = 2.61$, $p < .10$. Disorganized infants as compared to nondisorganized ones

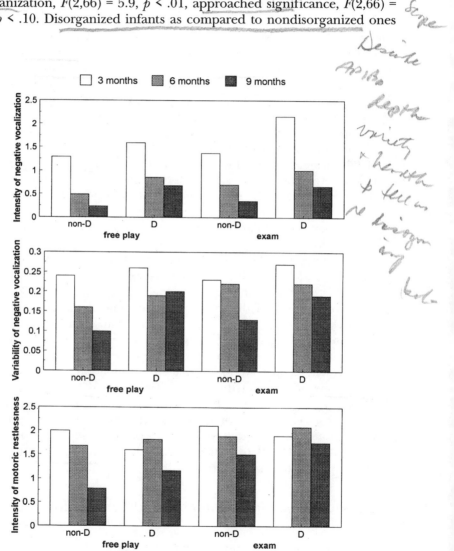

FIGURE 4.5. Intensity and variability of negative vocalization and intensity of motoric restlessness in two different situations during the first year of infants clas-sified disorganized (D) and nondisorganized (non-D) in the strange situation.

had a higher mean score in emotional variability (Figure 4.5). As with the intensity measure, a decrease of emotional variability from 3 to 9 months was observed in both situations. This decrease, however, was observed predominantly in infants without disorganization.

For intensity of motoric restlessness, the three-way MANOVA revealed main effects for age, $F(2,72) = 14.16$, $p < .001$, and situation, $F(1,36) = 16.34$, $p < .001$, and interaction effects between age and situation, $F(2,72) = 4.89$, $p < .01$, and between age and disorganization, $F(2,72) = 3.40$, $p < .05$. As revealed by post hoc tests, a significant decrease in motoric restlessness from 3 to 9 months was observed only in nondisorganized infants, whereas the changes in motoric restlessness observed in disorganized infants were not systematically related to age (Figure 4.5). Variability of motoric restlessness was not associated with infant disorganization.

In summary, infants classified as disorganized at 12 months expressed higher amounts of negative emotional behaviors and were more emotionally labile in interaction with mother and an examiner during their first year. Moreover, there was no decrease in motoric restlessness and emotional lability in these infants, which would be expected in the course of normal development during the first year (Spangler et al., 1994). This was actually observed in infants without later disorganization. The findings suggest a restricted ability for emotional regulation and a continuing restlessness during the first year in disorganized infants. This adds further support to the demonstrated link between disorganization in attachment strategies and a deficit in newborn behavioral organization. Our results indicate that individual differences independent of the attachment relationship contribute to a later status of disorganization of the infant. Of course, emotional regulation during the first year is not a sole individual characteristic but is also influenced by the caregiver's behavior. However, for the present sample, we found that within-situation changes of infants' negative emotion, but not the overall level, were influenced by maternal sensitivity (Spangler et al., 1994). Thus, variance of the emotional measures can be explained by individual characteristics as well as by social processes. It should be noted that while for the present sample emotional regulation was also related to maternal sensitivity, disorganization was not associated with maternal sensitivity.

Cross-Situational, Cross-Parental, and Longitudinal Stability of Disorganization

If infant disorganization is to a substantial degree a feature of the individual, we would expect to observe indices of disorganization in infants in more than one situation and across caregivers. A number of data sets from our Regensburg Longitudinal Sample I (see Table 4.1) were well suited to test this hypothesis.

Cross-Situational and Cross-Parental Concordance of Infant Disorganization

Infants of the Regensburg Longitudinal Sample I were observed during the strange situation (SS) with mother and with father at 12 and 18 months of age. One month prior to the respective strange situations, each infant–parent pair was observed in the clown session (CS) (Fremmer-Bombik & Grossmann, 1991), a procedure devised by Main and Weston (1981). The CS is a special parent–infant situation that includes a dressed-up adult play partner for the infant. The clown induces mild stress to the infant in the presence of the parent first by hiding behind a mask, then by the sudden interruption of ongoing playful interactions: The clown cries as he is called to leave the room. Main and Weston (1981) devised a scale for "conflict" behavior during the CS that was a precursor to the scale for disorganization as described by Main and Solomon (1990). "Conflict" behaviors were defined *"as having a disordered, purposeless, or odd appearance and they seem to lack an immediate explanation, such as rocking back and forth while staring into space, assuming odd postures, engaging in inappropriate affect, lying immobilized on the floor in fetal posture and huddling to the wall"* (Main & Weston, 1981, p. 935). Today, in the SS, these behaviors would be termed disorganized. For this sample, infant disorganization with mother as well as father was rated in the CS (analyses were performed separately and independently for mothers and fathers in Regensburg by Mary Main and Donna Weston). In addition, although many years later, infant attachment disorganization in the SS with mother was analyzed from the available tapes by Erik Hesse (see Wartner et al., 1994, for details). In the strange situation with mother, 14 out of 47 infants (29.8%) were classified as disorganized. Classification of disorganization of the infants in the strange situation with father has not yet been conducted.

Using these data, we first tested whether infants classified as disorganized in the SS with mother also had received higher ratings of disorganization in the CS with mother. Statistical comparison revealed a significant effect, Mann–Whitney $Z = -2.49$, $p < .05$ (see Figure 4.6). Thus, assessment of disorganized infant behaviors led to comparable results in these two different situations. In a second step, we calculated the correlation between the scores for disorganization during the CSs with mother and with father. Spearman rank correlation was $r = .54$ ($p < .001$). This correlation is particularly noteworthy, because five different interactive scales were applied for the CS (infant concerned attention, parental aversion to contact, infant relatedness, parental lack of affect, and infant disorganization). Infant disorganization was the only scale for which there was a significant cross-parent correlation. In a third step, infants with and without disorganization in the SS with mother were compared with respect to disorganization in the CS with father. There was a significant effect, Mann–Whitney $Z = -2.36$,

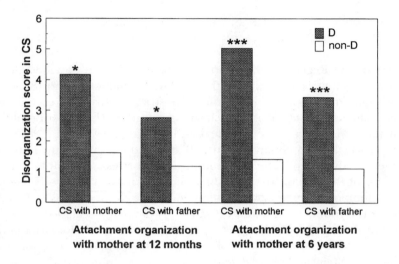

FIGURE 4.6. Mean scores for disorganization in the clown session in infancy in children classified disorganized (D) or nondisorganized (non-D) in the strange situation with mother in infancy and in the reunion procedure with mother at 6 years. *p < .05; ***p < .001.

p < .05 (see Figure 4.6), which remained so even when disorganization with mother in the CS was controlled for statistically.

Longitudinal Stability of Disorganization over 6 Years

At 6 years, children from the Regensburg Longitudinal Study I were classified with respect to their quality of attachment to mother using Main and Cassidy's (1988) reunion procedure and classification system. At 6 years, 12 out of 41 children (29.3%) were classified as insecure–controlling or insecure–unclassified (Wartner et al., 1994). According to Main and Cassidy (1988), these two classes of children were combined to the disorganized/controlling group. A high stability of pattern of attachment (A, B, C, D) from infancy to the 6-year attachment assessment was found, corroborating the findings of Main and Cassidy (1988). Specifically, 9 out of 13 children classified as disorganized in infancy were also given the status of disorganization at 6 years, whereas only 3 out of 26 children with no early disorganization were classified as disorganized at 6 years, χ^2 = 14.1, p < .001.

Additional longitudinal analyses were performed to find further predictive factors for child disorganization at 6 years. Disorganization in infancy during the CS with mother as well as with father significantly predicted the child's disorganization at 6 years, Mann–Whitney, mother: $Z = -4.16$, $p < .001$; father: $Z = -3.36$, $p < .001$. Figure 4.6 demonstrates the results: Children classified as disorganized at 6 years had significantly higher disorganization scores during the CS with mother and the CS with father. The relation between the infant's disorganization score with father in the CS and status of disorganization with mother at 6 years remained statistically significant even after controlling for disorganization in the CS with mother.

The findings of this section are summarized in Table 4.2. All relations between the different measures of disorganization are presented as correlations (i.e., phi correlation for dichotomous measures). Infants who showed marked signs of disorganization in the CS with one parent also received higher scores for disorganization in the CS with the other parent; that is, infant disorganization was concordant across parents. For the infant–mother attachment relationship, we found a high convergence of disorganization between the CS and the SS. This finding adds to the validity of the concept. Moreover, disorganization with mother during the SS significantly predicted disorganization with father during the CS, evidencing cross-situational, along with cross-parental, stability. In the longitudinal analyses, disorganization at 6 years with mother was predicted by disorganization in the CS with mother as well as with father. These findings suggest again a strong influence of individual characteristics on a child's status of disorganization in infancy or at 6 years.

DISCUSSION AND CONCLUSION

Three different issues regarding the physiological and individual correlates of attachment disorganization in infancy were addressed in this chap-

TABLE 4.2. Cross-Situational, Cross-Parental, and Longitudinal Stability of Disorganization

| | Infant disorganization | | 6-year disorganization |
	Clown session with M	Clown session with F	Reunion with M
Infant disorganization			
Strange situation with M	.41*	.39*	.59***
Clown session with M		.54***	.75***
Clown session with F			.60***

Note. Correlations: $N = 32$–40; $*p < .05$; $***p < .001$.

ter. First, by using a psychobiological research approach, we could provide evidence for the validity of the concept of behavioral disorganization on a physiological level. For most of the behavioral symptoms used for classification of disorganization in the system of Main and Solomon (1990), simultaneous cardiac activation as an index of a defensive response was observed. In addition, a greater increase in cardiac activity in disorganized infants as compared to nondisorganized infants during the second separation, when the child was alone, signified a more intense alarm reaction of disorganized infants in the SS. Main and Hesse (1990) had proposed that in disorganized infants, an intense alarm is elicited by the conflict between seeking proximity to the caregiver (elicited by the attachment system) and fear of the caregiver (due to the experience of frightened or frightening behavior with the caregiver). As a consequence, the cardiac activity should peak during reunion. But such an effect was not reflected in our data. (For a more extensive discussion of the issue of alarm see Lyons-Ruth, Bronfman, & Atwood, Chapter 2, this volume; Schuengel, Bakermans-Kranenburg, van IJzendoorn, & Blom, Chapter 3, this volume; and Solomon & George, Chapter 1, this volume.)

Another source of psychobiological evidence for the maladaptive nature of the behavioral response set exhibited by infants classified as disorganized was our finding of an association between disorganization and adrenocortical activity. High cortisol increases were found in disorganized infants irrespective of their underlying attachment behavior strategy, corroborating the evidence of Hertsgaard et al. (1995). In contrast to Hertsgaard et al., however, in the Spangler and Grossmann (1993) sample, a high cortisol increase was also found in insecurely attached infants with no status of disorganization during the SS compared to securely attached infants, but this finding awaits further replication. These results prompt us to interpret disorganized behaviors as ineffective responses of infants toward the attachment figures arising from intense alarm during separation.

Next, we reported that the infant's behavioral organization in the neonatal period was a significant determinant of disorganization at 12 months. Two longitudinal studies provided data for this analysis. The findings of the Spangler et al. (1996) study, like many other studies, confirmed the expected predictive link between maternal sensitivity during the first year and security of infant–mother attachment. But this study also demonstrated a specific association between newborn behavioral organization and disorganization of the infant in the SS. For this aggregated sample, attachment security at 12 months was not predicted by newborn behavioral organization. Infants exhibiting a disorganized attachment strategy or disoriented behaviors at the end of the first year, however, as newborns were conspicuous for their restricted ability to achieve behavioral organization to external stimuli and internal arousal. This result may seem to contradict findings reported by Grossmann et al. (1985) and Waters, Vaughn, and Egeland (1980), who found associations between traditional patterns of attachment and newborn orienting ability or optimal behavioral organization, or the studies by Crockenberg (1981), Miyake et al. (1985), and van den Boom (1994), who found a heightened proportion of the insecure–ambivalent and insecure–avoidant attachment pattern, respectively, in infants with high irritability during the newborn period. But in all of these studies, disorganization of the infants in the SS was not assessed or not reported. Thus, differences between infants showing the secure, avoidant, or ambivalent pattern in the SS as reported in these studies could have been due to a greater number of disorganized infants within the avoidant or ambivalent attachment groups. Such a confound was avoided by aggregating the Bielefeld and Regensburg III data, which resulted in a comparable proportion of disorganized infants within the secure and insecure (avoidant or ambivalent) groups.

Several types of pathways linking maternal behavior to infant disorganization have been reported in the literature. Ainsworth and Eichberg (1991) reported a substantial concordance between infant attachment disorganization and unresolved traumatic attachment experiences of the mother. Murray (1992) found a substantially higher proportion of disorganized infants in a sample of postnatally depressed mothers. And in studies of mother–infant interactions in families at high risk for mothering disorders, infant disorganization was associated with hostile and/or neglectful behaviors in mothers (Carlson et al., 1989; Lyons-Ruth et al., 1991). Even under cultural conditions of communally approved nocturnal separation of infants from their parents, such as in some Kibbutzim, the proportion of disorganized infants was more than half of the sample (Sagi, van IJzendoorn, Aviezer, Donnell, & Mayseless, 1994). Our findings from middle-class samples suggest still another pathway to infant disorganization, a fairly stable individual characteristic that could be predicted by individual differences in behavioral organization after birth.

Our findings are not in opposition to the proposed pathways but add a further line of reasoning. First, although infant attachment disorganization at 12 months could not be predicted by maternal sensitivity during the first year, this could have a methodological reason. In our two studies, maternal interactive behaviors were rated globally for the whole session or home visit according to Ainsworth's maternal sensitivity scale. Maternal behavior was not coded in terms of specific behaviors such as frightened or frightening behaviors. Main and Hesse (1990) have suggested that these kinds of behaviors could be associated with infant disorganization in the SS. Although we assume that the occurrence of frightening maternal behavior during interaction would lead to lower sensitivity scores, the probability of detecting these specific behaviors in nonrisk samples may be very low. And maternal behaviors indicative of the mother's own fearfulness might have been overlooked during the ratings.

Second, newborn behavioral organization is not necessarily a reflection of genetically determined individual differences in the infants. Individual differences in behavioral organization observed during the neonatal period can also be of environmental origin. There may be additional or different experiential processes working already before birth that contribute to the link between parental traumatic experiences and infant disorganization. Mothers with traumatic attachment experiences may experience their pregnancy and pending new attachment relationship as more stressful than mothers with gratifying attachment histories. Thus, their unborn infants could be exposed to much chronic prenatal stress, which, according to Schneider and Coe (1993), may lead to restricted behavioral and physiological organization in the newborn.

Still another pathway was suggested by Main and Solomon (1990). They addressed this issue by noting that factors such as neurological difficulties may operate in a substantial minority of disorganized subjects. Thus, disorganization may be biased toward individual origin in some cases but toward social origin in other cases. In addition, individual risk may be heightened by inappropriate social experiences. On the other hand, high quality of external organization brought about by a sensitive caregiver may function as a social buffer against individual risk.

The findings reported here indicate two independent dimensions of infant attachment classification in the SS following different lines of development. Infant security within an attachment relationship is facilitated by the infant's social experience of an attachment figure that is willing to respond appropriately to the infant's attachment needs. Thus, the security dimension may represent the history of interaction between the infant and the attachment figure. In contrast, signs of disorganization during the SS may be due to a somewhat restricted behavioral regulation ability within the infant, which can already be observed during the newborn period and throughout the first year.

Finally, our findings on the cross-situational, cross-parental concordance of infant disorganization adds additional evidence to this argument. Disorganization in the SS with mother was predictable from ratings of disorganization in another situation, the CS, with mother as well as with father, which in turn, were significantly interrelated. Infant disorganization in the CS with either parent predicted child disorganization at 6 years in the child–mother reunion procedure. In contrast to the findings of Main and Solomon (1990) and Steele et al. (1996) of their reported independence of infant disorganization with mother and father in the SS, our findings result in a concept of disorganization being as much an individual disposition construct as it is a relationship construct. From the perspective of the several-pathway model of development of disorganization mentioned earlier, some children may exhibit disorganized behavior in different situations, thereby contributing to the cross-situational stability of individual differences. For other children, the occurrence of disorganized behavior should be restricted to situations in which the specific, fear-eliciting caregiver is present. For the former group, the SS would tap an individual feature of the infant rather than assess a disorganized attachment relationship. A valid assessment of attachment disorganization in the latter group would have to include different situations or interactive behavioral analyses. These should include indications of frightened or frightening behavior in the caregiver present, as has been demonstrated in part by Schuengel et al. (1997).

In summary, the findings of our studies clearly suggest that when looking for determinants of infant attachment disorganization, individual qualities of the infant should be given as much attention as experiential factors resulting from the caregiver's behaviors. As a consequence, disorganization in infancy and later on should be seen as a construct that includes individual components rather than being purely a relational concept.

absolutely

ACKNOWLEDGMENTS

The various research projects were supported in part by Deutsche Forschungsgemeinschaft (GR299 to Klaus E. Grossmann), by Köhlerstiftung (Munich, Germany, to Gottfried Spangler), and by the Stiftung Volkswagenwerk (to Klaus E. Grossmann, 1977–1982). We are very indebted to Inge Bretherton, Erik Hesse, Mary Main, and Donna Weston for their assistance in training and evaluation of the various observational methods. We wish to thank our many dedicated Diplom students who did the assessments and data analyses, and especially Claudia Kramer and Fabienne Becker-Stoll, for her never ending patience in evaluating the attachment disorganization of infants in the strange situation. We further want to thank Klaus E. Grossmann for his steady support and valuable advice. And, of course, special thanks to the most cooperative families, who made these studies possible. Finally, we want to thank the editors of the book, Judith Solomon and Carol George, and an anonymous reviewer for their very helpful comments which substantially contributed to the quality of this chapter.

NOTE

1. The MANOVAs were also conducted by comparing the three attachment groups, D, A, and B, instead of D and non-D. There were no substantial differences between infants classified A and infants classified B.

REFERENCES

Ainsworth, M. D. S. (1973). The development of infant–mother attachment. In B. M. Caldwell & H. N. Riciutti (Eds.), *Review of child development research* (Vol. 3, pp. 31–96). Chicago: University of Chicago Press.

Ainsworth, M. D. S., Bell, S. M., & Stayton, D. J. (1974). Infant–mother attachment and social development: "Socialization" as a product of reciprocal responsiveness to signals. In P. M. Richards (Ed.), *The integration of a child into a social world* (pp. 99–135). Cambridge, UK: Cambridge University Press.

Ainsworth, M. D. S., Blehar, M. C., Waters, E., & Wall, S. (1978). *Patterns of attachment. A psychological study of the strange situation.* Hillsdale, NJ: Erlbaum.

Ainsworth, M. D. S., & Eichberg, C. (1991). Effects on infant–mother attachment of mother's unresolved loss of an attachment figure, or other traumatic experience. In C. M. Parkes, J. Stevenson-Hinde, & P. Marris (Eds.), *Attachment across the life cycle* (pp. 160–183). London/New York: Tavistock/Routledge.

Belsky, J., Rovine, M., & Taylor, D. G. (1984). The Pennsylvania infant and family development project, 3: The origins of individual differences in infant–mother attachment: Maternal and infant contributions. *Child Development, 55,* 718–728.

Bowlby, J. (1969/1982). *Attachment and loss: Vol. 1. Attachment.* New York: Basic Books.

Brazelton, T. B. (1984). *Neonatal Behavioral Assessment Scale.* London: Spastics International Medical Publications.

Carlson, V., Cicchetti, D., Barnett, D., & Braunwald, K. (1989). Disorganized/disoriented attachment relationships in maltreated infants. *Developmental Psychology, 25,* 525–531.

Cicchetti, D., Cummings, E. M., Greenberg, M. T., & Marvin, R. S. (1990). An organizational perspective on attachment beyond infancy: Implications for theory, measurement, and research. In M. T. Greenberg, D. Cicchetti, & E. M. Cummings (Eds.), *Attachment in the preschool years* (pp. 3–50). Chicago: University of Chicago Press.

Crittenden, P. M. (1985). Maltreated infants: Vulnerability and resilience. *Journal of Child Psychology and Psychiatry, 26,* 85–96.

Crittenden, P. M. (1988). Relationships at risk. In J. Belsky & T. Nezworski (Eds.), *Clinical implications of attachment.* Hillsdale, NJ: Erlbaum.

Crockenberg, S. B. (1981). Infant irritability, mother responsiveness and social support influences on the security of infant–mother attachment. *Child Development, 52,* 857–865.

Egeland, B., & Farber, E. A. (1984). Infant–mother attachment: Factors related to its development and changes over time. *Child Development, 55,* 753–771.

Fowles, D. C. (1980). The three arousal model: Implications of Gray's two-factor learning theory for heart rate, electrodermal activity, and psychopathy. *Psychophysiology, 17,* 87–103.

Fox, N. A., Kimmerly, N. L., & Schafer, W. D. (1991). Attachment to mother/attachment to father: A meta-analysis. *Child Development, 62,* 210–225.

Fremmer-Bombik, E., & Grossmann, K. E. (1991). Frühe Formen empathischen

Verhaltens. *Zeitschrift für Entwicklungspsychologie und Pädagogische Psychologie,* *23,* 299–317.

George, C., & Solomon, J. (1996). Representational models of relationships: Links between caregiving and attachment. *Infant Mental Health Journal, 17,* 198–216.

Goldsmith, H. H., & Alansky, J. A. (1987). Maternal and infant temperamental predictors of attachment: A meta-analytic review. *Journal of Consulting and Clinical Psychology, 55,* 805–816.

Graham, F. K., & Clifton, R. K. (1966). Heart-rate change as a component of the orienting response. *Psychological Bulletin, 65,* 305–320.

Grossmann, K., Fremmer-Bombik, E., Rudolph, J., & Grossmann, K. E. (1988). Maternal attachment representations as related to child–mother attachment patterns and maternal sensitivity and acceptance of her infant. In R. A. Hinde & J. Stevenson-Hinde (Eds.), *Relations within families* (pp. 241–260). Oxford, UK: Oxford University Press.

Grossmann, K., & Grossmann, K. E. (in press). Parents and toddlers at play: Evidence for separate functioning of the play and the attachment system. In P. M. Crittenden (Ed.), *The organization of attachment relationships: Maturation, culture, and context.* Cambridge University Press.

Grossmann, K., Grossmann, K. E., Spangler, G., Suess, G., & Unzner, L. (1985). Maternal sensitivity and newborns' orientation responses as related to quality of attachment in northern Germany. In I. Bretherton & E. Waters (Eds.), Growing points in attachment theory and research. *Monographs of the Society for Research in Child Development, 50*(1–2, Serial No. 209), 233–278.

Hertsgaard, L., Gunnar, M., Erickson, M. F., & Nachmias, M. (1995). Adrenocortical responses to the strange situation in infants with disorganized/disoriented attachment relationships. *Child Development, 66,* 1100–1106.

Hinde, R. A., & Stevenson-Hinde, J. (1990). Attachment: Biological, cultural, and individual desiderata. *Human Development, 33,* 62–72.

Levine, S. (1983). A psychobiological approach to the ontogeny of coping. In N. Garmezy & M. Rutter (Eds.), *Stress, coping, and development in children* (pp. 107–131). New York: McGraw Hill.

Levine, S., Wiener, S. G., Coe, C. L., Bayart, F. E. S., & Hayashi, K. T. (1987). Primate vocalization: a psychobiological approach. *Child Development, 58,* 1408–1419.

Lundberg, U., & Frankenhaeuser, M. (1980). Pituitary-adrenal and sympathetic-adrenal correlates of distress and effort. *Journal of Psychosomatic Research, 24,* 125–130.

Lyons-Ruth, K., & Block, D. (1996). The disturbed caregiving system: Relations among childhood trauma, maternal caregiving, and infant affect and attachment. *Infant Mental Health Journal, 17,* 257–275.

Lyons-Ruth, K., Repacholi, B., McLeod, S., Silva, E. (1991). Disorganized attachment behavior in infancy: Short-term stability, maternal and infant correlates, and risk-related subtypes. *Development and Psychopathology, 3,* 377–396.

Main, M. (1981). Avoidance in the service of attachment: A working paper. In K. Immelmann, G. Barlow, L. Petrinovich & M. Main (Ed.), *Behavioral develop-*

ment: The Bielefeld interdisciplinary project (651–693). New York: Cambridge University Press.

Main. M. (1996). Introduction to the special section on attachment and psychopathology: 2. Overview of the field of attachment. *Journal of Consulting and Clinical Psychology, 64,* 237–243.

Main, M., & Cassidy, J. (1988). Categories of response to reunion with the parent at age six: Predictable from infant attachment classification and stable over a one-month period. *Developmental Psychology, 24,* 415–426.

Main, M., & Goldwyn, R. (1985/1991/1994). Adult attachment scoring and classification system. Unpublished classification manual. University of California, Berkeley.

Main, M., & Hesse, E. (1990). Parents' unresolved traumatic experiences are related to infant disorganized attachment status: Is frightened and/or frightening parental behavior the linking mechanism? In M. T. Greenberg, D. Cicchetti & E. M. Cummings (Eds.), *Attachment in the preschool years* (pp. 161–184). Chicago: University of Chicago Press.

Main, M., Kaplan, N., & Cassidy, J. (1985). Security in infancy, childhood, and adulthood: A move to the level of representation. In I. Bretherton & E. Waters (Ed.), Growing points in attachment theory and research. *Monographs of the Society for Research in Child Development, 50*(1–2, Serial No. 209) 66–106.

Main, M., & Solomon, J. (1986). Discovery of an insecure disorganized/ disoriented attachment pattern: Procedures, findings and implications for the classification of behavior. In T. B. Brazelton & M. Yogman (Eds.), *Affective development in infancy* (pp. 95–124). Norwood, NJ: Ablex.

Main, M., & Solomon, J. (1990). Procedures for identifying infants as disorganized/ disoriented during the Ainsworth strange situation. In M. T. Greenberg, D. Cicchetti, & E. M. Cummings (Eds.), *Attachment in the preschool years. Theory, research and intervention* (pp. 121–160). Chicago: University of Chicago Press.

Main, M., & Weston, D. R. (1981). The quality of the toddler's relationship to mother and to father: Related to conflict behavior and the readiness to establish new relationships. *Child Development, 52,* 932–940.

Matas, L., Arend, R., & Sroufe, L. A. (1978). Continuity of adaptation in the second year. The relationship between quality of attachment and later competence. *Child Development, 49,* 547–556.

Miyake, K., Chen, S. J., & Campos, J. (1985). Infant temperament, mother's mode of interaction, and attachment in Japan: An interim report. In I. Bretherton & E. Waters (Ed.), Growing points in attachment theory and research. *Monographs of the Society for Research in Child Development, 50*(1–2 Serial No. 209), 276–297.

Murray, L. (1992). The impact of postnatal depression on infant development. *Journal of Child Psychology and Psychiatry, 33,* 543–561.

Radke-Yarrow, M., Cummings, E. M., Kuczynski, L., & Chapman, M. (1985). Patterns of attachment in two- and three-year olds in normal families and families with parental depression. *Child Development, 56,* 884–893.

Sagi, A., van IJzendoorn, M. H., Aviezer, O., Donnell, F., & Mayseless, O. (1994). Sleeping out of home in a Kibbutz communal arrangement: It makes a difference for infant–mother attachment. *Child Development, 65,* 902–1004.

Schneider, M. L., & Coe, C. L. (1993). Repeated social stress during pregnancy impairs neuromotor development on the primate infant. *Developmental and Behavioral Pediatrics, 14*, 81–87.

Schuengel, C., van IJzendoorn, M. H., Bakermans-Kranenburg, M. J., & Blom, M. (1997, April). *Frightening, frightened and dissociated behavior, unresolved loss and infant disorganization.* Paper presented at the biennal meeting of the Society for Research in Child Development, Washington DC.

Seifer, R., Schiller, M., Sameroff, A. J., Resnick, S., & Riordan, K. (1996). Attachment, maternal sensitivity, and infant temperament during the first year of life. *Developmental Psychology, 32*, 12–25.

Spangler, G., Fremmer-Bombik, E., & Grossmann, K. (1996). Social and individual determinants of attachment security and disorganization during the first year. *Infant Mental Health Journal, 17*, 127–139.

Spangler, G., & Grossmann, K. E. (1993). Biobehavioral organization in securely and insecurely attached infants. *Child Development, 64*, 1439–1450.

Spangler, G., & Scheubeck, R. (1993). Behavioral organization in newborns and its relation to adrenocortical and cardiac activity. *Child Development, 64*, 622–633.

Spangler, G., Schieche, M., Ilg, U., Maier, U., & Ackermann, C. (1994). Maternal sensitivity as an external organizer for biobehavioral regulation in infancy. *Developmental Psychobiology, 27*, 425–437.

Sroufe, L. A. (1979). The coherence of individual development: Early care, attachment, and subsequent developmental issues. *American Psychologist, 34*, 834–841.

Starr, R. H. (1988). Pre- and perinatal risk and physical abuse. *Journal of Reproductive and Infant Psychology, 6*, 125–138.

Steele, H., Steele, M., & Fonagy, P. (1996). Associations among attachment classifications of mothers, fathers, and their infants. *Child Development, 67*, 541–555

Suess, G., Grossmann, K. E., & Sroufe, L. A. (1992). Effects of infant attachment to mother and father on quality of adaptation in preschool: From dyadic to individual organization of self. *International Journal of Behavioral Development, 15*, 43–65.

Ursin, H., Baade, E., & Levine, S. (1978). *Psychobiology of stress: A study of coping men.* New York: Academic Press.

van den Boom, D. C. (1994). The influence of temperament and mothering on attachment and exploration: An experimental manipulation of sensitive responsiveness among lower class mothers with irritable infants. *Child Development, 65*, 1457–1477.

van IJzendoorn, M. H., & Bakermans-Kranenburg, M. J. (1996). Attachment representations in mothers, fathers, adolescents and clinical groups: A meta-analytic search for normative data. *Journal of Consulting and Clinical Psychology, 64*, 8–21.

van IJzendoorn M. H. (1995). Adult attachment representations, parental responsiveness, and infant attach ment: A meta-analysis on the predictive validity of the adult attachment interview. *Psychological Bulletin, 117*, 387–403.

Volling, B. L., & Belsky, J. (1992). Infant, father, and marital antecedents of infant–father attachment security in dual-earner and single-earner families. *International Journal of Behavioral Development, 15*, 83–100.

von Holst, D. (1986). Vegetative and somatic components of tree shrews' behavior. *Journal of the Autonomic Nervous System, Suppl.*, 657–670.

Wartner, U. G., Grossmann, K., Fremmer-Bombik, E., & Suess, G. (1994). Attachment patterns at age six in South Germany: Predictability from infancy and implications for preschool behavior. *Child Development, 65*, 1014–1027.

Waters, E., Vaughn, B. E., & Egeland, B. R. (1980). Individual differences in infant–mother attachment relationships at age one: Antecedents in neonatal behavior in an urban, economically disadvantaged sample. *Child Development, 51*, 208–216.

PART 2

Social and Cognitive Sequelae of Attachment Disorganization

CHAPTER 5

Developmental Pathways from Infant Disorganization to Childhood Peer Relationships

DEBORAH JACOBVITZ
NANCY HAZEN

For two decades, attachment theory has served as a unifying construct for the study of social and emotional development in infancy. A burgeoning array of studies has demonstrated continuity from organized patterns of infant–caregiver attachment to the development of social and emotional competencies in early childhood and beyond (Bretherton, 1985; Belsky & Cassidy, 1994). However, the developmental trajectories of infants who are disorganized/disoriented in the strange situation have not been studied and are still not well understood. The primary purpose of this chapter is to develop a model of how infants who display disorganized and disoriented behavior in attachment-relevant situations develop strategies for interacting with parents and peers over the course of early childhood.

Main and Solomon's (1986, 1990) landmark discovery of the "disorganized/disoriented" attachment category was based on a recognition that some infants were difficult or impossible to classify in the strange situation using Ainsworth's three-category attachment classification system (Ainsworth, Blehar, Waters, & Wall, 1978). They concluded that what these infants had in common was contradictory and conflicting behavioral tendencies (e.g., turning in circles, approaching mother with head averted) suggesting attachment disorganization and signs of apprehension (putting their hands to the mouth; falling huddled to the floor upon their mother's entrance) or disorientation (postural stilling and dazed affect and/or mistimed and anomalous movements). Main and Hesse (1990) have proposed that disorganized infant behaviors can be traced to frightening–frightened parental behavior. Infants who are frightened by their caregivers are placed in a paradoxical situation. The caregiver is at once the source of comfort and the source of fear, resulting in a collapse of behavioral strategies for dealing with stress.

Only a handful of studies have investigated the developmental pathways that disorganized/disoriented infants follow through childhood, as they develop internal working models of self and other, and how they may carry these forward to later relationships, both within and outside of the family (see Lyons-Ruth & Jacobvitz, 1999, for review). Although disorganized children appear to lack organized strategies for meeting their attachment needs as infants, this literature suggests that they do develop consistent strategies for interacting with their caregiver by age 6. These children act in a controlling fashion toward the caregiver, using either a punitive or caregiving strategy (Main & Cassidy, 1988; Solomon, George, & De Jong, 1995; Wartner, Grossman, Fremmer-Bombik, & Suess, 1994). However, because of a lack of longitudinal data following disorganized children over the course of early childhood, little is understood about how disorganized children develop these strategies.

Only a few longitudinal studies have examined early peer relationships of children classified as disorganized in the strange situation; the majority of these have used at-risk samples. Studies examining peer relations indicate that these children are at risk for developing behavior problems, including externalizing behaviors (Shaw, Owens, Vondra, Keenan, & Winslow, 1996; Lyons-Ruth, Easterbrooks, & Cibelli, 1997; Solomon et al., 1995) and internalizing behaviors with peers (Carlson, 1998; Solomon et al., 1995). Again, however, the developmental pathways from disorganized infant-mother attachment to interactions with peers remain unclear.

Building on this emerging literature, we present a preliminary working model of how the disorganized child's internal working model may develop over the course of early childhood from interactions with the caregiver and influence subsequent interactions with both parents and peers. We use case studies of three disorganized children to illustrate when and how preschool children classified disorganized in infancy develop strategies for interacting with others. This descriptive pilot study is presented for the heuristic purpose of developing hypotheses concerning the development of parent–child and peer relationships in young disorganized children that should be systematically examined in future research.

Consistent with previous research, we expect disorganized infants to develop controlling behavior with their mothers. The parent, in turn, is expected to show less overtly frightened and/or frightening behavior and settle into an out-of-control or helpless pattern, abdicating the parental role (George & Solomon, 1996; Solomon & George, 1996). We propose that the more disturbed the mother's caregiving, the more delayed the child's development of controlling behaviors.

We further propose that the types of controlling behavioral patterns children develop with the caregiver (e.g., controlling–punitive vs. controlling–caregiving) are likely to reflect the particular dynamics of the caregiver–child relationship and the way that the relationship functions within the whole family system. Consistent with family systems theory, we believe that the father–child, mother–child, and marital relationships are interdependent. Specifically, some disorganized children have been shown to take on the parental role, becoming either punitive or caregiving. Since emotional distance or conflict in the marriage has been linked to parent–child alliances, including role reversal (Jacobvitz & Bush, 1996; Jurkovic, 1998), we explore the possibility that disorganization in the mother–child relationship may predispose the disorganized child to form an alliance with either the mother or father. We also sought to understand how all of the relationships within the family (mother–child, father–child, and marital), relate to the disorganized child's development of peer relationships.

Finally, consistent with other longitudinal studies, we expect that children's early relationship experiences will influence their relationships with peers. Specifically, preschool children who are disorganized in infancy will be the least competent with peers, becoming aggressive, fearful, or displaying odd, contradictory behavior when initiating play (e.g., smiling and laughing while shining a flashlight in the peer's eyes). We further propose that only after children develop a strategy for interacting with their parents will they carry over such patterns of interaction to their relationships with peers.

The case studies that we use to illustrate our ideas are taken from a larger longitudinal study of the links between parent–child relationships and children's early peer relationships (Hazen, 1994). Sixty-six middle-class intact families were recruited from high-quality child care centers when their children were young toddlers. At 18 months, children were assessed for security of mother–child attachment in the strange situation. Data on children's interactions with their parents and peers were collected at five phases, when the children were 20, 26, 32, 44, and 56 months old. At each phase, mother–child and father–child interactions were videotaped in play, cleanup, and problem-solving situations in the family's home. During the last three phases, the whole family was videotaped while interacting at dinnertime. Peer interactions also were observed in the child's child care center at all five phases. Each child was videotaped in dyadic play and cleanup interactions with two different peers identified by their teachers as "friends," or children with whom the target child played frequently. At 44 and 56 months (i.e., the last two phases), they also completed problem-solving tasks with the peer. One of the problem-solving tasks was a task that the child had previously completed with the parents during the home visit. Target children were also videotaped in their classrooms with their whole peer group during free play during each phase of data collection. We are not reporting the empirical results of the longitudinal study here, but instead, focus on case studies of three children in this larger study.

THE CENTRAL ROLE OF FEAR IN ATTACHMENT THEORY

Understanding the central role of fear in attachment theory is critical to understanding caregiving correlates and outcomes of attachment disorganization. Over the first year of life, the infant-caregiver relationship becomes an increasingly sophisticated behavioral system whose adaptive function is to protect the infant from harm (Bowlby, 1969/1982). Although the infant continually monitors his or her caregiver's whereabouts, an infant's attachment system is activated at higher intensities in response to signs of danger or potential danger to the infant. Such signs include separation from the caregiver, strangeness, hunger, fatigue, and anything that frightens or distresses the infant.

Separation from an attachment figure, although not necessarily truly dangerous, arouses anxiety and activates the attachment system in virtually all 1-year olds because it signals an increase in the risk of danger. The three-category attachment system described by Ainsworth, Blehar, Waters, and Wall (1978) has demonstrated, however, that infants vary in their capacity to use the caregiver to regulate arousal when distressed. Infants whose mothers were sensitive and contingently responsive to their signals over the first year of life are most often classified as "secure." They seek comfort and contact with little or no avoidance or angry resistance toward the mother, express emotions directly, and readily accept physical contact and reassurance from their caregiver. Infants whose mothers consistently ignored their signals for comfort are most often classified as "avoidant." They show minimal displays of emotion, ignoring the mother and shifting attention to toys. Finally, caregivers that are inconsistently available when their infant seeks comfort and interfering when the infant does not want contact most often have infants classified as "resistant" in the strange situation. They mingle proximity and contact seeking with angry behavior when alarmed and show heightened expressions of distress, such as sitting close to mother or clinging to her, even under conditions of mild threat.

Disorganized children, on the other hand, do not appear to have an organized strategy for coping with the stress of separation and reunion. Recent studies have shown that mothers classified as unresolved with respect to trauma or loss during their own lives were more likely than the other mothers to engage in frightening and frightened caregiving behavior such as baring teeth, sudden looming movements, or a sequence of pursuit movements (Jacobvitz, Hazen, & Riggs, 1997; Schuengel, van IJzendorn, Bakermans-Kranenburg, & Blom, 1997; Thalhuber, Jacobvitz, & Hazen, 1998) that, in turn, has been related to disorganized infant attachment behavior in the strange situation (Lyons-Ruth, Bronfman, Parsons, & Griffin, 1997; Schuengel et al., 1997). According to Main and Hesse (1990), experiencing the caregiver as frightening places the infant in an unresolveable paradox. Fear activates the attachment system, but the primary attachment figure is herself a source of fear for the infant. These infants experience a collapse of behavioral strategies for dealing with stress with the mother, resulting in disorganized and disoriented attachment behaviors.

Infants classified as disorganized are also given the best-fitting alternate classification—secure, avoidant, or resistant. For example, disorganized infants that show a preponderance of avoidance are assigned a secondary classification of avoidant, and those showing a preponderance of resistance receive a secondary classification of resistant.

The case studies presented in this chapter are based on three children, Sam, Kate, and Tim, who were classified as disorganized in the strange situation.

In the first reunion, Sam approached his mother with his eyes cast down. When he was about two feet away, he looked up at her, rising suddenly to his toes and making gasping noises with sharp intakes of breath as he did so. He quickly looked down again, bared his teeth in a half-grimace/half-smile, and turned away. Hunching his shoulders and holding his arms and legs stiffly, he tiptoed to the chair on the other side of the room. He sat motionless in the chair for 30 seconds, grasping the armrests and staring straight ahead with a dazed expression.

In the second reunion, Kate approached her mother with her arms outstretched toward her mother. When she was about two feet away from making contact, she moved her arms to the side and abruptly circled away from her mother like a banking airplane. As she moved away, she had a dazed, blank expression on her face.

When his mother returned after a brief separation, Tim ran to greet her with outstretched arms, then immediately fussed and squirmed to be put down. She put him down, and he became very quiet and subdued. He walked to every electrical outlet in the room, pointed to each and said, "Hot." He then wandered around aimlessly for 55 seconds, periodically crying and fussing.

All three children showed signs of disorganization. Sam showed conflicting behavioral tendencies (e.g., approached his mother with his head averted), apprehension, (e.g., a half-grimace/half-smile and hunched shoulders), and disorientation (e.g., dazed expression). In fact, he received the highest possible score on Main and Solomon (1990) disorganization scale, a "9" (see Appendix). Kate showed conflicting behavioral tendencies (e.g., approached her mother while simultaneously creating a pathway that involved moving away). Finally, Tim also showed conflicting behavioral tendencies (e.g., keeping a distance from his mother when distressed and yet crying for help) and disorientation (e.g., wandering around the room aimlessly). Both Sam and Kate were assigned an alternate avoidant classification and Tim was given an alternate "resistant" classification. Although we did not find any disorganized infants in this sample with a secondary classification of secure, such infants do exist, and it may be that their patterns of parent–child and peer interaction are less problematic than those described in the following case studies.

THE SHIFT FROM INFANT DISORGANIZATION TO CONTROLLING BEHAVIOR

As a consequence of the quality of early infant–caregiver interactions, the infant acquires a sense of security or insecurity. Bowlby (1980) proposed that this sense of security lays the groundwork for the development of representational models of the self and others, and forms the basis of the behavioral strategies that the child develops for interacting with caregivers in later years. In infancy, internal working models of the child's relationship with the parent can be inferred from the organization of attachment behavior in the strange situation. As children become capable of language and symbolic representations during the preschool years, they will begin to develop internal working models that are more abstract and differentiated. Thus, during childhood, internal working models of attachment may be inferred through observing children's symbolic representations of the family and of attachment themes depicted in language and pretend play (Solomon, George, & De Jong, 1995).

Prospective longitudinal studies show that children classified as disorganized during infancy develop a controlling strategy with their caregivers by age 6 (Main & Cassidy, 1988; Wartner et al., 1994). In these studies, children's behavioral and verbal response patterns to a reunion with the parent after an hour-long separation were classified into four categories, corresponding to four infant attachment classifications—secure–confident, insecure–avoidant, insecure–ambivalent, and insecure–controlling. Children classified insecure–controlling "seem to actively attempt to control or direct the parent's attention and behavior, and assume a role which is usually considered more appropriate for a parent with reference to a child" (Main & Cassidy, 1988, p. 418). Controlling children consistently try directly or indirectly to manipulate the caregiver, using either a punitive or a caregiving strategy. The controlling–punitive child acts bossy toward the caregiver, typically in a rejecting or humiliating way. In contrast, controlling–caregiving children act overbright, cheerful, or solicitous, attempting to meet their caregivers' needs by humoring and assisting them.

Recent studies that have examined how controlling children symbolize attachment-relevant family situations through symbolic means confirm that the working models of controlling children seem dominated by themes of fears without solution and a helpless self (Kaplan, 1987; Main, Kaplan, & Cassidy, 1985; Solomon et al., 1995). In one study, 6-year-old children classified as disorganized at age 1 responded to the photographs of parent–child separations with fear and helplessness (Kaplan, 1987). Some children appeared afraid and yet unable to do anything about it, while others remained silent throughout the task. Still others engaged in catastrophic fantasies, indicating that the attachment figure would be hurt or killed. In a study conducted by Solomon et al. (1995) children used dolls to enact a story in which parents leave the child overnight in the care of a babysitter and later return. Some controlling children enacted themes of danger in which dangerous events were left unresolved, leading to chaos and disintegration of the self or family. Others appeared uncomfortable, inhibited, and frightened about enacting the story at all. Although the development of controlling strategies illustrates the child's attempt to overcome his or her sense of helplessness, the fear that controlling children experienced as infants does not appear to be resolved.

Solomon and George (1996; George & Solomon, 1996, 1999) have studied the nature of the caregiving system among parents of children considered controlling. In semistructured interviews about mothers' relationships to their 6-year-olds, they found that a helpless parental stance was related significantly to controlling attachment behavior on the part of the child. In some cases, this helpless stance involved failing to provide reassurance and protection to their child, while in other cases, the helpless stance included fear either of their child or fear of themselves losing control in some way. Other mothers of controlling children described feeling that the child was in control of the relationship, either because of the child's precocious positive capabilities or unmanageability. Although links between disorganization in infancy and controlling behavior at age 6 have been reported, few studies have examined how such controlling patterns develop.

THE DEVELOPMENT OF CONTROLLING BEHAVIORS IN DISORGANIZED CHILDREN

The case of Sam illustrates the considerable time and effort that a disorganized child may need to construct a more effective way to cope with a frightening parent. Our observations of mother–child interactions at 20 months suggested to us that Sam had not yet developed controlling behavior patterns. Sam's interaction with his mother looks similar to his strange situation behavior. He tried to avoid his mother but could not effectively do so, and instead collapsed and showed signs of disorganization.

> Sam's mother was building with foam shapes while Sam sat a few feet away, facing away from her, playing with a tool set. She took no notice of Sam's interest in the tool set. Instead, she picked up a foam shape she was playing with and asked Sam, "I wonder what this is for? Look here. Look here, Sam. Look, look Sam!" Sam did not respond. Sam's mother still showed no interest in Sam's behavior. Instead, she picked up a doll on the other side of the room and said, "Sam, look at the sweet baby. Here, hold her for me." Again, he did not respond. As part of the research protocol, Sam's mother asked Sam to help put away the toys. Sam's mother asked, "Will you help me put these in here?" Sam continued to play with the tools and ignored her request until she took a toy from his hand. He made a high-pitched scream, looked at her and yelled, "No!" He then grabbed the container and dumped out the shapes. She said, "Sam, sweetie, we gotta put these up," in a sweet, wheedling tone. He pulled more toys back out of the toy chest, and screamed. His mother's voice deepened to a sharp tone, She said, "Hm. This isn't working very well, is it?" Sam ignored her and continued to remove toys from the box. She restrained him physically, and said in the same low, sharp voice, "No! No! No!", then immediately shifted to a high singsong voice and said, "I'm sorry, sweetheart," while trying to hug him. Sam squirmed away, screaming and crying. Suddenly, she grabbed his arm roughly and yanked him back while making a loud, harsh, growling sound. Sam collapsed on the floor in a hunched position, crying hard and making gasping noises.

Similarly, in the next task at this 20-month visit, Sam's mother gave many instructions, which Sam ignored. Sam insisted on doing a shape-sorting task his own way rather than putting the shapes in the correct slots. Sam's mother showed a sudden voice shift from a high, singsong tone to a sharp, deep-voiced tone as she said, "That isn't right. You're not even trying." Sam tried to leave the room and his mother grabbed him roughly. Again, the session ended with Sam collapsing on the floor in a hunched position, crying and making gasping noises.

There appeared to be a total lack of mutual regulation in these interactions. Mothers of most 20-month-olds take the lead in reciprocal interaction, while following their child's interests. Sam's mother, on the other hand, played independently and the two engaged in parallel play similar to that of toddler peers. Most children are disappointed when it is time to clean up the toys. Power struggles are likely to ensue, particularly in the toddler years. What is notable in this situation, however, was the mother's unusual and frightening growl followed by a sudden shift in voice tone, considered frightening on Main and Hesse's (1995) frightening–frightened caregiving scale, and Sam's collapse to the floor, gasping noises, and huddled position (signs of disorganization). Perhaps, the mother's frightening behavior was a result of the helplessness she felt. Sam, however, still looked disorganized at 20 months—too frightened to successfully avoid his mother, resulting in a collapse of behavioral strategies.

Later, during a play session at 26 months, Sam no longer engaged in power struggles but he still lacked a more effective strategy for interacting with his mother.

> Sam's mother appeared dreamily absorbed with the toys herself, paying little attention to Sam or Sam's interests. Sam still did not play with his mother but he watched her much more and was more attentive to her moods and interests. Near the end of the play session, his mother became inexplicably very still, staring into space with a dazed expression for over 30 seconds. Sam looked concerned, and tried to snap her out of this state by going up to her face and saying, "Hi!" This was his only utterance during the entire interaction session and his mother still could not respond.

Thus, as early as 26 months, Sam may have been showing the precursors of a later pattern of mother–child role reversal as he tried to alter what appeared to be a trance-like state (or symptoms of dissociation) on the part of his mother. The caregiving behavior Sam displayed, however, was brief. Sam was withdrawn, vigilant, and anxious for the rest of the session. His mother, who was unresponsive to Sam's current mood and interests, ordered him in a sharp, demanding voice to obey her and to complete each task as she commanded.

Sam moved from avoiding his mother at times and asserting his autonomy at other times during the 20-month visit to showing pathetic and pleading behaviors at 32 months.

Sam spent almost the entire family dinner (about 30 minutes) huddled and crouching in his chair, pleading and begging to be excused from the table so he could play with the toys. He repeated over and over in a pathetic, breathless, whining voice, "Please Mommy, please Mommy, please Mommy, please." His mother responded to his pleading with sarcasm and exasperation. During the toy cleanup sessions, Sam also pleaded, whined, and begged for more playtime. Sam's mother did not grant his requests, laughed at his whining, and spoke to him in a cold and sarcastic tone of voice.

Finally, by 42 months, Sam developed a pattern of mother–child role reversal. He no longer avoided and ignored his mother, nor did he engage in power struggles or act immature and pleading. As in all of the play sessions, Sam's mother was judged to dominate the play interactions. She played with the toys in a childlike fashion, showing no interest in Sam or in Sam's interests, demanding instead that he show an interest in her play. In contrast to the previous interactions in which Sam simply watched his mother and ignored her attempts to draw him into her play themes, Sam appeared highly vigilant to his mother's interests. He was quick to follow her suggestions, as illustrated in the following example:

> The toys available for free play included a tea set. Sam's mother suggested that he prepare lunch for her. Sam prepared all the pretend drinks and food for his mother at her request. When his mother pointed to the tea set and said, "Can I have some tea, please?" Sam picked up the cup and suggested, "How 'bout coffee?" She agreed that coffee would be fine.

This pattern seemed to allow him to be close to her and gain her approval and, at the same time, gave him some control over his mother's moods. As long as he pleased her, she seemed to accept him and to grant him some autonomy. If he allied himself with her, they could be close. For the first time, Sam laughed and talked with his mother; he appeared to relax somewhat. Yet we observed that Sam needed to be constantly vigilant about pleasing his mother or she could again become frightening:

> During a structured task at 42 months in which Sam's mother asked Sam to come up with a list of things that have wheels, Sam gave some correct answers, but then could not come up with any more ideas. He then tried to be cute, giving silly answers. His mother became visibly tense, her voice harsh. Sam's voice softened. His shoulders tensed as he said to his mother in a soft, pleading tone, "I don't know any more, Mommy. I don't know any more, Mommy." His mother stared ahead and stilled for a full 42 seconds. Sam twisted his foot and arm, appearing anxious, and he repeated over and over in the same soft, pleading

voice, "I don't know, Mommy," while leaning up against her and patting her knee several times to move her out of what appeared to be a dissociated state. Sam's mother did not respond at all to Sam.

By the time Sam was 56 months old, his pattern of pleasing and caregiving with his mother appeared firmly established. As before, the play revolved around his mother's interests and ideas, but Sam now watched her almost constantly and responded quickly to her suggestions. Furthermore, this pattern seems to have proven successful in providing Sam with a way to be close to his mother. During the entire play interaction, Sam sat close to his mother, and they whispered and giggled together like child peers:

> Sam's mother asked Sam to bring over a box of dress-up clothes. She then proceeded to dress herself up with hats, jewelry, and a feather boa, asking Sam to help her, which he did. She said, "I love this! How do I look?" When Sam just smiled, she took a duck puppet and made it bite his ear. He looked down and said, "Stop, Mommy," in his soft, wheedling voice, still smiling. His mother smiled back and complied with his request.

The extent to which mother and child reversed roles in this interaction is striking. Sam's mother played and dressed up like a child, and expected her child to attend to her interests and needs, rather than the reverse. Thus, by the time Sam was 4 years old, he had learned a way to keep his mother happy and meet her needs. It is interesting to note that Sam also increased his use of what Crittenden has called "coy, disarming behaviors," such as tipping his head to one side, gazing up with his head lowered, and smiling shyly (Crittenden, 1992).

The case of Sam, who scored the highest on disorganization in the sample, illustrates the length of time it may take a disorganized child to develop a strategy of interacting with his mother. Solomon and her colleagues (1995) have described controlling behavior as a "brittle behavioral strategy" that children use to control the parent who is the source of their fear, allowing them to regulate their own internal state and behavior. The case of Sam also illustrates the brittle nature of controlling behavior, since it broke down when Sam was under stress or could not effectively control his mother. Finally, Sam's case illustrates the interdependent nature of the child's development of a controlling strategy. As Sam developed a caregiving style with his mother, she increasingly acted childish and encouraged him to take responsibility for her feelings.

We expect that children who do not score extremely high on the disorganization scale during infancy may develop patterns of interacting with their caregiver more quickly. This was the case for both Tim and Kate, who showed controlling behavior with their mothers by the time they were 32 months old, more than a year before Sam became controlling with his mother. In the next section, we explore the issue of how and why some disorganized children develop a punitive controlling style, while others develop a caregiving style.

ANTECEDENTS OF CAREGIVING VERSUS PUNITIVE STRATEGIES

Why some disorganized infants eventually adopt a caregiving strategy to control the caregiver, whereas others adopt a punitive strategy, is not well understood. One possibility is that children like Sam, whose mother was domineering, are likely to show pleasing and caregiving behavior, whereas children whose mothers appear more withdrawn may become bossy and punitive with them. Of course, we can only speculate about such pathways, particularly since the children in this sample were not formally classified as controlling–caregiving or controlling–punitive. In the case of Sam, it seems clear that his mother would strike back harshly if Sam dared to control her through punitive rejection or humiliation. Indeed, when he showed a normal 2-year-old's negativity, she would not tolerate it. The case of Tim and Kate illustrate how children can become bossy and punitive with a mother who withdraws from the parental role.

At the 26-month home visit, Tim's mother tried to be punitive but was helpless in carrying out her threats.

> Tim's mother instructed him on how to complete a shape-sorter puzzle, and when he did so incorrectly, she said in a mocking voice, "Not that way, silly." For the most part, Tim followed her directions, but eventually he tried to move away from his mother and ignore her. She threatened, "I won't buy you a truck. I'll make your fire truck be all gone." She then pleaded with him to do the puzzle, saying, "Oh, please? Oh, please? Oh, please, show me where the elephant goes." When he refused to comply, she said, "All the toys are gonna go away and Tim's gonna go to bed." Tim continued to lie on the floor, and his mother did not carry out any threats.

But by the time Tim was 32 months old, he showed signs of having developed a controlling-punitive style with his mother. As long as his mother did not try to make him do anything he did not want to do, their play interaction proceeded smoothly. His mother was very directive, as before, but now he often purposely ignored her directions. When he did, she yawned, moved away, and lay down on the floor to watch. Conflict between Tim and his mother occurred when Tim did not follow his mother's orders and his mother did not withdraw, as illustrated in the following example:

> After a few brief attempts to complete a puzzle, Tim tried to leave. His mother said, "Hey! I thought you were going to help me, you little . . ." Tim then hurled the puzzle pieces around the room. His mother made several escalating threats: "Then you won't get your train back with this behavior, and you won't get your puzzles, either"; and later, "Say bye-bye, camera, bye-bye, friends, Tim has to go to sleep." Tim ignored the threats, then ordered his mother to pick up the pieces ("Mama do it"). His mother began to pick them up, then whined in a childlike tone, "I have to do this all by myself? Mama is not happy!" Lying on the floor, Tim smiled up at her and said in a mocking voice, "No, Mama *is* happy!" His mother picked up all of the puzzle pieces, while saying, "No more puzzles! Tim has to go to bed!"

In fact, Tim's mother never carried out any of the threats that she made. Perhaps Tim learned over time that his mother's threats and anger, which may have frightened him in infancy, would not hurt him. He could control her by simply refusing to comply, and by becoming angry and hostile himself.

Similar to Tim's mother, Kate's mother also appeared helpless during the free-play and interactive tasks filmed at 24 months. However, she did so in a way that differed from Sam's or Tim's mother. She frequently stared off into space, periodically appearing to enter into trancelike states (i.e., stilling, staring straight ahead). Her affect was flat; other than a small "pasted on" smile, she rarely expressed positive or negative feelings. Kate tried to leave the room several times during one of the teaching tasks. Her mother sat quietly for a while and finally called plaintively to her, "Kate, come play with me." After trying this several times without success, her mother shrugged and said helplessly to the home visitor, "I guess she doesn't like this puzzle."

By the time Kate was 32 months old, she was bossy with her mother:

> During the play interaction, Kate chattered about what she was playing. Her mother was silent and sat at a distance during most of the session. Next, the mother was instructed to help Kate complete a set of tasks. On three different occasions when Kate completed one of the tasks incorrectly, her mother moved a piece to illustrate the correct procedure. Each time Kate screamed, "No!", and ordered in a threatening tone, "Put it back!" On each occasion, her mother obeyed.

Whereas Tim appeared to develop a punitive strategy as a way of gaining power and autonomy with a controlling but ultimately helpless mother,

Kate seemed to develop a controlling and bossy strategy that appeared punitive with her uninvolved, depressed-looking mother. Indeed, the strategy may have been effective, since her mother became much more involved with her by 44 months. During the play and cooperative tasks, Kate's mother sat closer to Kate and was more responsive to her questions.

We can only speculate about why some controlling children become caregivers, while others are punitive. Perhaps, children are afraid of a domineering punitive parent and try to please and show caregiving behaviors. It is interesting to note that Sam, like Tim, tried to be noncompliant and outwardly displayed his anger when he was 20 months old. But Tim was able to control his mother using power assertion and hostility, whereas Sam could not. Rather, it seemed that Sam was punished and treated harshly by his mother when he asserted himself, which may be why he ultimately adopted a controlling–caregiving strategy. Children like Kate and Tim, whose mothers were more submissive and withdrawn, on the other hand, were more bossy or punitive with them. It is also possible that because caregiving requires a certain amount of role-taking skill and affect regulation, it may be a later developing strategy than controlling–punitive behavior. Longitudinal research following a larger sample of children is needed to test these ideas empirically. To more fully understand how controlling behaviors develop, it may be important to look beyond the parent–child relationship to the whole family system.

THE DEVELOPMENT OF CONTROLLING STRATEGIES IN THE CONTEXT OF THE FAMILY SYSTEM

Family systems theorists have argued that it is not just isolated patterns of behavior that are internalized and carried forward from family to peers, nor even roles within a given relationship, but instead, entire relationship systems are internalized and carried forward (Sroufe & Fleeson, 1986; Minuchin, 1974). According to this view, the child internalizes all of the roles learned within each relationship system; for example, an abused child learns to be not only a victim (his or her own role), but also the role of victimizer. In addition, roles within the family are interdependent; they mutually constrain and influence each other. For example, unhealthy parent–child alliances, often involving role reversal, are likely to develop in families in which the marital relationship is distant or conflictual (Jacobvitz, Riggs, & Johnson, 1999). We propose that it may also be the case that unhealthy parent–child relationships (such as those involving disorganized attachment) will also increase the likelihood that role-reversed or peer-like parent–child alliances may develop.

The families of our case study children consisted of a single child, mother, and father. Observations of these families interacting at dinner illustrate how the father–child and marital relationship may contribute to the development of controlling strategies.

> Kate's father said to Kate, "Mommy is trying to be so polite, eating her eggroll with a knife and fork. We don't do it that way, do we, Kate?" Kate says, "No!", and they both laugh derisively at her mother. Later, Kate purposely opened her mouth full of chewed food to show her mother. Her mother said seriously, "Don't show food." Her father smiled and said, "Hey Kate, show food!" He then said, "Eww!", and laughed appreciatively at her display. Throughout the dinner, Kate and her father playfully teased each other, and most of the interchanges were between the two of them.

Sam showed a similar pattern of aligning with one parent while demeaning the other, but with gender roles reversed. At the family dinners observed when Sam was 44 and 56 months old, he was controlling with both his parents. Interestingly, while he was pleasing and caregiving toward his mother, he was punitive and derogating toward his father. Sam and his mother contradicted or ridiculed nearly everything his father said and did, speaking to him in a hostile and demeaning voice. Sam joined in the ridicule using the same demeaning voice tone. One such incident occurred while his father was eating his potatoes mixed with peas. Sam said, in a mocking voice, "You've got a pea in that!" His mother uttered, "Yeah, that's really gross!" Many times during dinner, Sam's mother spoke to her husband through Sam, and Sam spoke to his father through his mother ("Tell daddy . . . "). Twice during dinner, Sam ran over to whisper a secret in his mother's ear, and the two of them giggled. When Sam wanted something, he asked his mother each time, never his father. He used a soft, sweet voice and a coy demeanor with her. In contrast, he made stern demands of his father, using a mocking, challenging, authoritarian tone. For example, pointing to a piece of pizza and shaking his finger at his father, Sam ordered him, "Don't you take this piece! It's for me!"

Thus, by aligning with his mother and modeling her hostile, controlling behavior with his father, Sam gained some measure of power and autonomy. He achieved closeness to his mother and, we infer, was able to control, to some degree, her frightening, unpredictable behavior. Kate showed a similar pattern, even though she and her father mocked her mother in a more playful and less hostile fashion compared with Sam and his mother's disparagement of Sam's father. In both cases, Sam and Kate aligned with the opposite-sex, more dominant parent and became punitive toward the more passive, same-sex parent. In both cases, the couple had strained marital interactions characterized by direct or indirect expressions of hostility. Certainly, more research is required to clarify the links between controlling parent–child relationship patterns, unhealthy parent–child alliances, and problematic marital relationships.

The case of Tim does not fit the same pattern of family alliance as clearly as Sam and Kate. However, looking at Tim's relationship with his father is important in understanding why Tim, as described earlier, is punitive with his mother. As suggested by the following observation, it is possible that Tim re-created with his mother the victim–victimizer relationship he experienced with his father:

> At dinner, Tim's parents discussed adult topics, ignoring Tim. Tim spit on his high chair. His mother tried to distract him, offering more food. Tim said, "No! I spit, Mama! I spit!" His mother replied sweetly, "Sweetie, the camera's taking a picture of you, and if you spit at the camera, everybody's gonna know you spit." His father ignored all of this and resumed discussing adult topics with his wife. Tim said a few words, but his parents ignored him. Tim spit again. This time, while his mother held up a warning finger, his father slapped Tim on top of his head, showing no emotion and saying nothing to him. Tim spit again. His father warned harshly, "You're gonna get smacked!" These were the first words he had spoken to Tim since the dinner began. He then offered Tim some food. At first Tim said, "No!", then he reached for the food. His father held the food out of his reach and gave him a cold, warning stare. His mother resumed adult conversation with her husband, as though everything was fine, but showed signs of nervousness and discomfort, fidgeting in her chair and moving around aimlessly in the kitchen. Tim continued to spit. His father gave him a threatening stare and raised his clenched fist, saying, "You're gonna get whacked!" Tim spit again, and his father slapped him on the head again. Tim did not react, and soon spit again. His mother decided dinner was over and removed Tim from his high chair.

Tim's father seemed to be a stern, cold man who wanted all of his wife's attention at dinner and was intolerant of any interruptions from his child. Tim was used to getting his mother's full attention; however, his mother seemed passive. Perhaps Tim learned to be controlling and punitive from his father, who acted in a similar way.

Observing the parent–child interactions in the family context illustrates the range of role relationships the child may have internalized. For example, by the time Sam was 5 years old, he may have internalized interaction patterns for at least three roles: pathetic and helpless victim; sweet, helpful "big boy," who can take care of his mother; and taunting bully who can belittle and control his father, thereby gaining his mother's favor. Any or all of these role relationships theoretically could be carried over into the context of later peer interactions. It is important to note that disorganized infant attachment does not inevitably lead children to controlling strategies of interacting with the parents, particularly when parents move away from the use of frightening or controlling caregiving strategies.

SUMMARY: THE DEVELOPMENT OF THE PARENT–CHILD RELATIONSHIP DURING EARLY CHILDHOOD

Disorganized children vary in the strategies they finally develop as well as how long it takes them to find a workable pattern of interacting with the caregiver. If the caregiver is intimidating and dominating, a punitive or bossy strategy may invite more frightening behavior, or even abuse. Children, like Sam, may learn to control such parents by acting pleasing and obsequious, and attending to the parents' needs and interests. Employing a punitive and bossy strategy may be more common when the mother acts powerless, or incompetent. In Tim's and Kate's cases, they could not count on their mothers to guide them or set safe limits. Although Tim's mother was overly controlling, whereas Kate's mother was withdrawn, in both cases, the children's defiant and derogating behavior toward their mothers allowed them to be close with their mothers and, at the same time, maintain their autonomy.

Most of the children we observed developed a strategy for interacting with their mother between 26 and 32 months. The case of Sam, who was given the highest possible rating on disorganization in the strange situation, suggests that children with extreme disorganization may have considerable difficulty developing such strategies. We believe that these children will be especially at risk for developing maladaptive peer relationships. As we illustrate in the next section, until children develop an integrated strategy with their attachment figures, we expect that they cannot carry over a strategy of interacting with their parents to their peers.

CARRYING FORWARD DISORGANIZED ATTACHMENT PATTERNS IN INFANCY TO PEER RELATIONSHIPS

Attachment theorists have shown that attachment security in infancy predicts competent adaptation across development with respect to developmentally salient issues (cf. Sroufe, Carlson, & Shulman, 1993). Considerable evidence has been amassed indicating a relation between the child's quality of attachment to the mother in infancy and peer competence in early childhood. Specifically, preschoolers who were securely attached as infants (vs. insecure) have been found to be more socially accepted and competent with peers (LaFreniere & Sroufe, 1985; Erickson, Sroufe, & Egeland, 1985), more involved in positive and synchronous friendships (Youngblade & Belsky, 1992), less aggressive, hostile (Renken, Englund, Marvinney, Sroufe, & Mangelsdorf, 1989), less socially withdrawn with peers (Kemple & Hazen, 1997), and less likely to become either a bully or a victim with their peers (Troy & Sroufe, 1987). Preschoolers who were securely attached as infants have also been found to be less hostile and more empathic than those classified avoidant (Elicker, Englund, & Sroufe, 1992), and less socially withdrawn than those classified resistant.

The development of peer relationships among disorganized children is poorly understood. Nearly all of the studies examining peer relationships among children classified as disorganized or controlling rely on behavior checklists completed by teachers or parents. Virtually no study has observed directly how disorganized/controlling children interact with peers. Furthermore, studies that have relied on behavior checklists have yielded mixed results. Some studies indicate that controlling children classified as disorganized in infancy show peer aggression or externalizing behaviors during the preschool years (Lyons-Ruth, Alpern, & Repacholi, 1993; Shaw, Owens, Vondra, Keenan, & Winslow, 1996) and at ages 6 (Greenberg, Speltz, DeKlyen, & Endriga, 1991; Solomon et al., 1995; Speltz, Greenberg, & DeKlyen, 1990) and 7 (Lyons-Ruth, Easterbrooks, & Cibelli, 1997). Lyons-Ruth et al. (1997), however, found that only 25% of disorganized infants were rated as highly externalizing at age 7, whereas 50% of disorganized infants were rated over the clinical cutoff score for overall maladaptive behavior at school age. This suggests that the forms of later maladaptation associated with early disorganization may not be entirely captured by conventional checklists for internalizing and externalizing symptoms. For example, odd, intrusive, controlling, or incompetent patterns of interactions may not be assessed on checklists that primarily cover aggressive or anxious/depressed behavior. Solomon et al. (1995) suggested that more subtle assessments may be needed to examine the social adaptation of children considered disorganized/controlling who do not display aggressive behavior.

Other studies of controlling children have reported associations between controlling behavior with the caregiver and high ratings on behavior problem scales, with either a direct association with internalizing behaviors (Carlson, 1998) or no clear pattern of internalizing or externalizing behaviors (Solomon et al., 1995; Moss, Parent, Gosselin, Rousseau, & St-Laurent, 1996). Impressive longitudinal data following children from birth to sixth grade demonstrated that teachers score children classified as disorganized during infancy higher on dissociative behavior and internalizing behavior, but not externalizing behavior, in grades 1, 2,

3, and 6 (Carlson, 1998). Finally, in one cross-sectional study of preschool children, the association between controlling behavior with the caregiver and externalizing behaviors was significant for girls but not boys (Hubbs-Tait et al., 1991). Thus, although it appears that attachment disorganization in infancy and controlling behavior in preschool forecast behavior problems at age 6, no single pattern of interaction with peers has emerged. Observational studies of the peer interactions of disorganized children are badly needed. Such observations, however, must be informed by theoretically based hypotheses concerning the processes by which the disorganized child's attachment history is expected to carry forward to later peer relationships.

Sroufe, Egeland, and Carlson (1999) have proposed four bases for predicting a relationship between a child's attachment history and later peer competency: (1) *motivational base*—the secure child believes that engaging with others will be rewarding; (2) *attitudinal base*—the secure child believes that he or she can master the challenges of engaging with others; 3) *instrumental base*—through smooth, reciprocal interactions with the caregiver, the secure child attains skills that promote successful interactive play; and 4) *emotional base*—the secure child is capable of effective regulation of emotions due to the smooth emotional regulation orchestrated by the parent during infancy.

The disorganized child appears to be at risk for poor peer relationships in all four areas. Because disorganized children view themselves as helpless and powerless, we expect them to see peers as a potential threat. They will not believe they can master the challenges of engaging with peers (*attitudinal* base), and therefore, lack a strong *motivational* base for peer interaction. A trapped, frightened animal is likely to alternate between extreme fight-or-flight behaviors. In a similar fashion, the peer behavior of disorganized children might be expected to shift between extreme social withdrawal and defensively aggressive behaviors (i.e., aggression accompanied by fearful affect in which the children aggress against peers to ward off perceived threats to themselves or their possessions). This may be why the research on the peer relationships of disorganized children is mixed, with some studies suggesting peer aggression and others indicating internalizing problems.

The *instrumental* base of the disorganized child's peer relationships is also likely to be compromised, since the disorganized child has not experienced smooth reciprocal interactions with the caregiver. Reciprocal communication skills are essential for establishing successful peer relationships, since the basis for preschool peer interaction is socially coordinated fantasy play (Gottman, 1983). Engaging in such play requires that children freely communicate their ideas for play and respond appropriately to the suggestions of others (Hazen & Black, 1989; Black & Hazen, 1990). Competent reciprocal communication implies a balance of power between interaction partners. When one interaction partner dominates or controls the other, communication becomes one-sided.

Children with a secure attachment history have experienced smooth, cooperative, noninterfering interactions with the caregiver, preparing them for balanced peer interactions in which they neither dominate and control their peers nor allow themselves to be manipulated or exploited (Troy & Sroufe, 1987). Disorganized children, in contrast, have generally experienced unbalanced mother–child interactions as a natural consequence of having a mother who perceives herself to be helpless (George & Solomon, 1996). As a consequence of this helpless stance, the mother may show withdrawn, apathetic behavior (like Kate's mother), overly controlling and interfering behavior (like Tim's mother), or alternate between the two (like Sam's mother). These caregiving patterns will inevitably be highly unbalanced, as the disorganized child tends to alternate between helplessly submitting to the mother's controlling behavior and trying to control such behavior (Lyons-Ruth & Jacobvitz, 1999). Thus, both the parent and child have internalized a helpless/controlling relationship system, in which both participants know both roles, and in different circumstances may enact either role. We would expect to see variations of the helpless/controlling pattern carried over to peer relationships: The disorganized child knows how to play the part of the controlling caregiver or the helpless baby, the victim or the bully, but he or she will not easily be able to be an equal partner in a balanced interaction.

Finally, the *emotional* base of a disorganized child's peer interaction is likely characterized by emotional undercontrol, such as excessive expression of verbal or physical aggression, and/or emotional overcontrol, whereby the child is uncomfortable expressing feelings and coping with conflict, and therefore withdraws from peers. In stressful peer interactions, these children may also show the type of odd "displacement" behaviors that ethologists have observed to be typical of animals in paradoxical situations (Tinbergen, 1951). For example, a frightened rabbit who faces conflicting impulses to fight and flee, but is powerless to do either, may begin to groom itself. As noted by Main and Hesse (1990) these odd, out-of-context conflict behaviors indicate a breakdown in affect regulation, similar to the indices of disorientation displayed in the strange situation, although the actual behavior is likely to differ in form as the child matures. Both preschool and elementary school teachers occasionally come across children they would describe as "odd" or "strange," but interestingly, there is almost no discussion of odd, strange, or contextually disconnected behavior with peers in the literature. Instead, most of the research on peer relationship problems in childhood has focused on aggressive or socially withdrawn children. Yet the inability to respond appropriately and contingently to peers, and to carry on a coherent play theme, is a very strong predictor of social rejection in the preschool years (Hazen & Black, 1989; Black & Hazen, 1990; Kemple, Speranza, & Hazen, 1992). In fact, in these studies, disconnected discourse was a much stronger predictor of a child's social rejection than was disagreeing with a peer. Children who behave in ways that have no connection with the ongoing peer play situation are likely to be identified by peers not as "mean," but as "weird" or "annoying."

Thus, based on theory and existing research, we expect disorganized/ controlling children to show maladaptive patterns in their peer relationships: (1) They are likely to view peers as threatening and to act wary with them, alternating between defensive aggression and apprehensive withdrawal. These patterns will be particularly apparent in the toddler years, before they develop consistent controlling strategies with their parents. (2) After developing controlling strategies to help control their fear, disorganized children will be able to engage in sustained peer interactions, but these interactions are likely to be markedly unbalanced, with the disorganized child alternating between controlling and helpless stances. (3) When the disorganized child is unable to cope with conflict in peer interaction, he or she may act in an odd, disoriented fashion that is unconnected to the ongoing peer interaction. This pattern is expected to be especially characteristic of children who have experienced very frightening care and have developed poor strategies for affect regulation. In the following sections, these three patterns of peer interaction are illustrated with our case study data.

Illustrations of Defensive Aggression and Withdrawal in the Peer Interaction of Disorganized Children

Sam showed a clear pattern of wariness and defensive withdrawal with peers in all of his interactions observed from 20 to 32 months, as illustrated in this example at age 20 months:

> Sam was very absorbed in playing with little people and a dollhouse, glancing warily on occasion at Jack, a bigger and more dominant peer. When Jack approached and also began to play with the dollhouse, Sam watched passively, then moved away and lay down on the floor. When Jack approached Sam again, Sam picked up some toys and started to walk away with them, but then hesitated, rising up on his toes, hunching his shoulders, and dipping up and down as he moved away. He tried to leave the room several times, but each time the camera person brought him back. Each time he tried to leave, he tiptoed with stiff legs, swinging his arm stiffly, and making odd, gasping noises (signs of disorganization).

At 26 months, Sam still showed no signs of enjoying peers, or even the ability to play in close proximity. He and Davy, a rather passive child, played apart during their entire play session. At one point, when Sam wanted a toy that was near Davy, he tried to "sneak" behind him, making roundabout, sidestepping movements on his tiptoes while staying close to the wall. Davy looked up as he approached, and Sam furtively scurried back to his spot, as though caught transgressing. Tim showed a similar pattern of fearful withdrawal at this age:

Tim hovered behind Rob, a larger, dominant boy, watching him play with a truck. With his hand in his mouth, Tim wandered back and forth behind Rob, swinging his arms and circling around aimlessly. Suddenly, he rushed up and furtively tried to grab the truck from Rob. Rob pushed him back forcefully and yelled, "Go 'way!" Tim continued to wander aimlessly behind Rob, kicking at the toys on the floor. Finally, he went to the toy piano and played with it. Rob soon came by and took the piano away. Tim then sidestepped up to Rob, on tiptoe, and furtively reached out to touch the piano. Rob yelled, "Don't do that!", and Tim pulled his hand away quickly.

By 32 months, Sam's peer interactions still had not improved. When paired with Greg, a friendly, talkative boy, Sam avoided physical proximity and engaged only in solitary play, even though Greg talked to him throughout the play session. Sam's defensive aggression is illustrated in this example:

Sam played for several minutes with a toy bus and ignored Greg's repeated requests for a turn with it. When Greg took the bus from him, Sam became extremely distressed, jumping around aimlessly and screaming in a panicked voice, "My car! My car!" The screaming did not seem to be directed to Greg or anyone else. Later, when Greg's back was turned, Sam quickly ran up to grab the bus, pushed Greg away, and ran to the other side of the room with it.

Like Sam and Tim, Kate as a toddler also seemed to fear peers and was overly possessive of toys. Indeed, at 20 months, Kate was not even willing to participate in the peer play session. When her teacher tried to bring her inside her familiar classroom to play with a familiar peer, Kate immediately tried to leave the room. She continued to try to leave and cried or whined throughout the session. At 26 and 32 months, Kate participated in the play sessions but did not interact at with any of the peers. Most of the time, she turned toward the wall while playing with the toys, her back toward the peers. Her only exchange with a peer at the 26-month visit involved an altercation over the toy piano. When a peer approached Kate to play the piano with her, she picked up the piano and took it to the wall, turning her back on him. When he moved to join her, she screamed, "Mine!", and pushed him away.

The patterns of defensively aggressive behavior displayed by Sam and Kate are qualitatively different from the patterns of instrumental and hostile aggression that characterize the normative peer interactions of toddlers and preschoolers in terms of the accompanying affect. Instrumental aggression, defined as aggression performed as a means to an end (e.g., to obtain a desired object), typically is not accompanied by a strong expression of negative affect (Hartup, 1974). Hostile aggression refers to aggression with the intention of causing hurt or injury to another (e.g., in response to a perceived transgression) and is typically accompanied by angry affect (Hartup, 1974). Thus, a young child who wants a toy truck that his peer is using simply grabs it dispassionately from the peer (instrumental aggression). The peer, angered by the transgression, grabs the truck back and also yells at the peer and pushes him away in anger (hostile aggression). In contrast, the defensive aggression displayed by Sam and Kate in protecting their property and pushing away the peer was accompanied by obvious expressions of fear and anxiety, sometimes almost bordering on panic and desperation. We do not claim that disorganized children do not engage in other types of aggression as well, only that defensive aggression is expected to be more prevalent in disorganized children relative to other children, and that defensive aggression may be viewed as the "flip side" of fearful withdrawal.

Thus, as toddlers, these children primarily seemed actively to avoid contact with peers. They viewed the peer as a threat, as someone who would take their toys and perhaps even hurt them, rather than share in play and have fun. These children acted aggressively only on occasion, and each time, only in desperation, to defend against the peer invading their space or taking their possession.

Illustrations of Unbalanced Peer Interactions in Disorganized Children

By 42 months, an unbalanced pattern of peer interactions was evident in all of the case studies of disorganized children. At 42 months, Kate was only able to engage in sustained peer interactions with a submissive peer who would permit her to assume control. Kate's general helplessness and passivity when paired with a dominant peer was evident during the cooperative task interaction during which the children needed to work together to stack several clowns on top of one clown, a task that the target children had completed at an earlier home visit with their parents' help:

> Kate started to show Cathy how to stack the clowns. Cathy said, "No, I think this is how to do it," and begin to stack them straight up (an

unworkable strategy). Kate turned away, pushed all of the clowns to Cathy, and rested her head on her hands, looking sad and resigned. Cathy turned to Kate with an expression of concern and said kindly, "It's okay, you can play." Kate turned away.

However, in the group peer interaction in the classroom observed at this phase, Kate looked like a different child, as shown when she played in the home living center with Trey, a small, quiet, passive boy:

> Pretending to bake a cake in a toy oven, Kate said in a very loud, bossy tone, "You can't have cake now! Go away; you can't have cake 'til I call you!" She then ordered Trey to get some dishes for her. She frowned when she saw what he brought and scolded him, shaking her finger, with her hands on her hips. Trey pretended to eat some of the pretend cake, and Kate yelled, "No! It's not done!" Appearing angry, she ordered him to go away, pointing, with her hand on her hip. When he didn't move, she pushed him roughly, and he fell to the floor. Trey lay on the floor for several seconds, holding his hand to his mouth. Kate asked, "What's the matter?", with a concerned tone. But when he did not respond, and crawled under a table, she went to him and repeated the question several times in an increasingly angry and annoyed tone.

Although Kate and Trey engaged in role playing, Kate was completely dominating, even bullying Trey. It seemed that Kate, as a preschooler, was able to engage in reciprocal pretend play if paired with a submissive peer who allowed her to make all the decisions and control the play. (It is interesting to note that Trey showed fearful behavior—holding his hand to his mouth and crawling under the table—suggesting he, too, may have been disorganized.) Kate was comfortable reenacting the role patterns she internalized from her interactions with her mother, choosing to interact with a passive peer who followed her lead, waited for her to make the decisions, and remained engaged (or became even more engaged) when she was punitive. Kate had difficulty maintaining interaction with a peer who was dominating or made decisions of her own. Her family interaction experiences did not prepare her for such an interaction partner.

Tim also showed a clear pattern of unbalanced peer interaction in which one peer generally dominated and sometimes even victimized the other. In this case, however, Tim generally put himself into the role of the victimized peer rather than the controlling bully, although he continuously struggled (albeit passively) for control. At both 42 and 54 months, Tim's preferred playmate was Bob, a very impulsive, bossy, aggressive boy.

> In the 42-month cooperative task, Tim started to stack the clowns as he had learned to do on the home visit. He tried haltingly to explain the procedure to Bob, but Bob ignored him and used his clown to

knock down Tim's clowns. Tim pretended to make his clown fight Bob's clown, and Bob fought back roughly and forcefully. Bob hurt Tim's cheek with the clown. Tim held his cheek but did not complain. Then Tim spit at Bob, and Bob spit back forcefully. The spitting back and forth continued for several minutes.

In the 54-month dyadic free-play situation, Bob kept control of the toy doctor kit and would not let Tim use it when he asked for a turn. Tim took the syringe when Bob was not looking and used it on Bob. Bob said, "Ow! Stop!", grabbed the syringe, and pushed Tim down. Tim repeatedly asked, "Let me see," but Bob ignored him and continued to play with the kit. Bob then hit Tim hard and repeatedly with the toy hammer from the kit several times. Tim did not respond to the hitting but continued to ask for a turn. Bob tried to look into Tim's ear with a toy . Tim lay on the floor and said, "Stop!" He then threatened to "bite" Bob with a chicken puppet if Bob continued to look in his ear. He started to "bite" Bob with the puppet, and Bob then attacked Tim with another puppet forcefully enough to knock him down. Tim said, "Sorry! Sorry!" but Bob continued to "bite" Tim with the puppet and to kick him as he lay on the floor.

Oddly, even though their play was so rough that the cameraperson intervened several times to prevent Bob from hurting Tim, Tim laughed and seemed to enjoy the interaction. It is interesting to note that Tim's pattern of interaction with Bob is similar to his interaction pattern with his father, in that Tim would mildly provoke Bob to get him to respond (even using similar behaviors, for example, spitting) even though Bob (like his father) responded with verbal and physical aggression. Tim responded to the aggression with passive resistance and continued provocation, ensuring continuation of the interaction.

Thus, both Tim and Kate were able to engage in reciprocal pretend play with peers, but only in the context of unbalanced, agonistic interactions in which one peer continually tried to dominate the other. Interestingly, in Kate's case, she had to dominate and so could only interact with submissive peers. In contrast, Tim seemed most comfortable interacting with dominating, aggressive peers, fighting back in response to his peer's aggressive overtures as though continually trying to gain control and get the upper hand, and other times submitting passively to the aggression and helpless to stop it.

A Case of Odd, Disconnected Peer Interactions in an Extremely Disorganized Child

All of the disorganized children we observed displayed noticeably high frequencies of odd and socially disconnected behaviors with peers relative to nondisorganized children. These behaviors included the following: (1) verbal responses that had no connection to the peer's preceding utterances; (2) quirky mannerisms or stereotypies (e.g., rolling the tongue around in the mouth, hunching the shoulders, characteristic facial distortions); (3) repeated annoying and intrusive behaviors that were unrelated to the ongoing play (e.g., repeatedly tugging on peer's shirt; shining a flashlight in peer's eyes); (4) odd or bizarre behaviors that were not connected to the ongoing play (e.g., licking the wall, spinning around; making strange noises); (5) behaviors in which the affect expressed was inappropriate to the context (e.g., crying out for no apparent reason; responding with anger or fear to the peer's neutral or positive initiation); and (6) juxtaposition of extreme positive and negative affect (e.g., hugging and then immediately beating a doll). All of these types of odd behaviors were particularly striking in Sam's peer interactions, suggesting that such patterns may be especially prevalent in preschool children assigned high disorganization ratings in infancy.

Sam's wary withdrawal from peers at 20 months illustrates his display of odd behaviors in the presence of peers at an early age. When Sam tried to move away from his peer, Jack, and leave the play environment, he tiptoed with stiff legs, swung his arm stiffly, and made odd, gasping noises. These odd behaviors were much more pervasive in both Sam's parent–child and peer interactions than in those of any other disorganized child, and persisted much longer. Some of the behaviors persisted unchanged (e.g., swinging his arm stiffly, gasping), while others appeared later in his development (e.g., whooping, spinning around).

Sam did not actually interact with peers in any of the observed interactions until 42 months. Even then, his interchanges with peers were very brief and usually involved struggles over objects. Usually, he played alone, often watching peers from a distance with a wistful expression. He still tended to jealously guard certain toys, as he did as a toddler. At times, he tried to join in play with peers, but his odd, disconnected, and often obnoxious behavior seemed to put peers off. Eventually, they would leave or ignore him, or tell him to stop or to go away, as illustrated in the following example:

> Sam (42 months old) is paired with Jenny, a friendly child who tries to get him involved in doll play with her. At first he ignores her overtures, but finally he takes the doll she offered. Ignoring the pretense plans Jenny suggests, Sam alternates between brushing the doll's hair tenderly and smashing it against the floor. Jenny tries to integrate Sam's behavior into her pretend play themes; as he beat up his doll, she pretends the doll is speaking in a squeaky voice, "Ow! Don't do that!" Sam does not respond, so Jenny tries again, making her doll say,

"I'm going on the bus." Sam grabbed the toy bus before Jenny could put her doll in it, crammed his doll in, and drove the bus away. Jenny gave up trying to play with Sam.

Sam (54 months old) grabbed a syringe from the toy doctor's kit Davy was holding and gave him a "shot." When Davy ignored this, he shined a flashlight right in Davy's eyes, while making strange whooping–gasping sounds. Davy also ignored this and suggested that they play with puppets. Sam took the puppet that Davy offered, then made his puppet "bite" Davy's nose while Sam grinned and giggled. He continued even after Davy repeatedly told him to stop. Davy then tried to initiate doctor–patient play with Sam. He put on the stethoscope and said, "I need to listen to your heart." Sam looked frightened and cowered on the floor, saying, "No way!" He picked up a "magic wand" and waved it at Davy, making a whooping noise and grinning. Sam continued to wave the wand and whoop at Davy for several seconds. Davy finally ignored Sam and turned his back on him.

Sam's second dyadic peer interaction with Mark was similarly immature and out of sync with the peer. In fact, he repeated many of the initiations he used with Davy: shining the flashlight in his eyes, "biting" him with a puppet, trying to give him a "shot," and waving the magic wand at him. Mark was also annoyed and ultimately turned away.

A preschooler who, like Sam, was disorganized during infancy may become disoriented when approaching or when approached by peers, feeling at once a conflicting desire to affiliate with peers, and in the midst of approaching them, an irrational and unconsciously derived fear that the peers will hurt him. This may explain the odd, defensive behaviors that Sam used, such as continually waving the magic wand at the peer as though to ward him off, and pretending to "bite" the peer with a puppet. (Interestingly, Sam's mother also used a puppet to "bite" Sam's face during play). We characterize these examples as "odd" rather than aggressive, because they did not appear to be performed with an intent to harm the peer. They were accompanied by silly smiles and giggles, and by coy body positions (e.g., a sideways tilt of the head), as though Sam felt that he would be perceived as cute or funny.

It is possible that children like Sam, who score high on disorganization in infancy, will take longer to carry over strategies for interacting with their parents to their peer relationships. Thus, a child who develops a caregiving strategy to deal with an intimidating parent may act in a conciliatory way toward peers perceived as threatening. It may be that Sam did not carry over this strategy to the peer context because he was not able to achieve a consistent behavioral strategy in his interactions with his mother until he was 56 months old. In addition, employing a controlling–caregiving strategy with peers may require more advanced social–cognitive skills than use of such a strategy with a mother who structures the interaction, actively eliciting caregiving behavior from the child. Although not as healthy as a balanced, open, and affectively positive style of peer interaction expected from a secure child, a controlling–caregiving strategy would probably be at least partially successful in getting Sam involved in reciprocal pretend play with peers. It is also possible that the odd, silly, annoying initiations that characterize Sam's peer interactions are precursors of controlling–caregiving interaction patterns, if performed with the intent of pleasing the peer by being cute and funny. (Indeed, Sam acted silly in the teaching task with his mother when he could not come up with an answer to please her.) It would be interesting to see if Sam later carries over the punitive relationship dynamics he uses with his father to peers that he perceives as weak and submissive.

CONCLUSIONS

Our case studies are consistent with the hypothesis that disorganized infants do adopt strategies during the preschool years that enable them to partially communicate with and get close to their caregivers. These strategies may later carry over to peer relationships, enabling them to join in some level of reciprocal interactions with peers, however unbalanced and agonistic. We have suggested that the carryover of strategies will develop later in extremely disorganized children, like Sam. Our case studies also suggest that disorganized children show individual differences in the pathways they take to their peer relationships, based in part on differences in the early relationship patterns they developed with their caregivers. Kate and Tim participated in aggressive exchanges with peers, whereas Sam withdrew or engaged in odd behaviors that were out of sync with the ongoing peer interaction. Most of Sam's peer sessions quickly fell apart as he buried his head under a pillow, tried to leave the room, or annoyed his peers with his persistent repetition of odd behaviors.

Our observations indicate that it may be important to look beyond broad assessments of "aggression" or "social withdrawal" to the different ways that aggression and withdrawal can be behaviorally manifested (e.g., punitive vs. defensive vs. instrumental aggression), the different functions these behaviors can serve, and the various pathways through which they can develop. Along with looking at aggressive and withdrawn behavior in more depth, considerably more attention should be given to odd, socially, and affectively disconnected behaviors and communication patterns that are out of sync with the ongoing peer interaction. We propose that these maladaptive patterns, although less commonly observed than aggression and withdrawal, may be even more strongly predictive of later peer isolation and rejection.

It is interesting to note that among our disorganized children, we found that the same child could show quite different behavioral styles with one peer versus another. This may stem, in part, from experiencing disparate relationships with their mothers and fathers. By the time peer relationships become important to children, when they are preschoolers, father–child relationships are likely to be increasingly influential in developing a child's relationship patterns. This may be particularly true in the arena of preschool peer relationships in which interactions center around play. Numerous studies have found that fathers, more likely than mothers, function in the role of playmates to their toddlers and preschool children, whereas mothers are more likely to function as caregivers (Lamb, 1996). It may be necessary to observe the child alone with each parent, with both parents together, and with several different peers to more completely understand what is transferred from parents to peers.

Although many disorganized children develop a singular, coherent way to interact with their parents and peers, there are serious drawbacks to the strategies they adopt. First, such strategies are quite rigid. Unlike secure children, who can flexibly interact with many different kinds of peers, and in different roles, disorganized children may be unwilling or unable to interact with children who do not fit the familiar relationship pattern they have known all their lives. They may also seek out peer playmates that reinforce their negative views of self and other, such as the bullies with whom Tim always seems to find himself, or the very passive peers that Kate prefers. It is unlikely that the types of peer relationships they had as preschoolers will lead to the development of competent peer relationships in middle childhood, when a critical developmental task is the formation of loyal, reciprocal friendships involving trust and self-disclosure.

REFERENCES

Ainsworth, M. D. S., Blehar, M., Waters, E., & Wall, S. (1978). *Patterns of attachment.* Hillsdale, NJ: Erlbaum.

Belsky, J., & Cassidy, J. (1994). Attachment: Theory and evidence. In M. L. Rutter, D. F. Hay, & S. Baron-Cohen (Eds.), *Development through life: A handbook for clinicians* (pp. 373–402). Oxford, UK: Blackwell.

Black, E., & Hazen, N. L. (1990). Social status and patterns of communication in acquainted and unacquainted preschool children. *Developmental Psychology, 26,* 379–387.

Bowlby, J. (1969/1982). *Attachment and loss: Vol 1. Attachment.* New York: Basic Books.

Bowlby, J. (1980). *Attachment and loss: Vol 3. Loss.* New York: Basic Books.

Bretherton, I. (1985). Attachment theory: Retrospect and prospect. In I. Bretherton & E. Waters (Eds.), Growing points of attachment theory and research. *Monographs of the Society for Research in Child Development, 50*(1–2, Serial No. 209), 3–35.

Carlson, E. A. (1998). A prospective longitudinal study of disorganized/disoriented attachment. *Child Development, 69,* 1107–1128.

Crittenden, P. M. (1992). Treatment of anxious attachment in infancy and early childhood. *Development and Psychopathology, 4,* 209–241.

Elicker, J., Egeland, M., & Sroufe, L. A. (1992). Predicting peer competence and peer relationships from early parent–child relationships. In R. D. Parke & G. W. Ladd (Eds.), *Family-peer relationships: Modes of linkage* (pp. 77–106). Hillsdale, NJ: Erlbaum.

Erickson, M. F., Sroufe, L. A., & Egeland, B. (1985). The relationship between quality of attachment and behavior in preschool in a high-risk sample. In I. Bretherton & E. Waters (Eds.), Growing points in attachment theory and research. *Mongraphs of the Society for Research in Child Development, 50*(1–2, Serial No. 209), 147–193.

George, C., & Solomon, J. (1996). Representational models of relationships: Links between caregiving and attachment. *Infant Mental Health Journal, 17,* 198–216.

George, C., & Solomon, J. (1999). Attachment and caregiving: The caregiving behavioral system. In J. Cassidy & P. R. Shaver (Eds.), *Handbook of attachment: Theory, research, and clinical applications* (pp. 649–670). New York: Guilford Press.

Gottman, J. M. (1983). How children become friends. *Monographs of the Society for Research in Child Development, 48*(3, Serial No. 201).

Hartup, W. W. (1974). Aggression in childhood: Developmental perspectives. *American Psychologist, 29,* 336–341.

Hazen, N. L. (1994). *Family interaction and young children's peer competence.* Final report submitted to the National Institute of Child Health and Human Development, Washington, DC.

Hazen, N. L., & Black, E. (1989). Preschool peer communication skills: The role of social status and interaction context. *Child Development, 60,* 867–876.

Hubbs-Tait, L., Eberhart-Wright, A., Ware, L. Osofsky, J., Yockey, W., & Fusco, J. (1991, April). *Maternal depression and infant attachment: Behavior problems at 54 months in children of adolescent mothers.* Paper presented at the biennial meeting of the Society for Research in Child Development, Seattle, WA.

Jacobvitz, D. B., & Bush, N. F. (1996). Reconstructions of family relationships: Parent–child alliances, personal distress and self-esteem. *Developmental Psychology, 32,* 732–743.

Jacobvitz, D., Hazen, N., & Riggs, S. (1997, April). *Disorganized mental processes in mothers, frightening/frightened caregiving, and disoriented/disorganized behavior in infancy.* Paper presented at the biennial meeting of the Society for Research in Child Development, Washington, DC.

Jacobvitz, D., Riggs, S., & Johnson, E. M. (1999). Cross-sex and same-sex family alliances: Immediate and long-term effects on daughters and sons. In N. D. Chase (Ed.), *Parentified children: Theory, research and treatment.* Thousand Oaks, CA: Sage.

Jurkovic, G. J. (1998). Destructive parentification in families: Causes and consequences. In L. L'Abate (Ed.), *Family psychopathology*. New York: Guilford Press.

Kaplan, N. (1987). *Individual differences in 6-year-olds' thoughts about separation: Predicted from attachment to mother at age 1*. Unpublished doctoral dissertation, University of California, Berkeley.

Kemple, K., & Hazen, N. (1997). *Family correlates of toddlers' shyness: Parent–child interaction, and mother–child attachment*. Unpublish manuscript, University of Texas, Austin.

Kemple, K., & Speranza, H., & Hazen, N. L. (1992). Cohesive discourse and peer acceptance: Longitudinal relations in the preschool years. *Merrill–Palmer Quarterly, 38*, 364–381.

LaFreniere, P. J., & Sroufe, L. A. (1985). Profiles of peer competence in the preschool: Interrelations between measures, influence of social ecology, and relation to attachment history. *Developmental Psychology, 21*, 56–69.

Lamb, M. (1996). *The role of the father in child development*. New York: Wiley.

Lyons-Ruth, K., Alpern, L., & Repacholi, B. (1993). Disorganized infant attachment classification and maternal psychosocial problems as predictors of hostile–aggressive behavior in the preschool classroom. *Child Development, 64*, 572–585.

Lyons-Ruth, K., Bronfman, E., Parsons, E., & Griffin, M. E. (1997). *Atypical forms of maternal responsiveness associated with disorganized attachment patterns in infancy*. Paper presented at the biennial meeting of the Society for Research in Child Development, Washington, DC.

Lyons-Ruth, K., Easterbrooks, A., & Cibelli, C. (1997). Infant attachment strategies, infant mental lag, and maternal depressive symptoms: Predictors of internalizing and externalizing problems at age 7. *Developmental Psychology, 33*, 681–692.

Lyons-Ruth, K., & Jacobvitz, D. B. (1999). The disorganized attachment pattern: Loss, trauma, and relationship violence. In J. Cassidy & P. R. Shaver (Eds.), *Handbook of attachment: Theory, research, and clinical applications* (pp. 520–554). New York: Guilford Press.

Main, M., & Cassidy, J. (1988). Categories of response to reunion with the parent at age 6: Predictable from infant attachment classifications and stable over a 1-month period. *Developmental Psychology, 24*, 415–426.

Main, M., & Hesse, E. (1990). Parent's unresolved traumatic experiences are related to infant disorganized attachment status: Is frightened and/or frightening parental behavior the linking mechanism? In M. T. Greenberg, D. Cicchetti, & E. M. Cummings (Eds.), *Attachment in the preschool years: Theory, research, and intervention* (pp. 161–182). Chicago: University of Chicago Press.

Main, M., & Hesse, E. (1995). *Frightening, frightened, dissociated, or disorganized behavior on the part of the parent: A coding system for parent–infant interactions* (4th ed.). Unpublished manuscript, University of California, Berkeley.

Main, M., Kaplan, N., & Cassidy, J. (1985). Security in infancy, childhood and adulthood: A move to the level of representation. In I. Bretherton & E. Waters (Eds.), Growing points of attachment theory and research. *Monographs of the Society for Research in Child Development, 50*(1–2, Serial No. 209), 66–104.

Main, M., & Solomon, J. (1986). Discovery of an insecure-disorganized/disoriented attachment pattern In T. B. Brazelton and M. Yogman (Eds.), *Affective development in infancy*. (pp. 95–124). Norwood, N. J. : Ablex.

Main, M., & Solomon, J. (1990). Procedures for identifying infants as disorganized/disoriented during the Ainsworth Strange Situation. In M. Greenberg, D. Cicchetti, & E. M. Cummings (Eds.), *Attachment during the preschool years: Theory, research, and intervention* (pp. 121–160). Chicago: University of Chicago Press.

Minuchin, S. (1974). *Families and family therapy*. Cambridge, MA: Harvard University Press.

Moss, E., Parent, S., Gosselin, C., Rousseau, D., & St-Laurent, D. (1996). Attachment and teacher-reported behavior problems during the preschool and early school-age period. *Development and Psychopathology, 8*, 511–526.

Renken, B., Egeland, B., Marvinney, D., Mangelsdorf, S., & Sroufe, L. A. (1989). Early childhood antecedents of aggression and passive-withdrawal in early elementary school. *Journal of Personality, 57*, 257–282.

Schuengel, C., van IJzendoorn, M., Bakermans-Kranenburg, M., & Blom, M. (1997). *Frightening, frightened and/or dissociated behavior, unresolved loss and infant disorganization*. Paper presented at the biennial meeting of the Society for Research in Child Development, Washington, DC.

Shaw, D. S., Owens, E. B., Vondra, J., Keenan, K., & Winslow, E. B. (1996). Early risk factors and pathways in the development of early disruptive behavior problems. *Development and Psychopathology, 8*, 679–699.

Solomon, J., & George, C. (1996). Defining the caregiving system: Toward a theory of caregiving. *Infant Mental Health Journal, 17*, 183–197.

Solomon, J., George, C., & De Jong, A. (1995). Children classified as controlling at age six: Evidence of disorganized representational strategies and aggression at home and at school. *Development and Psychopathology, 7*, 447–463.

Speltz, M. L., Greenberg, M. T., & DeKlyen, M. (1990). Attachment in preschoolers with disruptive behavior: A comparison of clinic-referred and nonproblem children. *Development and Psychopathology, 2*, 31–46.

Sroufe, L. A., Carlson, E. A., & Shulman, S. (1993). Individuals in relationships: Development from infancy through adolescence. In D. C. Funder, R. D. Parke, C. Tomlinson-Keasey, & K. Widaman (Eds.), *Studying lives through time: Personality and development* (pp. 315–342). Washington, DC: American Psychological Association Press.

Sroufe, L. A., Egeland, B., & Carlson, E. (1999). One social world: The integrated development of parent–child and peer relationships. In W. A. Collins & B. Laursen (Eds.), *Relationships as developmental contexts: The 30th Minnesota Symposium on Child Psychology*. Hillsdale, NJ: Erlbaum.

Sroufe, L. A., & Fleeson, J. (1986). Attachment and the construction of relationships. In W. Hartup & Z. Rubin (Eds.), *Relationships and development* (pp. 51–71). Hillsdale, NJ: Erlbaum.

Thalhuber, K., Jacobvitz, D. J., & Hazen, N. L. (1998, March). *Effects of mothers' past traumatic experiences on mother–infant interactions*. Paper presented at the biennial meeting of the Southwestern Society for Research in Human Development, Galveston, TX.

Tinbergen, N. (1951). *The study of instinct.* New York: Oxford University Press.

Troy, M., & Sroufe, L. A. (1987). Victimization among preschoolers: Role of attachment relationship history. *Journal of the American Academy of Child and Adolescent Psychiatry, 26,* 166–172.

Wartner, U. G., Grossman, K., Bremmer-Bombik, E., & Suess, G. (1994). Attachment patterns at age six in South Germany: Predictability from infancy and implications for preschool behavior. *Child Development, 65,* 1014–1027.

Youngblade, L. M., & Belsky, J. (1992). Parent–child antecedents of 5-year-olds' close friendships: A longitudinal analysis. *Developmental Psychology, 28,* 700–713.

CHAPTER 6

Disorganized Attachment and Developmental Risk at School Age

ELLEN MOSS
DIANE ST-LAURENT
SOPHIE PARENT

Disorganized/disoriented infants have been distinguished from those with more "organized" secure or insecure attachment strategies by their apparent failure to show a coherent behavioral strategy for dealing with separation and reunion with their mothers (Main & Solomon, 1990). These infants display bouts or sequences of behaviors that seemingly lack a goal and, in contrast to infants of other attachment classifications, appear to experience a collapse of strategy (Main, 1995). School-age (age 6) follow-up studies of children who had earlier been classified as disorganized/disoriented revealed that these children often attempted to control parental behavior during reunions in a caregiving or punitive manner (Main & Cassidy, 1988). Preschool or school-age children showing this role-reversed pattern with the caregiver were referred to by Main and Cassidy as disorganized/controlling.

It is becoming increasingly clear that disorganized attachment is associated with risk in a number of developmental domains. Disorganized/controlling attachment is predictive of the development of behavior problems at preschool and school age in both high-risk and normal samples (Lyons-Ruth, Alpern, & Repacholi, 1993; Lyons-Ruth, Repacholi, McLeod, & Silva, 1991; Moss, Parent, Gosselin, Rousseau, & St-Laurent, 1996; Solomon, George, &

De Jong, 1995; Speltz, Greenberg, & DeKlyen, 1990). Studies indicate that both externalizing and internalizing symptoms characterize the behavior problems of disorganized school-age children between 5 and 9 years of age. Although at preschool and early school age, it is primarily an aggressive, disruptive behavior pattern that is associated with disorganization (Lyons-Ruth et al., 1993; Speltz et al., 1990), anxieties and fears related to performance, abilities, and self-worth become more pronounced in middle childhood (Cassidy, 1988). The child's internal working models of the interactional history with caregivers influence perceptions of self and other, thus coloring interpretations of social events and expectations regarding relationships (Bowlby, 1969, 1973; Bretherton, 1985; Sroufe & Fleeson, 1986). These motivational and self-dimensions have important implications for a wide range of developmental tasks, both social and academic.

In attachment theory, affective relationships are believed to have an impact on social and cognitive functioning through the mediation of caregiver–child interactive patterns that give rise to internal working models of self and one's relationship to others (Bowlby, 1973). The internal working model is defined as a dynamic structure containing affectively charged cognitions that give rise to different patterns of self-esteem and self-effectance (Bretherton, 1985; Cassidy, 1988). On an empirical level, we have studies exploring partial linkages between attachment, parent–child interactive patterns, self processes, and social or cognitive outcomes (Cassidy, 1988; Jacobsen, Edelstein, & Hofmann, 1994; Jacobsen & Hofmann, 1997; Moss, Humber, & Roberge, in press; Vershueren, Marcoen, & Schoefs, 1996). However, there are few multidimensional studies that have examined models linking pathways between these components. In this chapter, we review relevant literature and report results of a longitudinal study that examined multiple components of developmental risk associated with attachment at school age. In addition to reviewing results of already published studies on socioemotional development issuing from this project (Moss et al., 1996; Moss, Gosselin, Parent, Rousseau, & Dumont, 1997; Moss, Rousseau, Parent, St-Laurent, & Saintonge, 1998), we incorporate new data concerning school performance.

In the current study, we examine the following research questions: Do mothers and disorganized children (age 6) show distinct collaborative patterns when compared with mothers and children with organized attachment patterns? Does disorganized attachment (age 6) predict deficits in academic self-esteem and school performance in middle childhood (age 8)? To what extent do collaborative patterns mediate (account for) any demonstrated relations between disorganized attachment and academic self-esteem? Finally, to what extent do both mother–child collaborative patterns and child self-esteem mediate any relation between disorganized attachment and school performance at school age?

CORRELATES OF DISORGANIZED ATTACHMENT IN INFANTS AND TODDLERS: AFFECTIVE AND COGNITIVE DIMENSIONS OF CAREGIVING

In attachment theory, mother–child interactive patterns contribute to both the development of qualitatively different attachment patterns (A, B, C, D) and to the prediction of child adaptation (Ainsworth, Bell, & Stayton, 1971; Bowlby, 1969; Bretherton, 1985). A few studies that have included observations of disorganized infants and their mothers suggest that dis-rupted interactive patterns may potentiate developmental risk for disorga-nized children. Mothers of infants classified D using separation–reunion measures have been described as highly insensitive with repeated episodes of hostile intrusiveness and/or emotional detachment (Lyons-Ruth et al., 1991). Main and Hesse (1990) have suggested that these behaviors, in addi-tion to others, such as maternal dissociative states, may frighten the infant and interfere with the processing of affective, social and cognitive informa-tion. Further expanding beyond the Main and Hesse hypothesis, George and Solomon (in press; Solomon & George, 1996) have suggested that maternal behavior (and internal working models) revealing helplessness and mother being out of control of herself, the child, or the situation, leaves the child in momentary or prolonged states of feeling abandoned or unprotected. Thus, they suggested that it is not scary behavior per se, but the experience of abdicated care on the part of the attachment figure that are frightening for the child.

This second hypothesis underscores the importance of studying the components of caregiving behavior that may distinguish disorganized mothers from those of children with organized attachment patterns. In attachment studies, measures of maternal sensitivity have been tradition-ally restricted to more socioemotional components of interaction. How-ever, the adequacy of caregiving behavior also has implications for chil-dren's academic performance. Parent–child communication patterns characterized by autonomy support, involvement, and reciprocal control have been shown to predict child self-perceived competence and academic achievement (Grolnick & Ryan, 1989). In addition, the extent to which par-ents encourage children to be self-regulating in learning tasks and progres-sively transfer responsibility for monitoring joint problem-solving activities also facilitates the development of executive or metacognitive functions such as planning, monitoring, and evaluation (Gauvain & Rogoff, 1989; Vygotsky, 1978). Deficits in these metacognitive functions have been asso-ciated with underachievement at school age (Loper & Murphy, 1985).

Difficulties in metacognitive monitoring and reasoning regarding loss and other traumatic experiences have also been identified in adolescents and adults with unresolved attachment status (Main, 1991). According to

Main (1991) and others (Flavell, 1979; Inhelder, Sinclair, & Bovet, 1974), metacognitive monitoring refers to activities involved in regulating cognition, including planning, monitoring, and checking outcomes, and is activated when a person becomes aware of contradictions between presently held ideas or beliefs. Recent studies indicate that problems in cognitive self-regulatory activity of disorganized children and adolescents may not be limited to the processing of attachment-related information but also extend to tasks of a more academic nature (Jacobsen et al., 1994; Jacobsen & Hofmann, 1997). However, no study has yet explored whether these deficits in cognitive regulatory activity are related to components of mother–child interaction.

Although attachment theory is primarily a theory of socioemotional development, Bowlby's (1969) formulation of security as an attachment–exploration balance has inherent implications for cognitive development as well (see also Jacobsen et al., 1994). During the infancy and toddler period, security of attachment is associated with both maternal facilitation of collaboration and children's more appropriate use of adult resources to complete difficult tasks (Frankel & Bates, 1990; Matas, Arend, & Sroufe, 1978). Secure children manifest greater mastery motivation and cognitive executive capacity in exploring the environment than do their insecure peers (Belsky, Garduque, & Hrincir, 1984; Harmon, Suwalsky, & Klein, 1979). Avoidant and ambivalent toddlers manifest deficiencies in exploratory patterns during joint play with the mother. The emotional restriction of avoidant dyads and the exaggerated interpersonal focus of ambivalent dyads appear to interfere with attainment of joint problem-solving goals (Belsky, Rovine, & Taylor, 1984; Cassidy & Berlin, 1994; Lewis & Feiring, 1989; Pederson & Moran, 1996).

Since these earlier studies of exploratory patterns as a function of attachment were carried out prior to the development of the D classification, little is known concerning early behaviors associated with motivational and self-effectance patterns for this group. However, it is likely that the considerable cognitive and attentional resources necessary to cope with a caregiver who induces fear or feelings of abandonment or threat in the infant should considerably restrict the mental resources available for learning and exploration (Aber & Allen, 1987; Main, 1991).

We have also suggested a more direct role for caregiver–child interactions in mediating the relation between attachment and exploratory deficits (Moss, 1992; Moss et al., 1997). In this model, based on consideration of both Bowlby's and Vygotsky's ideas, knowledge of how to analyze problems is internalized along with models of how to engage social resources in facilitating one's cognitive efforts and expectations about the outcomes of such collaborative endeavors. According to Vygotsky (1978), the adult optimally leads the child toward greater self-regulation by making demands within the child's zone of proximal development. Adults need to raise the level of cognitive exchange slightly beyond children's actual level by providing more structuring for difficult tasks and allowing greater autonomy to children when competence is demonstrated. By the preschool period, the zone of proximal development shifts to the dyadic coordination of representations within problem definitions, plans, and subsequent evaluations (Moss & Strayer, 1990).

In attachment theory, as the preschooler's representational and communicative skills improve, caregiver–child interactions become increasingly focused on mutually affecting one another's plans (Marvin, 1977). An effective goal-corrected partnership (Bowlby, 1969) requires the ability to verbally negotiate shared plans that may conflict with individual motives. Dysfunctional patterns of mother–child collaboration may thus interfere with the development of child metacognitive abilities, which, in turn, reduces the chances of successful classroom adaptation. The abdicated caregiving style that characterizes mothers of disorganized children (Solomon & George, 1996) may be incompatible with the careful monitoring of, and adjustment to, the child's state required, not only for adequate development of child affective-self functions, but also to facilitate the emergence of developing cognitive and metacognitive functions.

Partial support for this idea comes from a few studies showing that, in addition to low levels of emotional support, mothers of D infants initiate less verbal communication, which may be associated with less cognitive support during joint play (Lyons-Ruth, Connell, Zoll, & Stahl, 1987; Lyons-Ruth et al., 1991). In a recent study by Lyons-Ruth, Easterbrooks, and Cibelli (1997), maternal depression and infant disorganization significantly predicted aggressive behavior at school age, while these two factors in conjunction with infant mental lag predicted clinical cutoff levels of externalizing problems. As these authors discussed, these data suggest that disrupted levels of cognitive as well as social engagement may characterize the interactive environment of those disorganized children most likely to be at risk, since both affective and cognitive development may be seriously compromised.

Support for this idea comes from studies that have examined concurrent associations between attachment classifications at preschool and school-age, and mother–child communication patterns. These studies used separation–reunion measures for preschool and school-age children (Cassidy & Marvin, 1992; Main & Cassidy, 1988) and examined mother–child interaction in both home and/or laboratory contexts. Main, Kaplan, and Cassidy (1985) observed the discourse style of 6-year-olds who had been classified secure in infancy and their mothers to be fluid, reciprocally balanced, and free-changing in focus. By comparison, dyads including 6-year-olds who had been classified insecure/controlling were the most dysfluent and role-imbalanced of all attachment groups in that the children often controlled the dialogue while the parent passively responded. Similarly, in another study, mothers of secure 4½-year-olds were observed to show relaxed, well-meshed interactions with their preschoolers at home and higher frequencies of planning, sensitivity, and positive affect in the laboratory when compared with insecures (Achermann, Dinneen, & Stevenson-Hinde, 1991; Stevenson-Hinde & Shouldice, 1995). Observations of the same sample showed that mothers of controlling 4-year-olds were the least affirming and provided a less sensitive framework than all other groups in laboratory tasks. In our sample of 120 families (Moss et al., 1998, in press), we compared the quality of dyadic interactive patterns among mothers and their children in the four attachment groups during an unstructured snacktime. Results indicated that controlling children were rated by observers as most poorly coordinated and showed the most incongruent verbal–nonverbal communication patterns of all dyads. A pattern of role reversal involving either coercive or oversolicitous child control of parental behavior was also evident. The quality of emotional expression was rated as least attuned and most negative and tense. Most importantly, further analyses indicated that these dysfunctional communication patterns partially mediated the relation between the D classification and concurrent clinical cutoff levels of behavior problems.

ATTACHMENT, MOTHER–CHILD COLLABORATION, AND CHILD SELF-ESTEEM AS PREDICTORS OF SCHOOL PERFORMANCE

Self-regulatory styles as well as caregiver–child collaborative patterns may, therefore, differentially potentiate developmental risk for attachment classification groups during the school-age period. Although no study has directly examined this hypothesis, several studies provide partial support. Solomon et al. (1995) found that 6-year-old children with fearful and disorganized representations of self and other were more likely to manifest a high level of behavior problems than any other attachment group. Other studies have found links between children's attachment pattern at early school age and measures of self-esteem and ego resiliency (Cassidy, 1988; Urban, Carlson, Egeland, & Sroufe, 1991; Verschueren et al., 1996). Concerning academic or cognitive outcomes, Jacobsen et al. (1994) found that attachment was related to differences in children and adolescents' (aged 7–15) cognitive regulatory activity, which, in turn, were mediated by feelings of self-confidence. In a more recent study of the same sample, Jacobsen and Hofmann (1997) found that school-age attachment predicted school behavior and academic competence in middle childhood and adolescence. In those studies that separately evaluated the effect of attachment classifications, the insecure/disorganized classification was most strongly associated with negative self-regulatory and/or self-concept outcomes. However, none of these studies examined concurrent associations between caregiver–child interactive patterns, self-processes, and adaptation to the school environment.

In this chapter, we present further analyses expanding on our earlier work linking controlling school-age attachment to the development of socioemotional problems by examining components of school-relevant functioning. We also expand the search for possible mediators in the association between the D classification and developmental risk in middle childhood by examining pathways between the controlling classification, cognitive and metacognitive components of mother–child interaction, child self-processes, and academic outcomes. We hypothesized that mothers and disorganized children (age 6) would have greater difficulty in a collaborative task when compared with mothers and children with organized attachment patterns. We also expected that disorganized attachment (age 6) would predict deficits in academic self-esteem and school performance in middle childhood (age 8). We then explored the extent to which mother–child collaborative difficulties mediated relations between disorganized attachment and academic self-esteem. Finally, we expected that both collaborative difficulties and low self-esteem would mediate the relation between disorganized attachment and school performance (age 8 math and language arts).

METHOD

Subjects

Subjects of this study were 63 French-speaking mother–child dyads (32 girls) who were drawn from a larger longitudinal project investigating the influence of parent–child relationships on developmental adaptation. Subjects were initially recruited through preschools in diverse socioeconomic areas of Montreal. This report includes data collected when the mean age of subjects was (1) 6 years ($SD = 1$), range between 5 and 7 ($n = 63$); and (2) 8.6 years ($SD = 0.6$), range between 7 and 9 ($n = 58$). For the purposes of this study which involved detailed and costly coding of joint problem solving, we selected a subsample of available subjects according to the following criteria: In order to be able to examine differences according to attachment subgroups, we randomly chose 12 subjects from each insecure group (A or D) for data analyses and all available C subjects ($n = 9$). We also randomly selected a comparison group of secure (B) subjects ($n = 30$) approximately equal to the total number of insecures from the wider sample. Of the 63 subjects selected at age 6 for observational coding of collaborative style, 5 did not return for the age 8 assessment (2 refused to participate and 3 could not be located). At age 8, owing to attrition, the sample included 58 subjects: 10 avoidant (A), 11 disorganized (D), 8 ambivalent (C), and 29 secure (B). This subsample did not differ from the original sample on background measures or attrition patterns.

The sample was heterogeneous with respect to income level, with 25% of families earning under $20,000, 40% between $20,000 and $50,000, and 35% earning $50,000 or more. Average maternal education was 13 years ($SD = 3.1$), with 56% of mothers experiencing 13 years or less education and the rest having some college- or university-level education. Seventy-three percent of sample children were firstborn, 24% second-born, and 3% third-born or later. Thirty-two percent of children were living in a mother-headed single-parent family, while the rest were living with both parents.[1] There were no significant differences between attachment groups on any of these measures.

Measures and Procedure

The data reported here were obtained during two laboratory visits, separated by approximately 2 years. Mother and child collaboration and child separation–reunion behavior were observed when children were age 6. Measures pertaining to child's self-esteem and academic achievement were collected when children were 8 years old. Child's Verbal IQ at each age was also assessed.

Mother–Child Collaborative Task (Age 6)

At the beginning of the 2-hour laboratory visit, each mother–child dyad participated in the Preschool Model Grocery Store Task (Moss, Parent, Gosselin, & Dumont, 1993), adapted from a task used by Gauvain and Rogoff (1989) with older children. Our version for younger children was introduced to the dyad as a game, the goal of which was to find a series of items from within the model grocery store using a plastic figurine. Grocery items to purchase were presented as a picture card set provided by the experimenter. The following rules were explained to the dyad: (1) The figurine must enter through the door, collect the grocery items, and exit through the door; (2) the figurine must walk along the aisles and not fly through the air; (3) after an item has been located, the figurine must be stationed in front of it while the item is placed in the basket; (4) the dyad, using the figurine, was instructed to take the shortest route in order to find the items; (5) the picture cards could be placed in any order to help find the shortest route. Mother and child were instructed to work together in solving the problem. Each dyad received a three-item and then a five-item list preceded by a short exploration period (2 minutes). No time limit was imposed on the problem-solving part of the task. However, no dyad exceeded 20 minutes. Mother–child collaboration was videotaped using a camera placed behind a one-way mirror.

Coding of Mother–Child Collaborative Activity

Filmed grocery store interactions were coded from videotape using a coding system that includes both verbal and nonverbal behavior. In coding behaviors, observers identified affective, cognitive, and metacognitive components of dyadic collaborative activity. Computations of the Cohen's kappa coefficient between trained observers ranged from .75 to .83. The following were used to describe mother–child collaboration:

Task-specific strategies were coded separately for both mother and child. They refer to the total of on-task activities including (1) the prior location of items to be purchased, (2) resource management, (3) division of labor, and (4) making contextual links between objects or events (e.g., "The popsicle goes with cold things"), or available material resources (e.g., "There are no bananas in the grocery store").

Maternal structuring is a measure of maternal regulation of child activity and is a composite score referring to the ratio of maternal structuring behaviors (instructing the child on task subgoals and actions to be performed) to child errors (actions that violate task rules).

Ratio of maternal positive–negative affect represents the ratio of maternal positive to negative affect expressed during collaboration. *Positive affect* includes expressions of joy, desire for contact (e.g., hugs), and approval of partner's person, task performance, or suggestions. *Negative affect* includes expressions of avoidance (e.g., mother ignores child's request for physical contact), aggression, annoyance or discontent, and disapproval of partner's person, performance, or suggestions.

Maternal corrective behavioral monitoring refers to total incidence of maternal criticism of child's behavior or task activity.

Child non-task-oriented behavior includes total number of child behaviors involving object manipulation or verbal descriptions that are unrelated to specific task goals or subgoals (e.g., opening shampoo bottle in grocery store or saying, "The shampoo is for washing your hair").

Child metacognitive activity refers to the proportion of behaviors assumed by the child for predefined local and global components of the planning process, which includes (1) rule definition, (2) planning, and (3) monitoring and evaluation. *Rule definition* refers to discussions and demonstrations related to task rules (e.g., "You need to leave by the door of the grocery store"). *Planning behaviors* include identifying the possible routes, ordering of cards, and predicting the consequences of these plans. For example, the child says, "I will first buy the apple because it is the closest." *Monitoring and evaluating behaviors* correspond to statements that contain information related to checking, controlling, and evaluating ongoing or already executed activities as a function of available resources or task constraints. For example, the child puts a card on the bottom of pile and says, "We've found this one, there are two left."

Separation–Reunion Procedure (Age 6)

Subjects were invited to a laboratory visit that included two separations and two reunions. On arrival at the laboratory, mothers and children participated in the grocery store task (approximately 20 minutes), followed by a separation (approximately 45 minutes) during which the child completed problem-solving tasks with an experimenter while the mother completed questionnaires in another room. After completing tasks, the child remained with the experimenter for a free-play session that lasted a minimum of 5 minutes (maximum 15 minutes) until the mother rejoined the child. Mothers received no specific instructions concerning the reunion. After the 5-minute reunion period, the mother and child remained in the room for a 10-minute snacktime. A second 30-minute separation and 5-minute reunion period (structured like the first) then took place. The child's attachment classification was given on the basis of behavior observed during both reunion periods.

Attachment Classification

Child reunion behavior was classified using criteria from both the Cassidy and Marvin (1992) and the Main and Cassidy systems (1988). Validation of the former system included more dyads of ambivalent–resistant children, while the latter offered detailed criteria for coding avoidance in 6-year-olds. Coding decisions in both systems were based on observer evaluations of physical proximity, affective expression, and verbal exchanges, with conversational patterns carrying increasingly greater weight according to child age. Both systems used a similar five-category (secure, avoidant, dependent, disorganized/controlling, insecure–other) coding scheme. When coding 5- to 7-year-olds, coding criteria and coding categories did not differ between the two systems (M. Greenberg, personal communication, March 1997). In support of this, Easterbrooks, Davidson, and Chazan (1993) reported 82% interrater reliability for a sample of 7-year-olds between coders who had been trained in the Cassidy and Marvin system and by an independent expert in the Main and Cassidy system.

The *secure* (B) pattern is categorized by relaxed, mutually enjoyable parent–child interaction. The secure child uses the caregiver as a base that facilitates exploration of the environment. The *insecure/avoidant* (A) pattern is characterized by the child's physical and affective avoidance of parent. The child will typically ignore parental verbal initiatives, and parent–child discussions are often short and "go nowhere," that is, there is little elaboration by one partner of topics initiated by the other. In the *insecure/ dependent* (C) attachment pattern, which corresponds to the anxious–ambivalent infant category, the child alternatively shows resistance and conflictual behavior patterns or excessive immaturity evidenced by passive behaviors. Interactions between parent and child often seem to interfere with child exploration. The child classified *disorganized/controlling* (D) attempts to control parent's behavior, often in a caregiving or punitive manner. The parent–child relationship is characterized by a pattern of role reversal. Children are classified *insecure–other* (IO) if they seem unable to use the caregiver as a secure base for exploration but either do not show the A, C, or D pattern of attachment or display a combination of these. As suggested by Cassidy and Marvin (1992), the D and IO groups were combined for data analyses on the assumption that both display disorganized (disordered or inconsistent strategies) in response to the attachment figure, as distinct from the more coherent, organized strategies of the A, B, and C groups.

Of the 63 tapes, half were coded by Moss and the remainder by a research assistant, with interrater reliability calculated on 35% of sample cases. Both coders were trained by Robert Marvin and achieved reliability with him on a separate sample. In order to support the applicability of the system to the 6- and 7-year-olds in our sample, we calculated reliability separately for this group and for the 5-year-olds. Kappa coefficient for the younger children was .86 and .88 for the older group, indicating excellent agreement for both groups.

Academic Self-Esteem (Age 8)

Child's academic self-esteem was assessed using the Scholastic Competence subscale of the well-known *Self-Perception Profile for Children* (Harter, 1985). This subscale consists of six items formulated in a structured alternative format to reduce problems with social desirability. Each item presents a choice between two legitimate answers such as, "Some kids have trouble figuring out the answers in school *BUT* other kids almost always can figure out the answers," and "Some kids feel like they are just as smart as other kids their age *BUT* other kids aren't so sure and wonder if they are as smart." The child has to decide first the kind of kid he or she is most like and then report if the description is sort of true or really true for him or her. Each item is scored from 1 (low perceived self-image) to 4 (high perceived self-image). The academic self-esteem score was obtained by averaging the scores on the six items.

School Achievement (Age 8)

School marks in language arts and in mathematics were obtained from end-of-year report cards. Since children attended different schools and systems of notation varied, literal and numerical notations were transformed using a 3-point scale level of performance: 1 = below average; 2 = average; and 3 = above average.

Child IQ (Age 6)

The children's intelligence at age 6 was evaluated using the well- validated Peabody Picture Vocabulary Test—Revised (PPVT-R; Dunn & Dunn, 1981).

Child IQ (Age 8)

An abbreviated version of the Wechsler Intelligence Scale for Children—Revised (WISC-R; Wechsler, 1974), consisting of the Block and the Vocabulary subtests, was used to assess the children's intellectual ability at age 8. These two subtests were selected because they are highly correlated with full-scale IQ (Sattler, 1982), and they constitute the best measure of "g" for the Performance and the Verbal scales, respectively (Kaufman, 1975).

RESULTS

In order to examine the research questions stated at the beginning of this chapter, two major sets of analyses were conducted. The first compared disorganized (D) and organized (A, B, and C) attachment classifications on mother–child collaborative patterns (age 6) and child academic self-esteem and achievement (age 8), using two-way analyses of covariance (ANCOVAs) followed by planned comparisons that specified differences between the disorganized–controlling group and each of the other attachment groups. Although preliminary analyses comparing the four attachment groups on all of the background measures, and child verbal IQ at both ages revealed no significant differences, we included child age and IQ as covariates in order to control for the moderately large age range in our sample and possible effect of child IQ on dyadic patterns and child academic competence.

The second set of analyses was designed to examine more closely mediational pathways between attachment, mother–child interaction, self- and academic performance. In other words, we examined to what extent collaborative patterns accounted for any demonstrated relation between disorganized attachment and academic self-esteem. We subsequently tested the extent to which collaboration and self-esteem functioned as explanatory mechanisms in relating disorganized attachment to school performance. Language arts and math marks were chosen to represent school performance, as these subjects are the core components of the elementary school curriculum. The multiple regression procedure outlined by Baron and Kenny (1986) was used to test each of the mediational pathways just described. According to these authors, to demonstrate mediation, one must establish strong relations between (1) the predictor (e.g., attachment classifications) and the mediating variable (e.g., collaboration and/or self-esteem), (2) the predictor and the dependent variable (e.g., self-esteem or school marks), and (3) the mediator and the dependent variable.

Mother–Child Collaboration as a Function of Attachment

In order to reduce the mother–child collaborative data to distinct patterns of goal-corrected partnership, we conducted a principal components factor analysis with Varimax rotation. Three factors (Table 6.1) with eigenvalues exceeding 1 emerged from this analysis. Factor 1 (30% of variance; eigenvalue 2.1) represents goal-directed cognitive participation with very high loadings of both mother and child strategy use. Factor 2 (26% of variance; eigenvalue 1.8) represents a dissynchronous interactive pattern in which child and mother show a lack of partnership with respect to task performance. This factor includes high loadings of child off-task behavior, maternal correction without restructuring, and negative affect. Factor 3 (16% of variance; eigenvalue 1.1) represents child metacognitive activity with maternal support, with significant loadings of both maternal positive affect and child metacognitive activity. Factor scores associated with each of these distinct patterns of collaboration were used in subsequent ANCOVAs. Results are presented in Table 6.2.

Results of the ANCOVA performed on Factor 1 scores of cognitive participation showed no significant differences between the disorganized group and others. However, very clear differences were evident on factors representing respectively dissynchronous interaction (Factor 2) and child metacognitive activity (Factor 3). Results of analyses of these factor scores indicated that dyads including disorganized children had significantly

TABLE 6.1. Rotated Factor Matrix

Measure	Factor 1	Factor 2	Factor 3
Maternal task-specific strategies	.92	.11	−.11
Child task-specific strategies	.86	−.02	.05
Maternal structuring	.28	−.73	−.06
Maternal corrective behavioral monitoring	.45	.70	−.18
Ratio of maternal positive/negative affect	−.06	−.62	.43
Child non-task-oriented behavior	.45	.61	.13
Child planning	−.01	−.03	.94

TABLE 6.2. Mother–Child Collaboration and Child Academic Measures as a Function of Child Attachment Classification: Significant Between-Group Differences and Adjusted Means

Measures	Disorganized vs. combined[a]	Disorganized vs. single groups	Attachment classification[b]			
			Avoidant	Secure	Ambivalent	Controlling
Mother–child collaboration (age 6)						
Factor 1: Cognitive participation	< 1		0.37 (1.65)	−0.18 (0.68)	0.35 (1.22)	−0.21 (0.46)
Factor 2: Dissynchronous interaction	5.99**	D > A**B*C*	−0.46 (1.11)	−0.01 (0.89)	−0.22 (0.83)	0.65 (1.10)
Factor 3: Child metacognitive activity	7.51**	D < B***	−0.16 (0.83)	0.40 (1.06)	−0.20 (0.89)	−0.69 (0.70)
Academic measures (age 8)						
Academic self-esteem	5.62**	D < B*C**	3.07 (0.72)	3.17 (0.56)	3.56 (0.34)	2.71 (0.70)
Language arts scores	< 1		2.01 (0.70)	2.13 (0.72)	2.22 (0.92)	2.02 (0.79)
Mathematics scores	4.71*	D < B*C*	2.16 (0.64)	2.26 (0.80)	2.28 (0.52)	1.78 (0.69)

[a]F-ratio (ANCOVA).
[b]Adjusted means. Standard deviations in parentheses.
*$p < .05$; **$p < .01$; ***$p < .001$.

173

higher scores than other groups combined on dissynchronous interaction and lower scores with respect to child metacognitive activity.

Self-Esteem and Achievement as a Function of Disorganized Attachment

Similar analyses were conducted to examine the effect of disorganized attachment on age 8 self- and academic measures. The results are presented in Table 6.2. Significant attachment effects were evident for academic self-perception and math school performance scores. As predicted, the disorganized group had significantly lower scores than others on both these variables, although no differences were found for language arts. These results suggest that disorganized children experience considerable difficulty at school. Their mean scores in academic self-esteem (Table 6.2) place them in the lowest quartile for the sample. In addition, the D group is the only attachment group with a mean score indicating below-average school performance in math.

Mediational Effects of Attachment and Mother–Child Collaboration in Predicting Child Academic Competence

As reported earlier, results indicated that attachment classification was related both to specific mother–child collaborative patterns (age 6) and to later measures of academic competence (age 8), thus fulfilling two essential preconditions for establishing a mediational pathway linking attachment, communicative patterns, and academic competence (Baron & Kenny, 1986). We further tested mediational models related to these findings by conducting a two-step test of mediation for each of the school adaptation measures, using hierarchical regressions with child age and IQ (entered first and second, respectively, in all equations) as control variables. In the first step, we evaluated the strength of association between attachment and each measure of academic competence. In the second step, we examined whether this association was attenuated when controlling for shared variance with mother–child communicative patterns. Results of these analyses are summarized in Table 6.3.

Disorganized Attachment and Academic Self-Esteem

In the first model, we examined whether the differences in academic self-esteem between disorganized children and other attachment groups were mediated by particular mother–child collaborative patterns. In this and subsequent mediational analyses, the disorganized group was compared to other attachment groups combined. This is justified by our theoretical interest in comparing disorganized to "organized" attachment, and the fact that ANCOVAs (Table 6.2) had empirically confirmed differences in disorganized versus organized comparisons, even though post hoc analyses showed stronger differences between the D group and certain attachment groups (especially B and C). As reported earlier, dyads including a disorganized child differed from other attachment groups on two factors:

TABLE 6.3. Summary of Regressions Examining the Relation of Attachment and Mother–Child Collaborative Patterns to Child Academic Measures

	R^2 ch.	F ch.	Beta
Dependent variable: Academic self-esteem			
Equation 1			
1. Child age	.00	< 1	−.05
2. Child IQ	.07	4.4*	.29*
3. Attachment (D vs. Non-D)	.10	6.3**	−.34**
Equation 2			
1. Child age	.00	< 1	−.05
2. Child IQ	.07	4.4*	.29*
3. Dissynchronous interaction			−.07
Child metacognitive participation	.05	1.6	.25
4. Attachment (D vs. Non-D)	.06	3.9*	−.31
Dependant variable: Mathematics performance			
Equation 3			
1. Child age	.04	2.1	−.19
2. Child IQ	.10	6.3*	.34*
3. Attachment (D vs. non-D)	.07	4.8*	−.29*
Equation 4			
1. Child age	.04	2.1	−.19
2. Child IQ	.10	6.3*	.34*
3. Dissynchronous interaction			−.23[+]
Child metacognitive participation	.12	4.3*	.31*
4. Attachment (D vs. Non-D)	.01	< 1	−.14
Equation 5			
1. Child age	.04	2.1	−.19
2. Child IQ	.10	6.3*	.34*
3. Academic self-esteem	.15	11.3**	.40**
4. Attachment (D vs. Non-D)	.02	1.7	−.17
Equation 6			
1. Child age	.04	2.1	−.19
2. Child IQ	.10	6.3*	.34*
3. Dissynchronous interaction		−.20[+]	
Child metacognitive participation		.23[+]	
Academic self-esteem	.22	6.0*	.34**
4. Attachment (D vs. Non-D)	.00	< 1	−.04

[+]p < .10; *p < .05; **p < .01; ***p < .001.

dissynchrony and child metacognitive participation. We tested the mediational role of each of these dimensions in predicting academic self-esteem using the two-step test described earlier (corresponding to Equations 1 and 2 in Table 6.3). In Equation 1, after having controlled for both child age and IQ, attachment (disorganized vs. organized) accounted for 10% of the variance in child academic self-esteem. In Equation 2, the collaborative variables, entered as a block, were not found to be significantly related to child academic self-esteem, accounting for only 5% of the variance. Attachment (D vs. non-D), which was entered last in the equation, still significantly predicted 6% of the variance. These results indicate that these collaborative patterns did not mediate the association between attachment (D vs. non-D) and child academic self-esteem.[2]

Disorganized Attachment and Math Performance

We further tested whether the association between attachment (disorganized vs. organized) and math performance was mediated by components of mother–child collaboration (Factors 2 and 3) and/or by child self-esteem. After having controlled for child age and IQ, attachment significantly predicted 7% of the variance in mathematics performance (Equation 3 in Table 6.3). In Equation 4, when factor scores (dissynchronous mother–child interaction and child metacognitive participation) were entered together as a block before attachment, they accounted for 12% of the variance in math scores, with metacognitive participation a significant predictor ($p < .05$) and dissynchronous interaction marginally significant ($p < .10$). As for attachment, it no longer accounted for a significant portion of the variance in academic performance. These results indicate that age-6 child metacognitive participation and (to a lesser extent) degree of dyadic synchrony mediate the attachment effect on age-8 math achievement.

In the last series of analyses, we explored the mediational role of child self-esteem in influencing performance (Equations 5 and 6 in Table 6.3). When child self-esteem was entered before attachment, it explained 15% of the variance in math scores, with attachment no longer a significant predictor, indicating that self-esteem was a mediator between attachment and math performance. To better understand the respective contributions of child self-esteem and collaboration to the association between attachment and math performance, we entered them together as a block before attachment. Together, dissynchronous interaction, child metacognitive participation, and child self-esteem predicted 22% of the variance in math scores, with child sense of self-esteem the strongest predictor. Attachment, when entered last, no longer accounted for any variance. These results suggest that the mediational effects of mother–child collaborative patterns and child self-esteem on math scores are largely independent of one another, since the predictive power was increased when they were combined together (accounting for 22% of variance in math, whereas child self-esteem by itself accounted for 15%, and collaborative patterns accounted for 12%).

DISCUSSION

In this study, we examined the influence of the disorganized/controlling attachment pattern on mother–child collaboration and on self and performance components relevant to school performance. We further explored relations between these dimensions according to hypotheses suggested by attachment theory. Our research strategy involved comparing patterns of mother–child collaboration as a function of attachment classification and then examining the predictive role of these patterns in determining self- and achievement outcomes.

As hypothesized, disorganized children and their mothers were least likely of all attachment groups to display a collaborative pattern facilitative of joint problem solving. The predominantly negative emotional climate and high levels of maternal criticism of child off-task behavior suggest a lack of joint focus in accomplishing the task. These results show continuity with studies indicating that mothers of D infants and preschoolers were lowest on involvement, teaching skill, positive parent–infant mutuality, and conversational skill (Lyons-Ruth et al., 1987; Main et al., 1985; Solomon & George, Chapter 9, this volume; Stevenson-Hinde & Shouldice, 1995). In the face of such a dissynchronous pattern, it is not surprising that disorganized children also had the lowest levels of metacognitive activity of all attachment groups. Since the development of metacognitive strategies is related to maternal monitoring and appropriate scaffolding of child efforts at task solution (Diaz, Neal, & Amaya-Williams, 1990; Moss & Strayer, 1990), the low level of maternal structuring and high level of child off-task behavior may impede the development of metacognitive skills. Children's demonstrations of their ability to apply strategies toward task solution are an important clue to the adult about how quickly to progress within the zone of proximal development.

These results, in conjunction with our previous findings concerning difficulties in socioaffective components of interaction (Moss et al., 1998, in press), support the idea that disrupted levels of cognitive as well as social engagement may characterize the interactive environment of disorganized children and their caregivers. In our previous studies, we demonstrated that the role reversal and lack of attunement that is characteristic of these dyads contribute to dysfunctional relationship problems in intra- and extrafamilial settings. Similarly, we discussed how negative and tense levels of emotional expression and lack of maternal affirmation in the interactive pattern of mothers and disorganized children play a role in the development of behavior problems of both an externalizing and internalizing nature. However, results of this study also suggest that this disrupted communication style further accentuates the level of developmental risk by failing to support the child's academic achievement. In failing to provide an adequate cognitive or emotional framework for structuring joint activity, this interactive pattern may interfere with the development of auxiliary ego functions needed for both the development of self-regulatory and socioempathic skills (Greenberg, Kusche, & Speltz, 1991).

Our second set of hypotheses concerned the influence of attachment on academic self-esteem. Since our subjects were followed until 8 years of age, we were able to reliably measure child academic self-esteem using self-report measures. The primary differences in child self-ratings on the Harter Scale of Academic Self-Competence were related to disorganized children's much poorer views of self when compared with other attachment groups. In fact, their scores fell within the lowest quartile of sample scores. This finding supports those of Cassidy (1988), indicating that disorganized 6-year-olds made the most overt negative statements about self-worth in a puppet interview self-esteem task, and those of Jacobsen et al. (1994), who reported a similar negative tendency for disorganized 7-year-olds in an interview task. However, analyses of the role of parent–child information-exchange patterns as mediators of this association did not reveal any significant pathways. More precise measures of the affective quality of parent–child interactions, such as degree of maternal hostility or role reversal, may have yielded significant results. As suggested by Main and Solomon (1990) and Solomon and George (1996), prolonged child exposure to a disorganized or frightening parent who does not assist the child in dealing with negative feelings may bring the child to view the self as unable to control untoward events. It is also possible that basic patterns of self-esteem represented in internal working models may already be formed by the preschool and school-age period, deriving from infant–mother interactive patterns.

With reference to academic performance, results showed significant differences between disorganized children and others in math scores but not in language arts. Only two other studies have examined links between attachment and cognitive or school performance. In the first (Jacobsen et al., 1994), disorganized children did particularly poorly on deductive reasoning tasks, while, in the second, the same children had an overall lower grade point average when compared with other attachment groups (Jacobsen & Hofmann, 1997). A possible explanation for the closer link between disorganization and math rather than language performance is the greater involvement of deductive and abstract reasoning processes in the former. These cognitive processes may be especially vulnerable to interference from anxiety and poor self-concept. Disorganized children's anxieties related to others' possible responses to them and their own competence or self-worth may inhibit the activation of high-level self-regulated thought processes (Main, 1991). These deficient evaluations of self and others' view of the self may influence math achievement by having an impact on the goals children may set themselves, abnormal cognitive oscillations, or difficulties in maintaining stable levels of reasoning, and expectations for support from parents, peers, or teachers (Inhelder, 1968; Jacobsen et al., 1994; Saxe, Guberman, & Gearhart, 1987). In support of this explanation are studies that suggest children who perceive themselves as having poor or uncertain ability are particularly susceptible to poor performance in math tasks as compared to other school subjects (Ginsburg & Asmussen, 1988; Reyes, 1984). Their focus on anxiety about possible failure may lead them to avoid math tasks or give up quickly when experiencing difficulty instead of increasing concentration. Deductive reasoning processes are less closely tied with language arts performance. Achievement may be more dependent on language exposure in the home setting, especially in our sample, which, like the current Montreal population, includes a large percentage of children educated in French schools, whose parents' mother tongue is not French.

A second possible explanation for this result is suggested by studies that demonstrate the important role of parent–child collaboration in mathematical learning. According to several studies (Pratt, Green, MacVicar, & Bountrogianni, 1992; Saxe et al., 1987), the development of mathematical abilities is dependent both on the numerical goals children initiate and adult support and challenging of children's efforts. In support of this hypothesis and previous findings (Jacobsen et al., 1994), our analyses revealed that the more negative self-evaluations of children with a disorganized classification mediated the relation between attachment and math marks. In fact, by school age, self-esteem and math performance probably constitute a reciprocal feedback loop—poorer performance scores of disorganized school-age children in math may also have an impact on their lower self-esteem. Our results further indicated that the quality of mother–child collaboration significantly added to prediction of math performance scores over and above the influence of self-concept. In particular, the low level of disorganized children's involvement in metacognitive operations and, to a somewhat lesser extent, their dissynchronous mother–child interactive patterns, predicted math difficulties.

Results of this study further demonstrate the predictive validity of separation–reunion measures of attachment for preschool and early school-age children. Classifications made using these measures have already been associated with differences in mother–child interaction patterns, maternal psychosocial self-reports, child mental representations, self-concept, and behavior problems (Cassidy, 1988; Easterbrooks et al., 1993; Greenberg et al., 1991; Moss et al., 1996; Solomon et al., 1995; see Solomon & George, 1999, for review; Stevenson-Hinde & Shouldice, 1995). This is the first study to show that postinfancy separation–reunion measures of attachment also predict school performance.

An important limitation of our study is the lack of attachment measures either preceding or following the 5–7 year age period, thus preventing confirmation of direct attachment–outcome associations at these ages. Owing to the fact that studies of stability of attachment between 1 and 6 years of age currently provide evidence for both stability (Main & Cassidy, 1988; Wartner, Grossman, Fremmer-Bombik, & Suess, 1994) and change (Goldberg, Washington, Myhal, & Janus, in submission), no assumptions can be made concerning pathways from early attachment to the school-age period. Moreover, since, in this study, attachment and collaboration were assessed concurrently at age 6, the "mediational" relation between these variables cannot be interpreted in a developmental sense. Delineating the developmental pathways between early attachment, collaboration, and later school performance is an important question for future studies. Although early maternal sensitivity may be a catalyst in the development of both attachment and collaborative abilities, there are likely age-specific dependencies in the development of socioaffective and cognitive processes that need to be understood in order to test specific-linkage hypotheses relevant to predicting overall adaptation.

CONCLUSION

This study is one of the few that has examined interactive patterns of mothers and disorganized children at school age and provides new information on cognitive and metacognitive components of these interactive patterns. Moreover, it is one of only a few previous studies that have established links between disorganization, self-processes, and school outcomes. The unique contribution of this study lies in its theoretical and empirical elaboration of the pathway between disorganized attachment and later developmental risk. This pathway appears to be mediated by both caregiving and self-patterns that may seriously compromise both affective and cognitive development.

On a theoretical level, we have advanced the idea that full understanding of the degree and type of risk associated with the D classification involves enlarging the traditional notion of maternal sensitivity to include scaffolding functions that are critical to the development of child self-regulatory or metacognitive skills. These skills play a key role in contributing to child success at school in both behavioral and academic domains. Although, in this study, we controlled for certain obvious determinants of academic performance—child IQ, maternal scolarity, family socioeconomic—it is important to consider other possible pathways linking disorganization to academic problems. For example, given the importance of supportive peer relationships in determining school success (Epstein, 1992), it is also possible that problems in peer social competence contribute to disorganized children's academic difficulties. Also, the parentified role of the disorganized child in the family system (Main & Cassidy, 1988; Marvin & Stewart, 1990; Moss et al., 1998) may contribute to school problems. For example, having to provide physical and emotional care for a "helpless" parent or other family members may leave little time and energy for concentrating on school.

Studies that further explore these processes and the school-age pathways discussed in this chapter are critical to linking the abundant literature on infancy with the accumulating evidence emphasizing the important metacognitive and affective differences associated with different attachment classifications at adulthood.

ACKNOWLEDGMENT

This research was supported by grants received from the Social Sciences and Humanities Research Council of Canada and the Conseil Québecois de la Recherche Sociale (CQRS). We thank Elise Chartrand, Catherine Gosselin, Denise Rousseau, Isabelle Guerra, and Roxanne Bergeron for their assistance in the research project.

NOTES

1. These statistics refer to the age-6 assessment, concomitant with the attachment measure.

2. The slight attenuation of the attachment effect on child academic self-esteem (from 10% to 6% of explained variance) can safely be attributed to the reduced power in Equation 2 due to the correlation between attachment and each of the factor scores resulting in multicolinearity, since examination of the beta weights associated with attachment in Equation 1 and Equation 2 indicated that they remained similar (respectively, beta = −.34, beta = −.31).

REFERENCES

Aber, J. L., & Allen, J. P. (1987). The effects of maltreatment on young children's socioemotional development: An attachment theory perspective. *Developmental Psychology, 23*, 406–414.

Achermann, J., Dinneen, E., & Stevenson-Hinde, J. (1991). Clearing up at 2. 5 years. *British Journal of Developmental Psychology, 9*, 365–376.

Ainsworth, M. D., Bell, S., & Stayton, D. J. (1971). Individual differences in Strange-Situation behavior of one-year-olds. In H. R. Schaffer (Ed.), *The origin of human social relations* (pp. 17–57). New York: Academic Press.

Baron, R. M., & Kenny, D. A. (1986). The moderator–mediator variable distinction in social psychological research: Conceptual, strategic, and statistical considerations. *Journal of Personality and Social Psychology, 51,* 1173–1182.

Belsky, J., Garduque, L., & Hrincir, E. (1984). Assessing performance, competence and executive capacity in infant play: Relations to home environment and security of attachment. *Developmental Psychology, 20,* 406–417.

Belsky, J., Rovine, M. J. & Taylor, D. G. (1984). The Pennsylvania Infant and Family Development Project: III. The origins of individual differences in infant–mother attachment: Maternal and infant contributions. *Child Development, 55,* 718–728.

Bowlby, J. (1969). *Attachment and loss: Vol. 1. Attachment.* New York: Basic Books.

Bowlby, J. (1973). *Attachment and loss: Vol. 2. Separation.* New York: Basic Books.

Bretherton, I. (1985). Attachment theory: Retrospect and prospect. In I. Bretherton & E. Waters (Eds.), Growing points of attachment theory and research. *Monographs of the Society for Research in Child Development, 50*(1–2, Serial No. 209), 3–35.

Cassidy, J. (1988). Child–mother attachment and the self in six-year-olds. *Child Development, 59,* 121–135.

Cassidy, J., & Berlin, L. (1994). The insecure/ambivalent pattern of attachment: Theory and research. *Child Development, 65,* 971–991.

Cassidy, J. & Marvin, R. S. (with the McArthur Working Group on Attachment). (1992). *Attachment organization in 2½ to 4½ year olds. Coding manual.* Unpublished coding manual, University of Virginia, Charlottesville.

Diaz, R. M., Neal, C. J., & Amaya-Williams, M. (1990). The social origins of self-regulation. In L. Moll (Ed.), *Vygotsky and education: Instructional implications and applications of socio-historical psychology* (pp. 127–154). New York: Cambridge University Press.

Dunn, L. M., & Dunn, L. M. (1981). *Peabody Picture Vocabulary Test–Revised: Manual for Forms L and M.* Circle Pines, MN: American Guidance Service.

Easterbrooks, M. A., Davidson, C. E., & Chazan, R. (1993). Psychosocial risk, attachment, and behavior problems among school-aged children. *Development and Psychopathology, 5,* 389–402.

Epstein, J. L. (1992). School and family partnerships. In M. Alkin (Ed.), *Encyclopedia of educational research* (6th ed., pp. 1139–1151). New York: Macmillan.

Flavell, J. (1979). Metacognition and cognitive monitoring: A new area of cognitive-developmental inquiry. *American Psychologist, 34,* 906–911.

Frankel, K. & Bates, J. (1990). Mother–toddler problem solving: Antecedents in attachment, home behavior and temperament. *Child Development, 61,* 810–819.

Gauvain, M., & Rogoff, B. (1989). Collaborative problem solving and children's planning skills. *Developmental Psychology, 25,* 139–151.

George, C., & Solomon, J. (in press). The development of caregiving: A comparison of attachment and psychoanalytic approaches to mothering. In D. Diamond, S. Blatt, & D. Silver (Eds.), Psychoanalytic Theory and Attachment Research: I. Theoretical Considerations. *Psychoanalytic Inquiry, 19* [Special issue].

Ginsburg, H. P., & Asmussen, K. A. (1988). Hot mathematics. In G. Saxe & M. Gearhart (Eds.), Children's mathematics. *New Directions for Child Development, 41*, 89–112.

Goldberg, S., Washington, J., Myhal, N., & Janus, M. (in submission). Stability and change in attachment from infancy to preschool.

Greenberg, M. T., Kusche, C. A., & Speltz, M. (1991). Emotional regulation, self-control, and psychopathology: The role of relationships in early childhood. In D. Cicchetti & S. Toth (Eds.), *The Rochester Symposium on Developmental Psychopathology: Vol. 2. Internalizing and externalizing expressions of dysfunction* (pp. 21–56). Hillsdale, NJ: Erlbaum.

Grolnick, W. S., & Ryan, R. (1989). Parent styles associated with children's self-regulation and competence in school. *Journal of Educational Psychology, 81*, 143–154.

Harmon, R., Suwalsky, J., & Klein, R. (1979). Infant's preferential response for mother versus unfamiliar adult. *Journal of the American Academy of Child Psychiatry, 18*, 437–449.

Harter, S. (1985). *Manual for the Self-Perception Profile for Children: Revision of the PCSC (1979)*. Unpublished manuscript, University of Denver, Denver, CO.

Inhelder, B. (1968). *The early growth of logic in the child*. New York: Basic Books.

Inhelder, B., Sinclair, H., & Bovet, M. (1974). *Learning and the development of cognition*. Cambridge, MA: Harvard University Press.

Jacobsen, T., Edelstein, W., & Hofmann, V. (1994). A longitudinal study of the relation between representations of attachment in childhood and cognitive functioning in childhood and adolescence. *Developmental Psychology, 30*, 112–124.

Jacobsen, T., & Hofmann, V. (1997). Children's attachment representations: Longitudinal relations to school behavior and academic competency in middle childhood and adolescence. *Developmental Psychology, 33*, 703–710.

Kaufman, A. S. (1975). Factor analysis of the WISC-R at 11 age levels between 6½ and 16½ years. *Journal of Consulting and Clinical Psychology, 43*, 135–147.

Lewis, M., & Feiring, C. (1989). Infant, mother, and mother–infant interaction behavior and subsequent attachment. *Child Development, 60*, 831–837.

Loper, A. B., & Murphy, D. M. (1985). Cognitive self-regulatory training for underachieving children. In D. Forrest-Pressley, G. McKinnon, & T. Waller (Eds.), *Metacognition, cognition and human performance: Vol. 2. Instructional practices* (pp. 223–266). Orlando, FL: Academic Press.

Lyons-Ruth, K., Alpern, L., & Repacholi, L. (1993). Disorganized infant attachment classification and maternal psychosocial problems as predictors of hostile–aggressive behavior in the preschool classroom. *Child Development, 64*, 572–585.

Lyons-Ruth, K., Connell, D. B., Zoll, D., & Stahl, J. (1987). Infants at social risk: Relations among infant maltreatment, maternal behavior, and infant attachment behavior. *Developmental Psychology, 23*, 223–232.

Lyons-Ruth, K., Easterbrooks, M. A., & Cibelli, C. D. (1997). Infant attachment strategies, infant mental lag, and maternal depressive symptoms: Predictors of internalizing and externalizing problems at age 7. *Developmental Psychology, 33*, 681–692.

Lyons-Ruth, K., Repacholi, B., McLeod, S., & Silva, E. (1991). Disorganized attachment behavior in infancy: Short-term stability, maternal and infant correlates, and risk-related subtypes. *Development and Psychopathology, 3,* 377–396.

Main, M. (1991). Metacognitive knowledge, metacognitive monitoring and singular (coherent) vs. multiple (incoherent) models of attachment: Findings and directions for future research. In C. Parkes, J. Stevenson-Hinde, & P. Marris (Eds.), *Attachment across the life cycle* (pp. 127–157). London: Routledge.

Main, M. (1995). Recent studies in attachment: Overview, with selected implications for clinical work. In S. Goldberg, R. Muir, & J. Kerr (Eds.), *Attachment theory: social, developmental, and clinical perspectives* (pp. 407–474). Hillsdale, NJ: Analytic Press.

Main, M., & Cassidy, J. (1988). Categories of response to reunion with the parent at age six: Predictable from infant attachment classifications and stable over a 1-month period. *Developmental Psychology, 24,* 415–526.

Main, M., & Hesse, E. (1990). Parents' unresolved traumatic experiences are related to infant disorganized attachment status: Is frightened and/or frightening parental behavior the linking mechanism? In M. T. Greenberg, D. Cichetti, & M. Cummings (Eds.), *Attachment in the preschool years* (pp. 161–182). Chicago: University of Chicago Press.

Main, M., Kaplan, N., & Cassidy, J. (1985). Security of attachment in infancy, childhood, and adulthood: A move to the level of representation. In I. Bretherton & E. Waters (Eds.), Growing points in attachment theory and research. *Monographs of the Society for Research in Child Development, 50*(1–2, Serial No. 209), 66–104.

Main, M., & Solomon, J. (1990). Procedure for identifying infants as disorganized/disoriented during the Ainsworth Strange Situation. In M. Greenberg, D. Cicchetti & M. Cummings (Eds.), *Attachment in the preschool years: Theory, research, and intervention* (pp. 121–160). Chicago: University of Chicago Press.

Marvin, R. (1977). An ethological–cognitive model for the attenuation of mother–child attachment behavior. In T. M. Alloway, L. Krames, & P. Piner (Eds.), *Advances in the study of communication and affect: Vol. 3. The development of social attachments* (pp. 25–60). New York: Plenum.

Marvin, R. S., & Stewart, R. B. (1990). A family systems framework for the study of attachment. In M. T. Greenberg, D. Cichetti, & M. Cummings (Eds.), *Attachment in the preschool years* (pp. 161–182). Chicago: University of Chicago Press.

Matas, L., Arend, R. A., & Sroufe, L. A. (1978). Continuity of adaptation in the second year: The relationship between quality of attachment and later competence. *Child Development, 49,* 547–556.

Moss, E. (1992). The socioaffective context of joint cognitive activity. In L. T. Winegar & J. Valsiner (Eds.), *Children's development within social context: Vol. 2. Research and methodology* (pp. 117–154). Hillsdale, NJ: Erlbaum.

Moss, E., Gosselin, C., Parent, S., Rousseau, D., & Dumont, M. (1997). Attachment and joint problem-solving experiences during the preschool period. *Social Development, 6,* 1–17.

Moss, E., Humber, N., & Roberge, L. (in press). Attachment at preschool and school-age and its relation to patterns of caregiver–child interaction. In G. M.

Tarabulsy, S. Larose, D. R. Pederson, & G. Moran (Eds.), *Attachment and development I: Infancy and the pre-school years.* Montréal: Les Presses de l'Université du Québec.

Moss, E., Parent, S., Gosselin, C., & Dumont, M. (1993). Attachment and the development of metacognitive and collaborative strategies. *International Journal of Educational Research, 19,* 555–571.

Moss, E., Parent, S., Gosselin, C., Rousseau, D., & St-Laurent, D. (1996). Attachment and teacher-reported behavior problems during the preschool and early school-age period. *Development and Psychopathology, 8,* 514–525.

Moss, E., Rousseau, D., Parent, S., St-Laurent, D., & Saintonge, J. (1998). Correlates of attachment at school-age: Maternal-reported stress, mother–child interaction and behavior problems. *Child Development, 69,* 1390–1405.

Moss, E., & Strayer, F. F. (1990). Interactive problem-solving of gifted and non gifted preschoolers with their mothers. *International Journal of Behavioral Development, 13,* 177–197.

Pederson, D., & Moran, G. (1996). Expressions of the attachment relationship outside of the Strange Situation. *Child Development, 67,* 915–927.

Pratt, M. W., Green, D., MacVicar, J., & Bountrogianni, M. (1992). The mathematical parent: Parental scaffolding, parental style, and learning outcomes in long-division mathematics homework. *Journal of Applied Developmental Psychology, 13,* 17–34.

Reyes, L. H. (1984). Affective variables and mathematics education. *Elementary School Journal, 84,* 558–580.

Sattler, J. M. (1982). *Assessment of children's intelligence.* Toronto: Allyn & Bacon.

Saxe, G. B., Guberman, S. R., & Gearhart, M. (1987). Social processes in early number development. *Monographs of the Society for Research in Child Development, 52*(2, Serial No. 216).

Solomon, J., & George, C. (1996). Defining the caregiving system: Toward a theory of caregiving. *Infant Mental Health Journal, 17,* 183–197.

Solomon, J., & George, C. (1999). The measurement of attachment security in infancy and childhood. In J. Cassidy & P. R. Shaver (Eds.), *Handbook of attachment: Theory, research, and clinical applications* (pp. 287–316). New York: Guilford Press.

Solomon, J., George, C., & De Jong, A. (1995). Children classified as controlling at age six: Evidence of disorganized representational strategies and aggression at home and at school. *Development and Psychopathology, 7*(3), 447–464.

Speltz, M. L., Greenberg, M. T., & DeKlyen, M. (1990). Attachment in preschoolers with disruptive behavior: A comparison of clinic-referred and nonproblem children. *Development and Psychopathology, 2,* 31–46.

Sroufe, L. A., & Fleeson, J. (1986). Attachment and the construction of relationships. In W. Hartup & Z. Rubin (Eds.), *Relationships and development* (pp. 51–71). New York: Cambridge University Press.

Stevenson-Hinde, J., & Shouldice, A. (1995). Maternal interactions and self-reports related to attachment classifications at 4. 5 years. *Child Development, 66,* 583–596.

Urban, J., Carlson, E., Egeland, B., & Sroufe, L. A. (1991). Patterns of individual adaptation across childhood. *Development and Psychopathology, 3,* 445–460.

Verschueren, K., Marcoen, A., & Schoefs, V. (1996). The internal working model of the self, attachment, and competence in five-year-olds. *Child Development*, 67, 2493–2511.

Wartner, U. G., Grossman, K., Fremmer-Bombik, E., & Suess, G. (1994). Attachment patterns at age six in South Germany: Predictability from infancy and implications for preschool behavior. *Child Development*, 65, 1014–1027.

Vygotsky, L. S. (1978). *Mind in society*. Cambridge, MA: Harvard University Press.

Wechsler, D. (1974). *Manual for the Wechsler Intelligence Scale for Children–revised*. New York: Psychological Corporation.

PART 3

Attachment Disorganization in Atypical Populations

Methdological and Definitional Issues

Indices of Attachment Disorganization among Toddlers with Neurological and Non-Neurological Problems

DOUGLAS BARNETT
KELLI HILL HUNT
CHRISTINE M. BUTLER
JOHN W. McCASKILL IV
MELISSA KAPLAN-ESTRIN
SANDRA PIPP-SIEGEL

Attachment theory has emerged as a dominant paradigm for understanding personality development (Ainsworth & Bowlby, 1991). According to attachment theory, children are predisposed to form an affectionate bond with a small number of caregivers whom they are motivated to seek as a source of joy and comfort when conditions are optimal and as a haven of safety during times of stress. Assessments of individual differences in the quality of these early relationships are based on the security and organization of behaviors children demonstrate toward their attachment figure. Infants and young children with anxious attachments demonstrate moderate to high levels of avoidance (Group A), ambivalence (Group C), or disorganization (Group D) toward their caregiver when distressed, such as following a brief separation (Ainsworth, Blehar, Waters, & Wall, 1978; Main & Solomon, 1990). Children with secure (Group B) attachments tend not to be conflicted in their approaches to their caregiver for comfort or interaction. Research suggests that individual differences in children's attachment security reflect the history of their attachment figures' behavior toward them, and with few exceptions, have not been shown to be a function of child characteristics such as temperament (De Wolff & van IJzendoorn, 1997; Goldsmith & Alansky, 1987). For instance, children with secure attachments tend to have caregivers who have responded sensitively and contingently to their signals.

Attachment theory emerged in opposition to perspectives that placed greater emphasis on child constitutional factors than social experiences in the genesis of psychopathology and dysregulation (Bowlby, 1988). Consequently, it has been important for the validation of attachment patterns to show that they are predicted from parenting factors and are not directly related to constitutional factors. Although most research on child factors in attachment has focused on child temperament, it is only one of many possible dimensions.

Congenital medical conditions and disabilities are child factors that have been receiving increased attention by attachment researchers. van IJzendoorn, Goldberg, Kroonenberg, and Frenkel (1992) compiled the distribution of attachment patterns from studies of parent or child problems. Their review included 13 samples from eight studies of children with chronic medical conditions or disabilities such as autism, Down syndrome, cystic fibrosis, and congenital heart disease. Although not significant statistically, the rate of security for samples of children with congenital problems (i.e., 50%) was lower than the nonproblem comparison samples (i.e., 65%). Table 7.1 lists attachment studies that have examined strange situations of children with organically based problems that have been reported subsequent to the van IJzendoorn et al. meta-analysis. Apparent from Table 7.1 is that, with the exception of children with craniofacial malformations, the percentage of secure attachments among children with congenital problems consistently averages less than 50%, a rate notably lower than the approximately 65% secure reported for low-risk samples.

Moreover, the rates of nontraditional attachments among children with handicaps involving collateral neurological problems (e.g., Down syndrome) are approximately two or more times those found among normative samples, which have about 15% on average in the disorganized group (van IJzendoorn et al., 1992). For instance, Capps, Sigman, and Mundy (1994) reported that 100% of their sample of children with autism demonstrated behavior consistent with a disorganized classification. However, because many of the observed indices of disorganization were viewed to be symptoms of autism rather than attachment behavior per se, only 20% (3 children) were considered disorganized in the final analyses. In a study of children with Down syndrome, Vaughn et al. (1994) reported 42% as disorganized or unclassifiable (Group U).

TABLE 7.1. Studies of Children with Congenital Medical Conditions Completed after 1992

Study	Condition	Secure	Group A	Group C	Group D	Group U	CA	DQ
Atkinson et al. (in press)								
Time 1	Down syndrome	40% (21)	8% (4)	4% (2)	2% (1)	47% (25)	26 mo.	50
Time 2	Down syndrome	48% (19)	8% (3)	0% (0)	13% (5)	33% (13)	42 mo.	n.r.
Capps et al. (1994)	Autism	40% (6)	7% (1)	13% (2)	20% (3)	20% (3)	24 mo.	46
Goldberg, Gotowiec, & Simmons (1995)	Congenital heart disease	43% (23)	22% (12)	9% (5)	26% (14)	n.r.	12 mo.	n.r.
	Cystic fibrosis	43% (17)	20% (8)	5% (2)	33% (13)	n.r.	12 mo.	n.r.
Ganiban, Barnett, & Ciccetti (in press)								
Time 1	Down syndrome	53% (12)	10% (3)	13% (4)	23% (7)	n.r.	19 mo.	62
Time 2	Down syndrome	43% (13)	23% (7)	3% (1)	30% (9)	n.r.	25 mo.	n.r.
Marvin & Pianta (1996)	Cerebral palsy	49% (34)	n.r.	n.r.	n.r.	n.r.	12 mo.	n.r.
Speltz, Endriga, Fisher, & Mason (1997)	Cleft lip and palate	75% (18)	13% (3)	8% (2)	4% (1)	n.r.	12 mo.	n.r.
	Cleft palate	59% (16)	19% (5)	22% (6)	0% (0)	n.r.	12 mo.	n.r.
Vaughn et al. (1994)								
Sample 1	Down syndrome	53% (20)	21% (8)	3% (1)	n.r.	24% (9)	37 mo.	57
Sample 2	Down syndrome	46% (20)	0% (0)	3% (1)	n.r.	52% (23)	25 mo.	58

Note. Numbers in parentheses represent number of children. CA, chronological age; DQ, developmental quotient; n.r., not reported. In the Capps et al. study, four children were judged to be unclassifiable, and are not represented in this table. All of the children were said to meet criteria for the type D pattern of attachment. The authors reported that in most cases this was due to the presence of neurological symptoms that overlap with Type D indices.

Children in this latter group were viewed as having no recognizable behavioral strategy that fit any existing classification. In another study of children with Down syndrome, neurological symptoms were removed from consideration in attachment classifications, resulting in somewhat lower, but nevertheless elevated, rates (~25%) for the disorganized group (Ganiban, Barnett, & Cicchetti, in press).

The findings on attachment among biologically compromised children raise two questions: First, why are children with medical conditions and disabilities at risk for forming insecure attachments? And second, can disorganized attachment classifications be made reliably and validly for children with neurological problems? By comparing two groups of children with congenitally based problems, one with neurological problems (e.g., cerebral palsy) and one without (e.g., cleft lip), the study presented in this chapter addresses these and related questions.

Having a child with a chronic medical condition or disability places unique emotional and physical demands on family members, often straining marital and other family relationships (Shonkoff, Hauser-Cram, Krauss, & Upshur, 1992). Parents have to adjust their expectations and hopes for their child in the face of substantial uncertainties likely to be inherent in their child's medical, psychological, and social prognosis. Emotionally and cognitively, parents must come to terms with their child's condition. Parents' reactions to their child's condition have been compared to grieving and mourning the hoped-for child (Emde & Brown, 1978). Marvin and Pianta (1996; Pianta, Marvin, Britner, & Borowitz, 1996; Pianta, Marvin, & Morog, Chapter 14, this volume) have examined this process and developed a technique for assessing whether parents have resolved their feelings about their child's diagnosis. Their research suggests that parental reactions are not a direct function of the severity of their child's condition. Like grief and mourning (Bowlby, 1980), parental reactions to diagnosis are thought to be determined by a complex set of processes related to parental personality and relationship histories. In the current study, we examined whether attachment insecurity among children with congenital problems was associated with parental resolution to their child diagnosis, as well as a variety of other indices of parental stress.

A basic assumption of attachment theory is that infants can develop the capacity to signal their needs, to make use of care to regulate themselves, to exhibit behaviors that reinforce the caregiver, and to maintain an ongoing social transaction. However, certain congenitally based developmental disorders may interfere with children's ability to elicit appropriate and effective care. For instance, children with conditions such as craniofacial deformities may present conflicting or inappropriate facial cues, making the establishment of a consistent signaling system more challenging than for children without this anomaly. Children with damage to their central nervous system can exhibit unusual behavior, such as seizures, making it difficult for caregivers to understand their children's behavior and respond appropriately. Children with congenital problems may be at increased risk for insecure attachments because they intensely challenge the limits of otherwise sensitive parents. Consequently, we also examined maternal sensitivity as a predictor of attachment security.

The increased rate of insecure attachments among children with congenital problems corresponds in part to the increase in the disorganized group in particular. There are several related explanations for the increased incidence of disorganized attachments in samples of children with these conditions. First, these children truly may be at increased risk for forming the disorganized or some other form of atypical attachment; that is, the processes contributing to their forming a disorganized attachment are similar to and consistent with those believed to play a role in the formation of a disorganized attachment among children without congenitally based problems. Disorganized attachment patterns are believed to result when the caregiver's behavior is disorganized and otherwise frightening, so that the child cannot respond to it in a coherent and adaptive manner (Main & Hesse, 1990). As has been noted, the presence of congenital problems and the development of chronic health conditions in offspring offer a significant test of most parents' coping ability. A breakdown in coping, or the adoption of atypical forms of coping, may undermine parents' ability to be sensitive and consistent when caring for their children. In some cases, unresolved grief reactions to a child's handicap may undermine parenting (Marvin & Pianta, 1996; Pianta et al., 1996 and Chapter 14, this volume). If the parent responds to the situation by becoming immobilized by depression or anxiety, or by becoming overwhelmed and helpless, caregiving behavior could become disorganized and thus disorganizing to the child (George & Solomon, 1999; Teti, Gelfand, Messinger, & Isabella, 1995; Solomon & George, 1996). Caregiving could also become disorganized if the parent is unable to understand the child's signals accurately and consistently, resulting in inappropriate responding.

On the other hand, the high rates of disorganized and other nontraditional attachments may be an artifact of these children's congenital problems, and may, therefore, not represent "true" disorganized attachments. The disabilities often associated with conditions such as cerebral palsy and epilepsy are often a result of congenital damage to the nervous system. As a result, children with these disorders are likely to exhibit a high incidence of neurological problems. Pipp-Siegel, Siegel, and Dean (in press) have discussed the numerous similarities between symptoms of neurological disorder and signs of a disorganized attachment pattern. They developed a system that classified indices of disorganized attachments as overlapping or not overlapping with symptoms of neurological disorder. For example, they noted that motor stereotypies, tense postures, and dazed facial expressions are symptoms of neurological disorder and signs of the disorganized pattern. Indeed, Pipp-Siegel and her colleagues catalogued a total of 53% overlap in neurological symptoms and indices of attachment disorganization. Perhaps researchers have not systematically and reliably discriminated signs of neurological disorder from signs of the disorganized pattern of attachment. This is the first validity study of Pipp-Siegel et al.'s system.

In this investigation, we expected toddlers with neurological defects to demonstrate more indices of the disorganized attachment pattern than children with non- neurologically based conditions. However, we hypothesized that using the system developed by Pipp-Siegel et al. to take into account neurological symptoms and disregard them as indices of disorganized attachment would result in normative rates (i.e., 10–20%) of attachment disorganization in these toddler groups. Moreover, as with normally developing youngsters, we expected insecurity, especially the disorganized pattern, to be associated with parental problems rather than aspects of the child's condition per se; that is, disorganized and other forms of insecure attachment would be related to factors that disrupt caregiving, including unresolved parental grieving.

METHOD

Sample

Fifty children comprising two diagnostic groups—neurological problems (e.g., cerebral palsy) and non-neurologically based congenital problem (e.g., cleft lip)—were recruited from medical specialty clinics in hospitals within the metropolitan Detroit area. Medical records were reviewed in order to select children between the ages of 12 and 36 months who represented these two diagnostic groups. Records also were reviewed to exclude families receiving Medicaid, in order to reduce the number of low-income families in the sample. Poverty is associated with a number of stressors that may increase the chances that a child forms an insecure and possibly disorganized attachment (Lyons-Ruth, Alpern, & Repacholi, 1993). By screening out families on Medicaid, the hope was to avoid a confound between poverty and parental stress. As noted in Table 7.2, these two groups were found not to differ on a range of family background factors.

Families were contacted by letter and telephone calls in which additional inclusion criteria were reviewed with the primary caregiver. These prerequisites were viewed as necessary for the child's participation in the strange situation, including (1) an estimated mental equivalency of 12 months; (2) no debilitating sensory impairment (i.e., able to apprehend and respond to mother, both visually and aurally, from a distance of 10–12

TABLE 7.2. Sample Demographics for the Two Diagnostic Groups

	Neurological (n = 25)	Non-neurological (n = 25)	Significance
Child age	M = 24.76 mo. (SD = 5.04)	M = 24.16 mo. (SD = 6.40)	n.s.
Child mental development equivalency	M = 17.60 mo. (SD = 4.58)	M = 23.32 mo. (SD = 6.22)	t(48) = –3.70**
Child motor development equivalency	M = 15.00 mo. (SD = 5.60)	M = 23.13 mo. (SD = 7.06)	t(48) = –4.42**
Number of child hospitalizations	M = 0.46 (SD = 1.06)	M = 0.20 (SD = 0.41)	n.s.
Time since diagnosis	M = 16.12 mo. (SD = 7.43)	M = 23.56 mo. (SD = 7.17)	t(50) = –3.60**
Family ethnicity			
African American	10 (40%)	3 (12%)	$\chi^2(1) = 4.67*$
Caucasian	14 (56%)	21 (84%)	
Other	1 (4%)	1 (4%)	
Mother age	M = 29.12 yr. (SD = 5.20)	M = 29.58 yr. (SD = 5.61)	n.s.
Mother education	M = 13.16 yr. (SD = 2.19)	M = 13.48 yr. (SD = 2.18)	n.s.
Father education	M = 12.91 yr. (SD = 1.91)	M = 14.08 yr. (SD = 2.34)	n.s.
Mother marital status			n.s.
Single, never married	7 (28%)	2 (8%)	
Married or with partner	18 (72%)	21 (84%)	
Separated or divorced	0	2 (8%)	
Receiving welfare	8 (32%)	3 (12%)	n.s.

*p < .05; **p < .01.

feet); (3) an ability to signal or interact across a distance (e.g., able to look and maintain eye contact, change facial expression and/or alter vocal intonation); and (4) at least partial mobility (e.g., able to roll or scoot). As a result of these criteria, it should be noted that the sample is limited to children with relatively mild impairments.

Half of the sample (n = 25) were diagnosed with a neurological disorder. Of these, 11 were girls, and 14 were boys. The majority (72%) was diagnosed with cerebral palsy, with the remaining children being diagnosed with hydrocephalus (16%), epilepsy (4%), myelomeningocele (4%), and brain anomaly (4%). Thirty-six percent also had a secondary medical diagnosis related to their primary diagnosis (e.g., hydrocephalus, epilepsy, and cerebral palsy). Twenty percent had been treated with inpatient hospitalization, with 12% being hospitalized more than once. The majority (56%) of the children had at least one surgery, with 28% having had more than one surgery (range = 0–11). The children's chronological ages ranged from 15 to 30 months. Based on the Bayley Scales of Infant Development–Second Edition (Bayley-II; Bayley, 1993), their mental and motor developmental ages ranged from 8 to 31 months and from 4 to 27 months, respectively. Mothers' age ranged from 18 to 39 years. Table 7.2 presents additional details about the children.

The remainder of the sample (n = 25) had a non-neurological diagnosis. Of these, 11 were girls, and 14 were boys. Children with craniofacial and/or limb malformations were selected as a comparison group because, although these parents face similar challenges arising from having a child with congenital anomalies, the child's impairments are not linked to impairments inevitably confounded with attachment behavior. Forty-four percent of these children had a primary diagnosis of cleft lip, with 28% having cleft lip and palate, 8% having cleft palate only, 8% having Pierre Robin syndrome, 8% having craniofacial anomaly not otherwise specified, and 4% having a limb deficiency. Twenty-percent of the children had a related secondary medical diagnosis (e.g., craniofacial anomaly not otherwise specified, Nager syndrome). Twenty-percent of the children had been treated with inpatient hospitalization, and 92% had had at least one surgery (range = 0–17). Toddlers in the non-neurological diagnostic group ranged in chronological age from 13 to 33 months. Based on the Bayley-II, their mental developmental ages ranged from 11 to 36 months, and their motor developmental ages ranged from 7 to 35 months. Mothers' ages ranged from 20 to 41 years. As reported in Table 7.2, this group had fewer toddlers of African American decent than the group with neurological problems, which is consistent with prior research indicating that craniofacial anomalies are more prevalent in white than in black children (Vanderas, 1987).

Procedures

Permission for identifying and contacting potentially eligible families was obtained from the clinic directors and Institutional Review Boards of the seven participating hospitals. Following a review of hospital records, families were contacted to describe the project, address any questions or concerns, and schedule assessments with interested and eligible mother–child dyads. Mothers were given the option of completing a single 4-hour visit to the university office or having the visit divided into two sessions. Mother and toddler initially completed the strange situation, followed by the 15-minutes of interactive and divided-attention play tasks. Next, mother and child remained together while the Bayley-II was administered. The mother then completed the interviews and questionnaires, while the child played with one of the examiners. If the mother chose to divide her participation into two visits, the interviews and questionnaires were completed at her home. Breaks were taken throughout the proceedings as needed, with snacks available for both mothers and children. Participants were paid a small honorarium.

Measures

Attachment Quality

All children were videotaped in Ainsworth's strange situation procedure. For children 12 to 29 months of age (n = 40), attachment classifications were based on Ainsworth et al.'s (1978) system for assessing avoidant, secure, and ambivalent attachments, and Main and Solomon's (1990) system for assessing attachment disorganization. For children 30-months or older (n = 10), attachment was assessed using Cassidy and Marvin's (1991) classification system for assessing, secure, avoidant, ambivalent, disorganized/controlling, or insecure–other (Group IO) attachments among pre-schoolers. Videotapes were reviewed by the first author to code attachment quality. He received training from expert coders of attachment and established reliability above 90% for the infant system, and above the established cutoff on an official set of test tapes for the preschool system. To establish reliability for the present sample, 15 tapes were randomly selected and coded by Butler, who was trained by Barnett on children from a variety of infant and preschool samples. No children in this sample were judged to demonstrate the controlling or Group IO classifications. The coders agreed at the level of major classification for 14 of the 15 cases (93%) with a kappa of .80. Because of the chapter's focus on attachment disorganization, Butler also reviewed the remainder of the tapes for assignment to the disorganized classification. Out of 50 cases, agreement as to the presence or absence of attachment disorganization was 98%, with a kappa of .96. Disagreements were resolved through discussion.

Neurological Indices of Disorganization

Butler also rated the strange situation tapes specifically for the number of indices of attachment disorganization seen in each episode. Indices of disorganization were then classified as potentially neurological or non-neurological in origin, according to a system devised by Pipp-Siegel et al. (in press). Neurological signs included behaviors specifically related to motor control and coordination, muscle tone, balance, and the presence of seizures. For example, in Main and Solomon's taxonomy, mild signs of potential disorganization include keeping arms and legs stiffly away from the parent when held; asymmetrical, jerky, start–stop or incomplete movements; dazed expression or "fearful" smile; circuitous, disjointed approach to the parent; slow, limp movements, motor stereotypies, and tense postures. A large number of these indices occurring together would be likely to result in assignment to the disorganized classification. Some single behaviors, such as freezing or stilling for a prolonged period, would in themselves result in assignment to the disorganized category. In Pipp-Siegel et al.'s system, any or all of these could be classified as a neurological symptom rather than a sign of disorganized attachment. For the purposes of the present study, we defined "neurological" disorganized behaviors as those included within Pipp-Siegel et al.'s taxonomy, which is comprised of simple motor-response items, and dazing and stilling in the case of a child with seizures. Butler attained interrater reliability with Pipp-Siegel on a random sample of 15 tapes. These included 52 behaviors that either or both coders viewed to be an index of the disorganized pattern. Of these, they agreed on 45 (88%) of the cases on whether the behavior was an index of disorganization or in the category of behaviors that overlapped with neurological symptoms.

Pipp-Siegel et al. stress the importance of interpreting the child's behavior with knowledge of the child's specific medical and functional condition and history. Given a key focus of our study was to determine whether neurological symptoms could be distinguished from signs of attachment disorganization, we chose to deviate from this particular guideline and classify indices of disorganization without specific knowledge of children's medical condition. In the absence of detailed information of the child's medical condition, we thought that making decisions about whether a behavior was neurologically or non-neurologically based would make for a more stringent test of the discriminant validity of the Pipp-Siegel et al. system. We chose to code the data in this fashion because we realized that in the contexts of most studies, researchers might not have access to detailed medical records concerning a child's condition. In addition, it has been our experience that information from medical records can vary widely in reliability and validity. Therefore, the coders of the disorganization indices were blind to the subjects' specific diagnostic category and medical history. Although in some cases the type of impairment was obvious, many of the children in both groups appeared normal, and some children in the neurological group also had facial or other physical anomalies in appearance. Consequently, guessing the diagnostic group of each child was not straightforward. All observed disorganized behavior that fell within Pipp-Siegel et al.'s grouping of neurological signs was counted as such, particularly if it was observed prior to the first separation.

Maternal Sensitivity

Maternal behavior was rated from videotaped recordings of mothers and their toddlers interacting in the laboratory in 15-minute play situations immediately following the strange situation. Each dyad participated in 5 minutes of unconstrained play in which the mother and toddler were given an attractive set of age-appropriate toys and instructed to play as they did at home. During the remaining 10 minutes of mother–toddler play activity, mothers were asked to complete a lengthy demographics questionnaire. This play interaction, designed after Smith and Pederson's (1988) mother–child interaction paradigm, was used to investigate mothers' sensitivity when they must comply with the investigator's instructions to complete the questionnaire while being responsive and attentive to their children. Theoretically, under the conditions of dividing attention between the questionnaire and the child's demands, individual differences in parenting sensitivity may be more likely to be observed than under less demanding conditions. Two coders trained to rate maternal behavior reviewed the play activity videotapes. A rating scale developed by Ainsworth, Bell, and Stayton (1974) was used to code the mothers' sensitivity to their child's communications from the 10-minute divided-attention segment. Mothers' attentiveness and responsiveness to their child are the primary foci of these ratings, which are behaviorally anchored and on a 9-point scale, ranging from 9 ("highly sensitive") to 1 ("highly insensitive"). Based on 15 randomly selected tapes, raters agreement was 60%, 87%, and 100% within 1, 2, and 3 points, respectively. The correlation between raters was .62, $p <$ .02.

Maternal Reaction to Child Diagnosis

The Reaction to Diagnosis Interview and Scoring System (RDI; Marvin & Pianta, 1996; Pianta et al., 1996 and Chapter 14, this volume) was used to assess resolution of maternal grief responses to children's congenital condition. The RDI is a semistructured interview specifically designed to assess parents' resolution of the emotional trauma related to the experience of learning about their child's medical diagnosis or disability. As part of the interview, parents were asked to recall their first perceptions that there might be a problem with their child's development, and their feelings about their suspicions. They also were asked about their emotional reactions to receiving a formal diagnosis for their child, any changes in their psychological status since the initial perception of problems, and subsequent diagnostic event, and attributions and/or personal explanations for their child's condition. The RDI was administered according to criteria developed by Marvin and Pianta (e.g., probes associated with specific topical questions, maintaining neutrality during the interview). All interviews were audiotaped, and later transcribed and scored according to criteria developed by the RDI authors.

The Reaction to Diagnosis Classification System (RDCS; Marvin & Pianta, 1996) is an organized scheme for assessing parents' general adaptation to their child's diagnosis (i.e., the extent of their resolution of emotional trauma related to learning of their child's condition). The system also yields more descriptive information about parents' adaptive patterns by assessing the extent to which integrative and dissociative strategies for coping with grief/loss are indicated in their responses to the RDI. Subjects' responses to the RDI are coded according to the presence or absence of predetermined elements suggesting resolution and lack of resolution of grief. Elements of both resolution and lack of resolution are expected to be present in most interviews. Resolution is characterized by the predominance of integrative mental strategies reflecting the overall adaptive operation of executive mental functions on the loss/trauma experience. A predominance of dissociative strategies and the inadequacy of executive functioning characterize lack of resolution. Descriptors of the interpersonal styles, emotional content and expressions, cognitive processes, and mental representations of self, child, and diagnosis-related events suggestive of Resolution and Lack of Resolution are described in the RDCS (see also Pianta et al., Chapter 14, this volume). Each interview is classified as either resolved or unresolved—reflecting the mother's general adaptation to her child's diagnosis. For purposes of reliability, 11 (22%) of the interviews were chosen at random and coded by McCaskill and Kaplan-Estrin. Initial agreement was 9/11 (82%). Six additional interviews were randomly selected and coded by Robert Pianta, with an agreement rate of 5/6 (83%) with McCaskill.

Maternal Attitudes Regarding Child Congenital Problems

The Dysfunctional Attitudes Regarding Child Congenital Problems Scale was designed specifically for this study to assess for parents' extreme positive or negative attitudes about their child's medical condition or disability. This 26-item scale is patterned after the Dysfunctional Attitudes Scale (Weissman & Beck, 1978) which has been found to identify attitudes associated with depression. Dysfunctional attitudes are considered to be trait-like phenomena reflecting negative, rigid, absolutistic, or overgeneralized thoughts that predispose an individual to depression (Beck, Rush, Shaw, & Emery, 1979). The Dysfunctional Attitudes Regarding Child Congenital Problems Scale was designed to assess parental appraisals of both the relational meaning (e.g., self-as-parent, child-in-relation-to-parent) and the long-term implications (for both self and child) of children's congenital problems. Sample items of the Negative Dysfunctional Attitudes scale include

"You have failed as a parent," "Your child will blame you," and "You will miss out on many of the joys of being a parent." Six items assessed mothers' Positive Dysfunctional Attitudes about their children's condition. A sample item from this scale is "You will become a stronger and wiser person as a result of having a child with a birth defect." Items were scored on a 5-point response scale, indicating the extent to which participants agree or disagree with each statement. For the current sample, internal consistency coefficient alphas were .91 and .74 for the negative and positive factors, respectively.

Parenting Hassles

The Parenting Daily Hassles Scale (Crnic & Greenberg, 1990) is a 20-item measure of typical, everyday events related to parenting and parent–child interactions that may be regarded as aversive or stressful to parents. For each item, parents rate the intensity of perceived hassle for the event (on a 5-point scale, ranging from "No hassle" to "Big hassle"). Cronbach's alpha for the current sample was .87.

Maternal Mental Health

Caregivers completed the Brief Symptom Inventory (BSI: Derogatis & Spencer, 1982), a 53-item self-report instrument covering the presence and severity of psychological problems, including depression, anxiety, hostility, and psychosomatic symptoms. For each item (e.g., "Suddenly scared for no reason"), caregivers were asked to report how much they are bothered by each symptom during the prior 2 months using a 5-point scale ranging from "Not at all" (0) to "Extremely" (4). Scores were totaled, with high scores indicating greater overall psychological distress. Internal consistency alpha was .97 for the current sample.

Stressful Life Events

Caregivers completed the Stressful Life Events Scale, a questionnaire designed for this investigation to assess occurrences of severe relationship stressors (e.g., death of family member, divorce, domestic violence) during the prior 12 months. The presence of eight potential stressful events was summed to compute a total score ranging from 0 to 8.

RESULTS

The results are presented in four parts. In Part 1, the potential effect of child neurological status on parent functioning is examined. Part 2 presents the relation between neurological status and indices of attachment disorganization, as well as neurological status and attachment classification. Part 3 addresses the prediction of the secure attachment grouping, and Part 4 examines the prediction of the disorganized attachment grouping. One parent did not have complete data on the Dysfunctional Attitudes Scale, and another was missing data on the Daily Hassles. Two children did not complete the Bailey-II. These participants were not included in analyses reflecting these measures.

To examine whether neurological status had a differential effect on parent functioning, two one-way multivariate analyses of variance (MANOVAs) with neurological status as the independent variable were conducted. The first included dependent variables viewed to be "distal" to the attachment relationship. These were maternal factors that characterized the mothers' well-being in a general sense, Daily Hassles, Symptoms, and Stressful Events. The second set of "proximal" dependent variables were those that had a more direct link to the mother–toddler relationship, Positive and Negative Dysfunctional Attitudes, and maternal sensitivity. Reaction to Diagnosis was not included in this analysis because it is a dichotomous dependent variable. Neither the MANOVA for distal factors, $F(3,45) = 1.02$, nor proximal factors, $F(3,45) = 2.15$, were significant. Also, none of the one-way follow-up analyses of variance (ANOVAs) was significant. However, child neurological status was related significantly to the Reaction to Diagnosis rating, $\chi^2(1) = 6.52$, $p < .05$. Specifically, mothers of children diagnosed with neurological problems were more likely to be rated as unresolved than mothers of children in the non-neurological group (64% vs. 28%, respectively). Because ethnicity, time since diagnosis, and mental and motor development significantly distinguished these two groups (see Table 7.2), a stepwise logistic regression was conducted predicting Reaction to Diagnosis from neurological group while controlling for the four background variables. Diagnostic group did not remain a significant predictor of Reaction to Diagnosis, nor was the overall model significant, $\chi^2(5) = 8.57$, n.s. The individual control variables also were not significant predictors of Reaction to Diagnosis. In summary, with the possible exception of Reaction to Diagnosis, child neurological status did not appear to have a differential impact on parent well-being. The possible effect of child neurological status on mothers' Reaction to Diagnosis did not appear to be robust, as it did not remain significant in the multivariate analyses. Important to the design of this study, these two groups of congenital anomalies can be viewed to have a comparable affect on maternal well-being and behavior.

Two one-way ANOVAs were conducted to examine the relation between neurological status and indices of attachment disorganization. As predicted, children with a neurological disorder exhibited significantly more neurological indices of disorganization (M = 2.12, SD = 2.42) than children with a non-neurological diagnosis (M = 0.76, SD = 1.19), $F(1,48)$ = 4.80, $p < .05$. However, the two groups did not differ significantly on the number of non-neurological indices of disorganization, $F(1,48)$ = 0.24, n.s., nor the overall number of indices of disorganization, $F(1,48)$ = 2.64, n.s. As reported in Table 7.3, neurological status was not related significantly to attachment group, $\chi^2(3)$ = 5.16, n.s. Because four of the cells had fewer than 5 children, we conducted two follow-up analyses examining whether neurological grouping was related to the secure–insecure distinction, and whether diagnostic status was associated with the disorganized attachment classification. The analyses for security and disorganization were not significant, $\chi^2(1)$ = 2.05, n.s., and $\chi^2(1)$ = 0.60, n.s., respectively. Taken together, the analyses examining the relation between neurological status and attachment support the following premises: (1) Some indices of disorganization overlap with neurological symptoms; (2) indices of disorganization can be distinguished from symptoms of neurological disorder; and (3) congenitally based neurological disorders, per se, do not predispose one to form a disorganized attachment.

Before addressing the prediction of attachment security from the maternal factors, the relation between security and parent–child background variables were examined. Except for mothers' age, security of attachment was not related to any other child or family demographic variables. According to a one-way ANOVA, mothers whose child was classified as insecurely attached were significantly older than mothers whose child had a secure attachment (M = 31.8, SD = 5.7, M = 27.8, SD = 4.5, respectively), $F(1,48)$ = 7.70, $p < .01$. Next, two stepwise logistic regressions were conducted predicting attachment security. The first included maternal age in the first step and variables viewed to be "distal" to the attachment relationship, Daily Hassles, Symptoms, and Stressful Events in the second step. The overall model was marginally significant, $\chi^2(4)$ = 9.10, $p < .06$. However, no individual variable other than mother's age was significantly related to attachment. The second logistic regression included maternal age and neurological status in the first step. Neurological status was

TABLE 7.3. Attachment Classification by Medical Diagnostic Group

	Attachment classification			
Diagnostic group	A Avoidant	B Secure	C Ambivalent	D Disorganized
Neurological	24% (6)	48% (12)	16% (4)	12% (3)
Non-neurological	8% (2)	68% (17)	4% (1)	20% (5)

included because of its significant relation to Reaction to Diagnosis, reported earlier. The second step included the proximal relationship variables: Positive and Negative Dysfunctional Attitudes, maternal sensitivity, and Reaction to Diagnosis. The overall model was significant, $\chi^2(6) = 26.93$. According to the Wald test, maternal age ($z = 8.46$, $p<.01$) and Reaction to Diagnosis ($z = 8.91$, $p < .01$), contributed individually to the prediction of security. In addition, there was a marginally significant trend for maternal sensitivity ($z = 2.79$, $p < .10$). Mothers who had resolved their grief over having a child with a congenital problem were more likely to have a child classified as secure than were mothers rated as unresolved, 76% versus 24%, respectively. Mothers of children classified as secure were rated as more sensitive than those classified as insecure ($M = 5.97$, $SD = 1.90$, $M = 5.00$, $SD = 1.90$, respectively).

The final set of analyses addressed the prediction of the disorganized attachment classification. First, the relation between disorganized attachment and parent–child background variables was examined. The disorganized classification was not related significantly to any child or family demographic variable. Next, two stepwise logistic regressions were conducted predicting whether or not the child was assigned to the disorganized group. The first included variables viewed to be "distal" to the attachment relationship, Daily Hassles, Symptoms, and Stressful Events. The overall model was not significant, $\chi^2(3) = 1.47$, n.s. Also, no individual variable was significantly related to the disorganized classification. The second logistic regression included neurological status in the first step. Neurological status was included because of its significant relation to Reaction to Diagnosis, reported earlier. The second step included the proximal relationship variables: Positive and Negative Dysfunctional Attitudes, maternal sensitivity, and Reaction to Diagnosis. The overall model was not significant, $\chi^2(5) = 7.15$, n.s. However, according to the Wald test, Reaction to Diagnosis ($z = 4.07$, $p < .05$) was a significant individual predictor of whether the child was assigned to the disorganized group. Mothers who had not resolved their grief over having a child with a congenital problem were more likely than were mothers rated as resolved to have a child classified as disorganized, 22% versus 7%, respectively.

Although disorganized attachment status was not significantly related to psychological risk factors, it appeared that mothers who had children with disorganized attachments were not reporting serious distress, but instead were reporting fewer and less intense parenting hassles and fewer symptoms compared to mothers who had children with other types of attachment (avoidant, secure, ambivalent). We hypothesized that such a response pattern might reflect a defensive coping pattern. To address this hypothesis, we examined the degree to which parents consistently denied negative reactions and affect to stressful situations. In particular, we examined whether mothers of children classified as disorganized compared to other classifications would be more likely to score within the lowest one-third of the sample on Symptoms, Negative Dysfunctional Attitudes, Daily Hassles, and scoring within the highest one-third of the sample on Positive Dysfunctional Attitudes. We considered such a positively biased profile to be evidence of defensive reporting of one's psychological state. Out of the four comparisons, Positive Dysfunctional Attitudes was significantly related to disorganized attachment. Specifically, mothers who had children with disorganized attachments were more likely to be in the top one-third of the sample on Positive Dysfunctional Attitudes than were mothers whose child was not classified as disorganized, $\chi^2(1) = 4.58$, $p < .05$. A final stepwise logistic regression was conducted predicting the disorganized classification. Neurological status was entered in the first step because of its significant relation to Reaction to Diagnosis. The second step included Negative Dysfunctional Attitudes, maternal sensitivity, Reaction to Diagnosis, and the dichotomous Positive Dysfunctional Attitudes variable. The overall model was significant, $\chi^2(5) = 11.92$, $p < .05$. According to the Wald test, Reaction to Diagnosis ($z = 4.80$, $p < .05$) and dichotomous Positive Dysfunctional Attitudes ($z = 4.01$, $p < .05$) were significant individual predictors of whether the child was assigned to the disorganized group. Neither of the findings could be accounted by other variables in the study such as parent ethnicity.

DISCUSSION

Taken as a whole, the results of this investigation provide preliminary support that congenital conditions involving damage to the nervous system, such as cerebral palsy, are associated with behaviors that overlap with those found among children without disabilities but who are classified as disorganized/disoriented in the strange situation. Attachment disorganization is thought likely to occur when children experience frightening forms of care from their attachment figure (Main & Hesse, 1990; Main & Solomon, 1990). Some of these parenting behaviors are overtly traumatic, such as in cases of abuse and neglect; others may be more subtly frightening, such as when parents are passively helpless and solicit care from their child (George & Solomon, 1999; Solomon & George, 1996). It may be that children with neurological disorders demonstrate indices of disorganization under lower levels of stress than are typically required to evoke such behaviors in children with normal nervous systems. It also may be the case that living under chronically stressful conditions in which comfort is rarely present contributes to congenitally healthy children developing neurological damage (Dawson, Grofer Klinger, Panagiotides, Spieker, & Frey, 1992; Levine, Johnson, & Gonzalez, 1985).

Despite the overlap in indices of neurological disorder and disorganized attachment, the results of this study indicate that it is possible to discriminate reliably between neurological symptoms and signs of relationship disturbance. In part, we recommend that attachment coders should be aware of, and familiar with, neurological indices. The organization and context within which neurological and non-neurological indices of disorganization occur should then be taken into account in assigning meaning to them.

The assessment of attachment among infants and preschoolers is based on careful observation of children's behavior across separations and reunions with their attachment figure. Based on observed behavioral patterns, inferences are made concerning the representational model presumed to guide each child's behavior. Children's behavior in the strange situation always has been interpreted in light of the social and emotional context of the behavioral occurrence (Ainsworth et al., 1978; Sroufe & Waters, 1977). In this regard, smiling provides information concerning the child's representational model of attachment only when it is viewed in the context in which the smile was expressed (e.g., to the mother or to the wall), and the temporal context, such as the event preceding the smile (e.g., showing a clown doll or throwing a toy hammer at the mother). Judgments about children's behavior in the strange situation also have to be made with consideration of children's developmental level. Control of motor output, including locomotion, vocalization, and affective displays, come under increasing control with development. Consequently, expectations change concerning the meaning of a child's behavior based on developmental level (Crittenden, 1992).

Theoretically, representational models of relationships play an increasing role in guiding and managing attachment affect and behavior. In this regard, children's models of caregivers' accessibility are believed to guide their communication with, and behavior toward, their caregivers. However, in cases of organically based pathology, children's expressions toward their caregivers might not clearly reflect their underlying representational model. In a small but significant percentage of infants, deficits and delays in emotional and behavioral expression are present. For example, children with autism have severe delays and deficits in affective expression, sharing, and social interest (Mundy, 1995). Children with Down syndrome typically have significant delays in cognitive and motor development. Developmental disorders often result from central or peripheral damage to the nervous system. For example, some infants lack the ability of locomotion due to spinal cord damage resulting in paralysis. Other children experience significant delays in motor development, and motor development is often a key indicator of overall developmental health in early infancy. Motor development, in turn, plays a key role in the organization and timing of development. Consequently, pathology and maturation of the nervous system (in addition to parenting) may have direct and indirect influences on the development of representational models of attachment (Atkinson et al., in press; Vaughn et al., 1994).

When there is reason to suspect damage to the central or peripheral nervous system, the interpretability of child behavior comes into question. Children may have difficulty coordinating intentions and inhibiting behaviors and emotions. Whenever the integrity of the child's neurological and motor systems is in question, we recommend that attachment raters consider how these impairments would influence children's behavior in the strange situation. Just as behaviors such as smiling have to be understood in the more general social context within which they occur, we believe that indices of disorganization must be interpreted within the context of the child's general neurological condition.

Nonetheless, questions remain on how much knowledge attachment coders should have about the health and developmental level of the children they are classifying in the strange situations. Clearly, researchers should carefully screen the children participating in their research and inquire about the their medical history. Moreover, careful assessments and examination of cognitive and motor delays may need to be included. In addition to data from medical records and standardized tests, it is important for coders to be sensitive to the child's cues and behaviors across conditions in the strange situation, using the child as their own standard, comparing behavior across the differing social contexts of this paradigm. Recommendations for classifying attachment among children with neurological conditions are elaborated in Pipp-Siegel et al. (in press).

Attachment security in the current sample was most strongly associated with parental reactions to diagnosis. Children whose parents were classified as resolved concerning their child's diagnosis were nearly three times more likely to be classified as secure than were those whose parents were judged unresolved. Conversely, children whose parents were classified as unresolved were more than three times as likely to be classified as insecure in the strange situation than those whose parents were resolved. The current study's findings among children with craniofacial anomalies and other conditions replicate and expand Marvin and Pianta's (1996) study of children with cerebral palsy. The fact that reactions to diagnosis were so strongly related to insecurity suggests that mothers' thoughts and feelings of grief and denial over their child's condition can be pervasively disruptive to their ability to serve as a secure base for the affected offspring. The processes that contribute to parents successfully coming to terms with their child's condition are currently unknown. Further research also is needed on how such challenges to parents are communicated to and thereby contribute to their child forming and insecure attachment (George & Solomon, 1999; Solomon & George, 1996).

A second independent contribution to insecurity was parental age. Children whose mothers were older were more likely to be insecurely attached. Risks for several congenital anomalies such as Down syndrome increase with parental age. Perhaps awareness of these risks may cause older parents to be more devastated by self-blame than younger parents when these worries become manifested in the birth of a medically compromised child. This is but one possible explanation for the significant link between parent age and child attachment. However, the effect for parental age was not predicted, and this and other interpretations should be considered tentative and examined in future research.

Maternal reaction to diagnosis also was a significant predictor of child attachment disorganization. Perhaps a reanalysis of these interviews may reveal clues as to why some parents rated as unresolved have children whose attachment patterns are disorganized. In this regard, one style that may be worth examining in the Reaction to Diagnosis Interview may be parental denial or defensive coping style. This is because a post hoc analysis of the Positive Dysfunctional Attributions scale revealed that the mothers in the sample with the most positive scores were significantly more likely to have children classified as disorganized. These parents appear to have taken on seemingly unrealistically positive views of their role as caregivers to a medically compromised child. When managing the challenges of parenting a child with medical problems or disabilities, such an optimistic view may be advantageous for staving off parental feelings of sadness and hopelessness. However, the significant link between overly positive attitudes and disorganized attachment suggests that such attitudes may be a sign that all is not right with the parent–toddler relationship. At the same time, these findings were evidenced in a relatively small number of dyads and replication is warranted. Indeed, few variables were significantly linked to security or disorganization, although it must be recognized that the small sample size limits the power to detect significant but modest effect sizes such as those that typically have been found for maternal sensitivity (De Wolff & van IJzendoorn, 1997).

It is unclear why parental stress and symptoms were not related to attachment disorganization. One possible explanation may pertain to the socioeconomic and psychiatric status of the families examined. Several studies have linked parental stress and symptoms to having a child judged to have a disorganized or nontraditional attachment (Lyons-Ruth et al., 1993; Spieker & Booth, 1988; Teti et al., 1995). However, these have been studies of families from low-income backgrounds and/or families selected for parental psychopathology. In nonpsychiatric and middle-class samples, others have found that the mothers of children judged to have disorganized attachments report the lowest levels of stress and symptoms (Moss, Rousseau, Parent, St-Laurent, & Saintonge, 1998; Stevenson-Hinde & Shouldice, 1995). Perhaps the attempt to screen out families living in poverty, along with the small cell sizes for attachment groups, explains the absence of a relation in the present sample.

In summary, the results of this study provide important discriminant validity for the disorganized attachment classification, suggesting that it is not a result of neurological damage. The study also provides important information about the development of attachment relationships among children with congenital problems. Because the current study did not include a normal comparison group, it is not possible to examine whether parent–child attachments are determined similarly for children with and without congenital disorders. For example, it could be that children with certain disabilities have a lower threshold to demonstrating signs of insecurity, although the same types of parenting behaviors are associated with infant attachment categories as have been found in studies of normal babies. This would demonstrate itself as an interaction of parenting by child diagnostic status (see Atkinson et al., in press). It also should be noted that this study was limited to children with relatively mild forms of congenital problems and associated impairment. It is therefore difficult to know to what extent these findings can be generalized to other forms of congenital problems or more severe forms of impairment.

ACKNOWLEDGMENTS

This study was supported by grants from the National Institute of Mental Health and the March of Dimes Birth Defects Foundation. We also wish to thank our research assistants: Josee Blais, Cindy Bui, Melissa Clements, Heather Chruscial, Deanna Dotterer, Sheila Harris Hicks, Jill Kofender, Katherine Lovell, Barbara Perrone, Kimberly Rogers, Karen Schieferstein, Raymond Small, Miriam Walton, and Shannon Waroway. We also acknowledge Brian Lakey for his contributions toward the development of the Dysfunctional Attitudes Regarding Child Congenital Problems Scale; Robert Pianta for training and assistance on the Reaction to Diagnosis Interview, and the editors of this volume for thoughtful comments throughout. We are especially grateful to the families who so generously have shared their time with us.

REFERENCES

Ainsworth, M. D. S., Bell, S. M., & Stayton, D. J. (1974). Infant–mother attachment and social development: "Socialization" as a product of reciprocal responsiveness to signals. In M. P. Richards (Ed.), *The integration of a child into a social world* (pp. 99–135). London: Cambridge University Press.

Ainsworth, M. D. S., Blehar, M. C., Waters, E., & Wall, S. (1978). *Patterns of attachment: A psychological study of the Strange Situation*. Hillsdale, NJ: Erlbaum.

Ainsworth, M. D. S., & Bowlby, J. (1991). An ethological approach to personality development. *American Psychologist, 46*, 333–341.

Atkinson, L., Chisholm, V.C., Scott, B., Goldberg, S., Vaughn, B., Blackwell, J., Dickens, S., & Tam, F. (in press). Maternal sensitivity, child functional level, and attachment in Down syndrome. In J. I. Vondra & D. Barnett (Eds.), Atypical attachment in infancy and early childhood among children at developmental risk. *Monographs of the Society for Research in Child Development.*

Bayley, N. (1993). *Bayley Scales of Infant Development* (2nd ed.). New York: Psychological Corporation.

Beck, A. T., Rush, A. J., Shaw, B. F., & Emery, G. (1979). *Cognitive therapy of depression*. New York: Guilford Press.

Bowlby, J. (1980). *Attachment and loss: Vol. 3. Loss*. New York: Basic Books.

Bowlby, J. (1988). *A secure base: Parent–child attachment and healthy human development*. New York: Basic Books.

Capps, L., Sigman, M., & Mundy, P. (1994). Attachment security in children with autism. *Development and Psychopathology, 6*, 249–261.

Cassidy, J., & Marvin, R., in collaboration with the MacArthur Working Group on Attachment. (1991). *Attachment organization in three- and four-year-olds: Coding guidelines*. Unpublished manuscript, Pennsylvania State University and University of Virginia, Philadelphia and Charlottesville.

Crittenden, P.M. (1992). Quality of attachment in the preschool years. *Development and Psychopathology, 4*, 209–241.

Crnic, K. A., & Greenberg, M. T. (1990). Minor parenting stresses with young children. *Child Development, 61*, 1628–1637.

Dawson, G., Grofer Klinger, L. G., Panagiotides, H., Spieker, S., and Frey, K. (1992). Infants of mothers with depressive symptoms: Electroencephalographic and behavioral findings related to attachment status. *Development and Psychopathology, 4*, 67–80.

Derogatis, L. R., & Spencer, M. S. (1982). *Administration and procedures: BSI Manual*. Baltimore: Clinical Psychometric Research, Johns Hopkins University.

De Wolff, M. S., & van IJzendoorn, M. H. (1997). Sensitivity and attachment: A meta-analysis on parental antecedents of infant attachment. *Child Development, 68*, 571–591.

Emde, R., & Brown, C. (1978). Adaptation to the birth of a Down's syndrome infant: Grieving and maternal attachment. *American Academy of Child Psychology, 17*, 299–323.

Ganiban, J., Barnett, D., & Cicchetti, D. (in press). Negative reactivity and attachment: Down syndrome's contribution to the attachment–temperament debate. *Development and Psychopathology.*

George, C. & Solomon, J. (1999). Attachment and caregiving: The caregiving behavioral system. In J. Cassidy & P. R. Shaver (Eds.), *Handbook of attachment: Theory, research, and clinical applications* (pp. 649–670). New York: Guilford Press.

Goldberg, S., Gotowiec, A., & Simmons, R. J. (1995). Infant–mother attachment and behavior problems in healthy and chronically ill preschoolers. *Development and Psychopathology, 7*, 267–282.

Goldsmith, H. H., & Alansky, J. (1987). Maternal and infant temperamental predictors of attachment: A meta-analytic review. *Journal of Consulting and Clinical Psychology*, *55*, 805–816.

Levine, S., Johnson, D. F., & Gonzalez, C. A. (1985). Behavioral and hormonal responses to separation in infant rhesus monkeys and mothers. *Behavioral Neuroscience*, *99*, 399–410.

Lyons-Ruth, K., Alpern, L., & Repacholi, B. (1993). Disorganized infant attachment classification and maternal psychosocial problems as predictors of hostile–aggressive behavior in the preschool classroom. *Child Development*, *64*, 572–585.

Main, M., & Hesse, P. (1990). Parents' unresolved traumatic experiences are related to infant disorganized attachment status: Is frightened and/or frightening parental behavior the linking mechanism? In M. Greenberg, D. Cicchetti, & M. Cummings (Eds.), *Attachment during the preschool years* (pp. 161–182). Chicago: University of Chicago Press.

Main, M., & Solomon, J. (1990). Procedures for classifying infants as disorganized/disoriented during the Ainsworth Strange Situation. In M. Greenberg, D. Cicchetti, & E. Cummings (Eds.), *Attachment in the preschool years* (pp. 121–160). Chicago: University of Chicago Press.

Marvin, R. S., & Pianta, R. C. (1996). Mothers' reaction to their child's diagnosis: Relations with security of attachment. *Journal of Clinical Child Psychology*, *25*, 436–445.

Moss, E., Rousseau, D., Parent, S., St-Laurent, D., & Saintonge, J. (1998). Correlates of attachment at school age: Maternal reported stress, mother–child and behavior problems. *Child Development*, *69*, 1390–1405.

Mundy, P. (1995). Joint attention and social–emotional approach behavior in children with autism. *Development and Psychopathology*, *7*, 63–82.

Pianta, R. C., Marvin, R. S., Britner, P. A., & Borowitz, K. C. (1996). Mothers' resolution of their children's diagnosis: Organized patterns of caregiving representations. *Infant Mental Health Journal*, *17*, 239–256.

Pipp-Siegel, S., Siegel, C. H., & Dean, J. (in press). Neurological aspects of the disorganized/disoriented attachment classification system: Differentiating quality of the attachment relationship from neurological impairment. In J. I. Vondra & D. Barnett (Eds.), Atypical attachment in infancy and early childhood among children at developmental risk. *Monographs of the Society for Research in Child Development*.

Shonkoff, J. P., Hauser-Cram, P., Krauss, M. W., & Upshur, C. C. (1992). Development of infants with disabilities and their families. *Monographs of the Society for Research in Child Development*, *57*.

Smith, P. B., & Pederson, D. R. (1988). Maternal sensitivity and patterns of infant–mother attachment. *Child Development*, *59*, 1097–1101.

Solomon, J. & George, C. (1996). Defining the caregiving system: Toward a theory of caregiving. *Infant Mental Health Journal*, *17*, 183–197.

Speltz, M. L., Endriga, M. C., Fisher, P. A., & Mason, C. A. (1997). Early predictors of attachment in infants with cleft lip and/or palate. *Child Development*, *68*, 12–25.

Spieker, S., & Booth, C. (1988). Maternal antecedents of attachment quality. In J.

Belsky & T. Nezworski (Eds.), *Clinical implications of attachment* (pp. 95–135). Hillsdale, NJ: Erlbaum.

Sroufe, L.A., & Waters, E. (1977). Attachment as an organizational construct. *Child Development, 48,* 1184–1199.

Stevenson-Hinde, J., & Shouldice, A. (1995). Maternal interactions and self-reports related to attachment classification at 4.5 years. *Child Development, 66,* 583–596.

Teti, D. M., Gelfand, D. M., Messinger, D. S., & Isabella, R. (1995). Maternal depression and the quality of early attachment: An examination of infants, preschoolers, and their mothers. *Developmental Psychology, 31,* 364–376.

Vanderas, A. P. (1987). Incidence of cleft lip, cleft palate, and cleft lip and palate among races: A review. *Cleft Palate Journal, 24,* 216.

van IJzendoorn, M. H., Goldberg, S., Kroonenberg, P. M., & Frenkel, O. J. (1992). The relative effects of maternal and child problems on the quality of attachment: A meta-analysis of attachment in clinical samples. *Child Development, 63,* 840–858.

Vaughn, B. E., Goldberg, S., Atkinson, L., Marcovitch, S., MacGregor, D., & Seifer, R. (1994). Quality of toddler–mother attachment in children with Down syndrome: Limits to interpretation of Strange Situation behavior. *Child Development, 65,* 95–108.

Weissman, A., & Beck, A. T. (1978). *Development and validation of the Dysfunctional Attitudes Scale: A preliminary investigation.* Paper presented at the annual meeting of the American Educational Research Association, Toronto, Canada.

CHAPTER 8

Conceptualizations of Disorganization in the Preschool Years
An Integration

DOUGLAS M. TETI

Main and Solomon's (1986, 1990) conceptualization of disorganization in infancy has forged new directions in attachment research. Disorganized infants, identified in strange situation assessments (Ainsworth, Blehar, Waters, & Wall, 1978) by manifestations of fear, contradictory behavior, and/or disorientation/dissociation in the caregiver's presence, may be the most insecure of all the insecure infant–mother attachment groupings, the products of highly pathological caregiving (Carlson, Cicchetti, Barnett, & Braunwald, 1989; Lyons-Ruth, Connell, Grunebaum, & Botein, 1990; Rodning, Beckwith, & Howard, 1991; Spieker & Booth, 1988; Teti, Gelfand, Messinger, & Isabella, 1995) and unresolved trauma or loss in the parent (Main & Hesse, 1990; Schuengel, 1997). Underlying this perspective is the view that behavioral manifestations of disorganization in infants reflect fear and/or confusion about whether or how to access the attachment figure in times of stress. These manifestations in turn make it more difficult to assign attachment classifications using Ainsworth et al.'s (1978) traditional tripartite scheme (i.e., Group A: avoidant, Group B: secure, and Group C: ambivalent, heretofore referred to as *traditional* or *standard* attachment classifications). Indeed, it was the inability of several research labs to classify some infants in the traditional Ainsworth et al. system that prompted Main and Solomon (1990) to search for thematic continuities among these originally "unclassifiable" infants. These efforts led to the development of the Group D disorganized/disoriented category.

Main and Solomon's (1990) formulations enjoy a preeminent position in discussions of the conceptualization, meaning, and assessment of disorganization in infancy. What constitutes disorganization in the preschool years (heretofore defined as 3 to 4 years of age), however, is a matter of considerable debate. The preschool years represent a rapidly developing transitional period, during which children move from sensorimotor to representational modes of functioning and, in turn, manifest greater behavioral diversity. Perhaps the most established perspective on attachment assessment in the preschool period is that of Cassidy, Marvin, and the MacArthur Working Group (Cassidy, Marvin, et al., 1987/1990/1991/1992), which identifies "disorganized/controlling" behavior patterns as outgrowths of disorganized attachment classifications (from the Main and Solomon criteria) in infancy. During strange situation assessments, these behavior patterns take two distinct forms. Controlling–caregiving behavior is identified by solicitous, overbright caregiving behavior directed by the child toward the caregiver. Controlling–punitive behavior, by contrast, is identified by attempts to punish or embarrass the caregiver. These patterns were first identified in 6-year-olds by Main and Cassidy (1988), who found significant linkages between caregiving and punitive behavior at age 6 with attachment disorganization in infancy. Disorganized/controlling preschool attachment patterns are thus assigned a Group D classification in the Cassidy–Marvin system.

An alternative interpretation of caregiving and punitive behavior patterns in the preschool years is offered by Crittenden (1992, 1995), whose Preschool Assessment of Attachment (PAA) views each pattern as an organized variant of what she termed defended (Group A) or coercive (Group C) attachment strategy, respectively. This argument is based on the premise that, unlike the incoherent, confusing nature of disorganized behavior, caregiving and punitive preschool behavior patterns appear to serve the child strategically in accessing the attachment figure in times of stress. It is important to note, however, that Main and Cassidy (1988) and the Cassidy–Marvin system also described the caregiving and punitive behavior patterns as *organized* vis-_-vis the parent. Thus Cassidy–Marvin's use of the term "disorganized/controlling" to identify caregiving and punitive patterns creates confusion as to whether Group D children in the Cassidy–Marvin system should be conceptualized as organized or disorganized.

A principal aim of this chapter is to address the differing conceptualizations and interpretations of caregiving and punitive behavior in the preschool years and the relation of these to the construct of disorganization. Equally at issue are conceptualizations of those preschool children whose attachment behavior follows no clear-cut strategy, and who sometimes manifest fear or confusion in the attachment figure's presence. These latter children are also classified differently by the two preschool attachment classification systems. The Cassidy–Marvin system would likely assign an "insecure–other" label to these children, and insecure–other children in turn are frequently combined with controlling (caregiving and punitive) children into a single "Group D" classification for analysis. By contrast, Crittenden might classify such children into any of a number of groups—compulsively compliant, feigned helpless, insecure–other, anxious depressed, or disorganized—depending on the behavior markers observed. This chapter critically examines the published work that has employed the Cassidy–Marvin and Crittenden attachment classification systems for preschoolers in the service of advancing an integrated conceptualization of disorganization during this important transitional period.

Before commencing, however, two preliminary points are in order. First, evidence in support of the construct validity of both systems is fragmentary at best. For example, although secure and insecure Cassidy–Marvin attachment classifications map significantly onto secure and insecure attachment classifications derived from measures of attachment representations (e.g., Bretherton's doll-play measure and Klagsbrun & Bowlby's [1976] Separation Anxiety Test), discrimination among the various insecure Cassidy–Marvin patterns with these representational measures could not be established (Bretherton, Ridgeway, & Cassidy, 1990; Shouldice & Stevenson-Hinde, 1992). Furthermore, Posada, Waters, Cassidy, and Marvin (in press) found weak relations between Cassidy–Marvin classifications and Waters's (1995) Q-sort assessment of secure base behavior in the home (the Attachment Q-set). The absence of such an association is of concern, since it was the correspondence between Ainsworth's traditional classifications in infancy and observations of infant secure base behavior in the home that was crucial to the establishment of the validity of this system (Ainsworth et al., 1978). Similar concerns can be raised regarding Crittenden's (1992, 1995) PAA. Teti and Gelfand (1997) found differences between mothers of secure versus insecure preschoolers, favoring the secure group, on indices of maternal sensitivity. Teti et al. (1995) did not find a significant secure–insecure difference, however, using a measure of maternal behavioral competence in a different context. Furthermore, there has been no attempt to relate PAA classifications to preschoolers' secure base behavior in the home.

Second, the PAA and Cassidy–Marvin systems employ different coding manuals and, to some extent, different coding criteria, with the PAA making greater use of maternal behavior to classify than does the Cassidy–Marvin system. There is only partial overlap between the two systems in what is recognized as Group A, Group C, Group D, and insecure–other. In addition, the PAA's classification system is expanded to include several insecure patterns (e.g., anxious-depressed [Group AD] and defended/coercive [Group A/C]) that are not recognized by the Cassidy–Marvin system. The concordance between the two systems is thus not clear. Additional work at establishing points of agreement and disagreement between the two systems with regard to classifications that each have in common would make an important methodological contribution to the field.

These two caveats render especially daunting any attempt to use Cassidy–Marvin and PAA data to develop an integrated perspective on preschool disorganization. The perspective developed in this chapter, however, relies heavily on Main and Solomon's (1986, 1990) original and seminal formulations about disorganization, specifically, that it is hallmarked by fear, contradiction, or disorientation. Empirical evidence is marshaled from work with the Cassidy–Marvin system, and from my own work with the PAA, to advance the hypothesis that two subgroups of disorganized children can be identified in the preschool years. The first is described by clearly identifiable, organized caregiving or punitive behavior patterns that are strategic, albeit compensatory, behavioral responses to parental insufficiency, although they continue to reflect disorganization at the representational level. The second is identified by behavioral signs of disorganization, as indexed by unclassifiable behavior patterns and perhaps by the presence of behavioral markers of disorganization originally outlined by Main and Solomon (1990). Both subgroups are considered to be at higher risk for subsequent maladaptations than children with traditional A, B, or C classifications. It is argued, however, that the caregiving environments of behaviorally disorganized preschoolers may be especially compromised. Finally, in light of the conceptual distinctions among caregiving, punitive, and behaviorally disorganized children, it is proposed that research on preschool attachment would benefit from efforts to examine the caregiving antecedents and developmental sequelae of these groups individually.

THE CASSIDY–MARVIN PRESCHOOL ATTACHMENT SYSTEM

The development of the Cassidy–Marvin preschool attachment behavioral system is rooted in Main and Cassidy's (1988) finding of strong developmental linkages between attachment classifications at 1 year of age, using the traditional strange situation classification systems of Ainsworth et al. (1978) and Main and Solomon (1990), and attachment classifications to the mother derived from a protracted separation–reunion laboratory protocol (1-hour separation followed by a 3 to 5-minute reunion) developed for the same children at six years of age (see also Main, Kaplan, & Cassidy, 1985). Four major attachment classifications at age 6 years were identified that formed the conceptual basis for the Cassidy–Marvin system for preschoolers: Secure, insecure–avoidant, insecure–ambivalent, and insecure–controlling. The latter group was composed of children showing a predominantly nurturing and caregiving or a punitive pattern, and also included two children with behavior patterns that did not conform to any of the predesignated categories and thus were labeled insecure–unclassified. An impressive concordance rate of 84% between infant and 6-year-old attachment classifications was obtained for children's attachments to the mother, with an analagous rate of 61% obtained between infant and 6-year-old attachment classifications to fathers. Centrally relevant to this chapter was the finding that, of the 12 children classified as disorganized to mother in infancy, 75% ($n = 9$) belonged to the insecure–controlling group at 6 years of age (the remaining member of the insecure–controlling group was classified in infancy as insecure–avoidant).

Main and Cassidy's (1988) study provided an empirical basis for the scoring guidelines of the Cassidy–Marvin preschool attachment classification system, developed for children 3 to 4 years of age, and which resulted from several years of collaborative effort on the part of the MacArthur Working Group (chaired by Mark Greenberg). The Cassidy–Marvin system typically employs the original strange situation procedure or a modified strange situation procedure that involves two 3-minute mother–infant reunions. Table 8.1 provides the basic Cassidy–Marvin categories and their descriptions. The Cassidy–Marvin system (Cassidy, Marvin, et al., 1987/1990/1991/1992) identifies three major attachment groupings for preschoolers that map conceptually and straightforwardly onto the traditional secure, insecure–avoidant, and insecure–ambivalent classifications of infancy. *Secure* (Group B) children are identified by their comfortable, relaxed interaction with the parent and the successful use of the parent as a base to explore the environment. *Insecure–avoidant* (Group A) children are characterized by a cool detachment and avoidance of the parent, both physically and affectively. *Insecure–ambivalent* (Group C) children show a mixture of babyish, coy behavior and/or subtle anger and resistance. A fourth insecure grouping, *disorganized–controlling* (Group D), is identified in terms of three subclassifications: *controlling–caregiving* (i.e., nurturant, solicitous, overbright behavior suggestive of a reversal in child and caregiver roles); *controlling–punitive* (i.e., blatantly hostile behavior, clearly intended to punish, humiliate, or reject the parent), and *controlling–general* (i.e., controlling behavior that is neither caregiving or punitive, or that contains elements of both). A fifth category, *insecure–other*, is reserved for insecure children whose behavior does not fit the insecure–avoidant, insecure–ambivalent, or insecure–controlling categories, and who give evidence of fear, depressed affect, or sexualized behavior. Interestingly, a few studies using the Cassidy–Marvin system identified some children as *disorganized* (but not necessarily controlling) (DeMulder & Radke-Yarrow, 1991; Shouldice

TABLE 8.1. Cassidy–Marvin Attachment Classifications

Classification	Identifiers

Secure (Group B)
    Secure–reserved (B1-2)
    Secure–comfortable (B3)
    Secure–reactive (B4)
	Relaxed, open child–parent communication and successful use of the parent as a base to explore. The three subclassifications differ in the degree of separation protest and proximity seeking, with secure–reserved showing the least and secure–reactive the most of each.

Insecure–avoidant (Group A)	Blunted communication and avoidance of the parent along physical and affective domains. There is typically little if any protest or distress during separation from the parent.
Insecure–ambivalent (Group C)	Mix of "cutesy," babyish behavior and subtle signs of resistance toward the caregiver, which in turn impedes the child's ability to use the parent as a base to explore.
Controlling (Group D)	Overt attempts to control the parent, typically through the use of caregiving or punishing behavior, or a mixture of both.
Controlling–caregiving	Overbright, solicitous caregiving behavior directed toward the parent, suggestive of a reversal of parental and child roles.
Controlling–punitive	Blatant angry behavior directed to parent, designed to punish, reject, or humiliate.
Controlling–general	Controlling behavior that is neither caregiving nor punitive, or that contains elements of both.
Insecure–other (Group IO)	Behavior that does not fit any of the above categories. Sometimes characterized by fearful, depressed, or sexualized behavior.

& Stevenson-Hinde, 1992; Stevenson-Hinde & Shouldice, 1995), applying Main and Solomon's (1990) coding guidelines for identifying disorganization in infancy.

As with disorganized infants, the following review provides some evidence that children identified as controlling–caregiving or controlling–punitive either in the preschool (e.g., 3 to 4 years of age) or early school years (e.g., 5 to 7 years of age) have experienced more pathogenic caregiving environments and evince greater maladaptation in other domains of child functioning than do children classified as secure, insecure–avoidant, or insecure–ambivalent. The evidence is not always clear-cut, however, and may depend upon whether or not children exhibiting controlling–caregiving and punitive behavior patterns have been combined with other children for whom no clear-cut behavioral patterns could be identified (e.g., children classified as insecure–other, or as disorganized, using Main and Solomon's [1990] criteria). Indeed, combining children without clearly identifiable attachment strategies with children who show controlling strategies may yield a group at considerably higher risk relative to a group of controlling children alone. This discussion reviews findings from studies that used either the Cassidy–Marvin system for preschoolers or Main and Cassidy's (1988) hour-long separation–reunion procedure and classification criteria for early school-aged children, without any attempt to differentiate findings of one system from the other. It is presumed, although not yet empirically demonstrated, that both systems are analagous (indeed, Cassidy–Marvin classification criteria overlap strongly with those of Main and Cassidy) and yield attachment classifications whose derivation and meaning are the same.

Studies Involving Controlling Children Alone

Studies that have apparently compared controlling children alone (i.e., a controlling group into which no other atypical attachment classifications have been added) to children with traditional classifications (secure, insecure–avoidant, and insecure–ambivalent) yield a rather equivocal picture regarding the risk status of the controlling classification. Perhaps the clearest evidence that controlling children, without the addition of other anomalous classifications, are at higher risk than other, more typical attachment groupings is provided by Speltz, Greenberg, and DeKlyen (1990), who studied fifty 3- to 6-year-old children, 25 of whom were referred to a child psychiatry clinic for behavior problems, and 25 of whom served as controls. Speltz et al. used the Cassidy–Marvin classifications guidelines for 3 to 4-year-olds and the Main and Cassidy (1988) guidelines for 5 to 6-year-olds. A significantly higher percentage of clinic-referred children were classified as insecure–controlling (40%) than in the control sample (12%). An additional 16% of clinic children were designated insecure–other, in comparison to none in the control group, and proportions of insecure–ambivalent and insecure–avoidant children were relatively similar in the two groups. Significant differences between secure and insecure children, favoring the secure group, were found on internalizing and externalizing symptoms. Unfortunately, no comparisons were reported between the more typical attachment groups and either the insecure–controlling or insecure–other groups. In a second study using an identical classification methodology and similar-aged sample, Greenberg, Speltz, DeKlyen, and Endriga (1991) essentially replicated their earlier findings, with 32% of clinic-referred 3- to 6-year-olds classified as controlling in comparison to 4% of controls and 16% of clinic children designated insecure–other versus 8% of controls.

By contrast, two additional studies that identified a controlling group of children without any apparent incorporation of other atypical classifications present more equivocal findings. Cassidy's (1988) study of relations between representations of self among 6-year-olds and security of attachment, using Main and Cassidy's (1988) classification criteria, revealed clear and theoretically predicted correlates for secure and insecure–avoidant children. Three interview measures were designed to tap differences in attachment representations reflecting either a flexible/open or an avoidant/ "perfect" stance. Greater proportions of insecure–controlling children (44% and 31%), however, were placed into a flexible/open (secure) category in two of the three interviews than were insecure–avoidant children (25% and 13%) or insecure–ambivalent children (33% and 17%). This is inconsistent with the premise that the insecure–controlling category reflects greater maladaptation than the avoidant and ambivalent categories. Easterbrooks, Davidson, and Chazan's (1993) investigation of relations among psychosocial risk, attachment security [using Main and Cassidy's (1988) classification criteria], and maternally reported behavior problems in a sample of 7-year-olds of low socioeconomic status reported the highest percentage of clinical-range problem behavior among insecure–controlling children (67%), with insecure–avoidant children a close second. However, teachers identified no insecure–controlling children with clinical-range problems, rendering the risk status of insecure–controlling children somewhat inconclusive.

Finally, two studies that identified an insecure–controlling group found no evidence that insecure–controlling children are at higher risk than other attachment groups. Cohn's (1990) study of attachment security and social competence in school among eighty-nine 6-year-olds, employing Main and Cassidy's (1988) classification criteria, identified 15% of the sample (n = 13) as insecure–controlling and another 10% (n = 9) as insecure–unclassified. The latter were eliminated from analyses. Secure boys, in contrast to insecure boys, showed greater school-based social competence. However, whereas significant differences were reported between secure children and insecure–avoidant and insecure–ambivalent children on selected measures of social competence, no differences on any measure were found between secure children and insecure–controlling children. Cicchetti and Barnett (1991) examined differences in attachment security between a maltreated group and a control group of preschoolers at 30, 36, and 48 months, using the Cassidy–Marvin system, splitting off insecure–controlling from insecure–other children. Significant (and large) differences in the proportion of secure attachments, favoring the control group, were found at all three assessment periods. However, similar proportions of controlling children were found in the maltreated and control groups (9.1% vs. 7.5% at 30 months, 11.4% vs. 10.5% at 36 months, and 13.9% vs.

13.3% at 48 months). Interestingly, higher proportions of insecure–other children were found in the maltreated group versus controls at all three time points, although a significant difference emerged only at 30 months. When insecure–controlling and insecure–other children were combined, significantly higher proportions of such children again were found in the maltreated group, with a significant group difference at 30 months.

Studies Combining Controlling with "Insecure–Other" and Other Atypical Children

When controlling children are combined with children designated insecure–other or disorganized (using Main and Solomon's criteria for infants), differences between this combined group and the more standard preschool/early school age classifications are more consistent. Wartner, Grossmann, Fremmer-Bombik, and Suess (1994), in a follow-up study of attachment security from infancy to age 6, used Main and Cassidy's (1988) criteria to classify twelve 6-year-old children into a "disorganized" group that combined insecure–controlling and insecure–unclassified children. The number of children in this combined group with clear-cut controlling patterns versus children deemed unclassifiable was not reported. When observed at 5 years of age in the school setting, secure 6-year-olds most often fell into a group designated as socially competent, whereas controlling–unclassifiable children fell into the incompetent preschool behavior group almost as often as the insecure–avoidant group. Solomon, George, and DeJong (1995) also examined security of attachment among 6-year-olds, using Main and Cassidy's (1988) procedure, in relation to the children responses to a separation–reunion completion task (Bretherton et al., 1990) involving doll play, and to behavior problems as reported by mothers and teachers. Their disorganized/controlling group (referred to here as "controlling + other") combined punitive, caregiving, and unclassifiable children, the latter of whom were described as exhibiting some behavioral signs of disorganization from Main and Solomon's (1990) criteria. Based on the manner in which children represented attachment relationships in their narrative responses to the doll-play procedure, Solomon et al. classified children into one of the following four groups: confident (confidence in the availability of one's caregivers), casual (avoidance of and casual disinterest in caregivers), busy (stories characterized by delay, distraction, and irrelevancies), or frightened (out-of-control fear and destruction, or marked fright and inhibition). Strong concordance was found between attachment classifications derived from the separation–reunion procedure (Main & Cassidy, 1988) and the classifications derived from the doll-play procedure (kappa = .74, $p < .001$), with 73% of secure children classified as confident; 56% and 44% of insecure–avoidant children classified as casual or busy, respectively;

86% of insecure–ambivalent children classified as busy; and 100% of "controlling + other" children classified as frightened. In comparison to secure, avoidant, and ambivalent groups, the "controlling + other" group's doll play was characterized either by marked danger and chaos (parents depicted as frightening, children as helpless) or by marked inhibition, in which the children themselves appeared frightened and unwilling to participate in the task. Interestingly, doll-play narratives in which themes of chaos predominated were more closely associated with controlling–punitive children (8 of 10 children), whereas doll-play narratives characterized by marked inhibition were more likely to be exhibited by controlling–caregiving children (5 of 7 children). *All* children in the "controlling + other" group thus had "disorganized" *mental* representations of attachment that reflected an inability to construct a coherent narrative. This group was also reported by mothers and teachers to have more behavioral problems at home and in the classroom than children with more traditional (secure, insecure–avoidant, insecure–ambivalent) attachment classifications.

Additional work on preschool and early school-age children that combined controlling children with children assigned other atypical classifications (insecure–other and/or disorganized, as identified by Main and Solomon's criteria) has found clear differences between the combined "controlling + other" children and children with more typical, organized classifications. Shouldice and Stevenson-Hinde's (1992) examined 4.5-year-old children's responses on an adaptation of the Klagsbrun and Bowlby (1976) Separation Anxiety Test (SAT) in relation to security of attachment (using the Cassidy–Marvin system). They found a combined group of controlling (*n* = 6) and disorganized (*n* = 2, using Main and Solomon infancy criteria) children to provide more incoherent responses to SAT items than did any other attachment group. In a more recent study of attachment security, using the Cassidy–Marvin system, and behavior problems among 5- to 7-year-old French Canadian children, Moss, Parent, Gosselin, Rousseau, and St-Laurent (1996) identified a combined group of 8 insecure–controlling and 3 insecure–other children who were more likely to be rated by teachers as problem children at ages 3 to 5 and 5 to 7 years than were children in any other attachment group. Stevenson-Hinde and Shouldice's (1995) study of 4.5-year-olds, using the Cassidy–Marvin system, identified 11 children classifed either as insecure–other or as behaviorally disorganized; 2 were forced into the avoidant group, 6 into the ambivalent group, and 3 into the controlling group (in contrast to the more typical strategy of combining all such children into an insecure–disorganized–controlling category). In a structured laboratory task, the maternal behavior of children in the "insecure–controlling" group (which also contained 3 anomalously classified children) was the least supportive and sensitive of all attachment groups, with mothers of secure children rated consistently higher than mothers in any other attachment group.

Finally, two studies of infants and preschoolers, which combined into one group controlling, insecure–other, and "disorganized" children, found this group to be more at risk in terms of mother–child psychiatric status and mother–child interaction than were the more traditional attachment groups (DeMulder & Radke-Yarrow, 1991; Manassis, Bradley, Goldberg, Hood, & Swinson, 1994). DeMulder and Radke-Yarrow (1991) employed Ainsworth et al.'s (1978) and Main and Solomon's (1990) classification criteria to derive attachment classifications for children under 30 months of age, and the Cassidy–Marvin system to classify children between 30 and 54 months of age. Manassis et al. (1994) employed the Ainsworth et al. and Main and Solomon criteria for children between 18 and 23 months of age, and the Cassidy–Marvin system for children between 24 and 59 months.

In summary, studies using the Cassidy–Marvin scoring guidelines for preschoolers or Main and Cassidy's (1988) conceptually similar scoring guidelines for early school-age children find inconsistent differences between controlling (Group D) children and other, more traditional attachment groupings (Groups A, B, or C). By contrast, when controlling children are combined with children designated as insecure–other or insecure–disorganized (i.e., children with atypical behavior patterns that do not conform to any of the traditional Group A, B, or C patterns, or the controlling patterns), more reliable differences emerge between the "atypical" group and other groups. It is acknowledged that compositing insecure–other and insecure–disorganized children with controlling children does not violate the integrity of the theory underlying the Cassidy–Marvin and Main and Cassidy (1988) systems. Controlling, insecure–other, and insecure–disorganized children collectively represent nontraditional attachment classifications, and thus are combinable under the assumption that it would be inappropriate to place them with the traditional organized groupings. It is also acknowledged that compositing insecure–other, insecure–disorganized, and controlling children into a single group has at times been necessary due to very small numbers of one or more of these groups, which renders impossible a separate examination of each. At the same time, the foregoing review suggests that children with incoherent attachment patterns may represent a different and perhaps higher risk group than children with clearly identifiable controlling patterns. Crittenden's (1992) conceptualization of caregiving and punitive patterns as organized variants of defended and coercive attachment strategies, respectively, is consistent with this premise. Moreover, in her formulations, caregiving and punitive behavior represent different attachment strategies and thus should be treated separately rather than combined into a larger group.

CRITTENDEN'S PRESCHOOL ASSESSMENT OF ATTACHMENT

Like the Cassidy–Marvin system, Crittenden's (1992, 1995) Preschool Assessment of Attachment (PAA) identifies three major organized attachment classifications for children 3 to 4 years of age: *secure/balanced* (Group B), *defended* (Group A), and *coercive* (Group C). Secure/balanced children are identified by free and open access to the parent, shared communication about feelings and desires, and successful use of the parent as a secure base. This group maps conceptually onto the Group B (secure) children within the Cassidy–Marvin system. The PAA's Group A and Group C categories include some subclassifications that overlap with Cassidy–Marvin's Group A and Group C classifications. However, other subclassifications are also included in PAA Groups A and C that do not overlap with Cassidy–Marvin's A and C groups. There are also several major categories that represent further points of departure from Cassidy–Marvin. Table 8.2 presents the PAA categories, subcategories, and their descriptors, and Table 8.3 indicates hypothetical points of conceptual convergence and divergence between the two systems.

The PAA's defended classification is defined in terms of a behavioral strategy that allows access to the parent while minimizing emotional involvement and engagement. Defended children strike a balance between physical availability and emotional distance, drawing attention away from the relationship and toward more neutral topics, such as play with toys. There are three subclassifications: inhibited (A1-2), analogous to the Cassidy–Marvin insecure–avoidant classification; compulsively caregiving (A3), analogous to the Cassidy–Marvin controlling–caregiving category; and compulsively compliant (A4), identified by immobilization, marked fear/wariness of the caregiver, and anxious compliance to caregiver directives. Based on the classification guidelines, compulsive compliance would likely be classified by Cassidy–Marvin as insecure–other. The PAA's coercive classification designates a strategy whose aim is to force the involvement of the parent using threatening, helpless, coy, or punitive behavior. Coercive children's enmeshment with their caregivers substantially curtails competent exploration of the environment. There are four subclassifications: threatening (C1) and disarming (C2), which coincide with Cassidy–Marvin's insecure–ambivalent category; aggressive (C3), coinciding with Cassidy–Marvin's controlling–punitive classification, and referred to henceforth as punitive for clarity, and feigned helpless (C4), designated by exaggerated signs of helplessness and timidity so as to coerce the caregiver's attention and responsiveness. Children who feign helplessness might be classified by Cassidy–Marvin as insecure–other. The PAA also includes a defended–coercive (Group A/C) classification, identified by a mix of defended and coercive patterns that can be straightforwardly linked

TABLE 8.2. PAA Attachment Classifications

Classification	Identifiers
Secure (Group B) Secure–reserved (B1-2) Secure–comfortable (B3) Secure–reactive (B4)	Free, open access to parents, competent exploration of the environment when security needs are met, and open, shared communication with the parent about feelings and desires. The three subclassifications differ in the amount of separation protest and proximity seeking, with secure–reserved showing the least and secure–reactive the most.
Defended (Group A)	Overall strategy that functions to allow access to the parent without emotional involvement or confrontation.
Inhibited (A1-2)	Inhibition and tight control of negative affect, avoidance of close interaction with the parent, and strong focus on toy play as a means of deflecting attention from the relationship.
Compulsively caregiving (A3)	Mixture of avoidance, inhibition of negative affect, and overbright bits to cheer and nurture the parent.
Compulsively compliant (A4)	Excessive tension, fear, and vigilance around the parent; strong gaze aversion, hyperalertness to parent's movements, facial expression, and body postures.
Coercive (Group C)	Overall strategy that forces the availability and involvement of the parent by threatening angry behavior and/or disarming, "helpless" behavior.
Threatening (C1)	Confrontational behaviors such as threats to gain the parent's attention and agreement to the child's demands.
Disarming (C2)	Coy, sweet, helpless behavior serving to seduce the parent into compliance with the child's wishes.
Aggressive (C3)	Harshly punishing, rejecting behavior serving to control and humiliate the attachment figure into submission and compliance with child's demands.
Feigned helpless (C4)	Exaggerated helpless behavior with the aim of soliciting the parent's nurturance and attention.
Defended/coercive (Group A/C)	Blend of defended and coercive behaviors, either simultaneously or sequentially that is linked with shifts in the parent's behavior.
Anxious depressed (Group AD)	No definite strategy, accompanied by sad affect; lethargy; dazed, unfocused behavior; and/or extreme panic during separations that is not alleviated by parent's presence.
Disorganized (Group D)	An underlying strategy (Group A, B, C, or A/C) that is not fully implemented for reasons unrelated to the caregiver's behavior.
Insecure–other (Group IO)	Behavior that does not fit into any of the categories above.

TABLE 8.3. Hypothetical Points of Convergence and Divergence between the PAA and Cassidy–Marvin Systems

PAA categories	Corresponding Cassidy–Marvin categories
Convergence	
Secure (Group B)	Secure (Group B)
Secure–reserved (B1-2)	Secure–reserved (B1-2)
Secure–comfortable (B3)	Secure–comfortable (B3)
Secure–reactive (B4)	Secure–reactive (B4)
Defended (Group A)	
Inhibited (A1-2)	Insecure–avoidant (Group A)
Coercive (Group C)	
Threatening (C1) and disarming (C2)	Insecure–ambivalent (Group C)
Divergence	
Defended (Group A)	
Compulsively caregiving (A3)	Controlling–caregiving (Group D)
Compulsively compliant (A4)	Insecure–other (Group IO)
Coercive (Group C)	
Aggressive (C3)	Controlling–punitive (Group D)
Feigned helpless (C4)	Insecure–other (Group IO)
Defended/coercive (Group A/C)	Insecure–other (Group IO)
Anxious depressed (Group AD)	Insecure–other (Group IO)
Disorganized (Group D)	Insecure–other (Group IO)
Insecure–other (Group IO)	Insecure–other (Group IO)

to changes in caregiver behavior. Cassidy–Marvin would perhaps classify the PAA's group A/C as insecure–other, or might force-classify it into insecure–avoidant, insecure–ambivalent, or insecure–controlling, depending on the specific behaviors observed.

Finally, The PAA assigns children without clear-cut secure–balanced, defended, coercive, or defended–coercive strategies to one of three categories: insecure–other (Group IO), anxious depressed (Group AD), or disorganized (Group D). All of these might likely be classified in the Cassidy–Marvin system as insecure–other. The PAA employs the insecure–other classification for children whose behavior does not fit into any of the organized, disorganized, or anxious depressed categories. Children classified as anxious depressed originally had the classification insecure–other/anxious depressed, because these children did not deploy behavior that clearly fit any of the organized PAA categories, but were later relabeled as anxious depressed (Crittenden, 1995), because they also manifested some combination of sad affect and lethargy; "dissociative" behavior such as dazed, blank staring; and extreme panic after the caregiver's departure. The dissociative behavior characteristic of anxious depressed preschoolers is similar to that previously identified by Main and Solomon (1990) and Main and Hesse (1990) in describing disorganized infants. Finally, children classified as disorganized in this system are identified by the presence of an underlying but uncoordinated strategy, the implementation of which is asynchronous with, and not logically tied to, the caregiver's behavior. The disorganized classification would be expected to be quite rare in the PAA system.

Two points about the PAA are especially noteworthy. First, at the behavioral level, classifying caregiving (subgroup A3) and punitive children (subgroup C3) as defended and coercive, respectively, rather than as disorganized, has face validity. Indeed, the strategies of caregiving and punitive children for accessing their attachment figures, and for maintaining these relationships over time, seem clear-cut, and it is not difficult to differentiate reliably between the two. Compulsively caregiving children, by virtue of their nurturance and overbrightness when interacting with their attachment figures, give the appearance of attempting to repair and/or maintain a damaged parent–child relationship that may have resulted from having a caregiver who is physically or psychologically withdrawn from the relationship. Punitive children, by contrast, function similarly to other coercive children (e.g., threatening and disarming children) but make special strategic use of a mix of punishment, humiliation, and coy/sweet behavior to keep their attachment figures off-balance as the latter strive to meet their children's demands. Caregiving and punitive children *look different* from each other and are identified by behavior that reflects an underlying logic. Under the assumption that the punitive and caregiving strategies show some degree of temporal stability, combining these two categories into a single group, which is typically done by Cassidy–Marvin users, may blur any caregiving antecedents or developmental sequelae that may be unique to one of these categories and not the other. It is important to note, however, that temporal stability of caregiving and punitive categories has not yet been demonstrated, nor has it yet been shown if the caregiving antecedents of each of these categories differ. Furthermore, both categories share important features with traditional avoidant or ambivalent attachment groups. If PAA assumptions that caregiving and punitive patterns represent distinctly different strategies are correct, however, this may in part explain the equivocal results that have been obtained when caregiving and punitive children are combined and contrasted with secure, insecure–avoidant, and insecure–ambivalent children. That punitive and caregiving children deserve separate recognition was underscored by Solomon et al.'s (1995) finding with 6-year-olds that qualitatively distinct doll-play themes were associated with punitive versus caregiving classifications. Furthermore, George and Solomon (1998) provide suggestive evidence that caregiving and punitive children may experience qualitatively distinct caregiving histories, a point to which we will return.

Second, an effective argument can be made for combining the more atypical PAA classifications such as insecure–other, disorganized, and anxious depressed into a composite group on the conceptual basis that such children have in common the inability to muster a coherent, organized behavioral strategy for dealing effectively with their attachment figures. It is argued that compositing these children in a separate group for analysis, given sufficient Ns, is more informative than combining them with controlling children, as many have done using the Cassidy–Marvin system. In their sample of 54 preschoolers (defined in this study as between 21 and 54 months of age) of clinically depressed and nondepressed mothers, Teti and his colleagues (e.g., Teti & Gelfand, 1997) formed a composite group of 11 such children, including 9 anxious depressed, 1 insecure–other, and 1 defended/coercive, on the conceptual basis that these children conspicuously lacked unitary and coherent strategies in the strange situation procedure during reunions with their mothers. Interestingly, 4 of these 11 children also exhibited some of the freezing/stilling and other behavioral anchors identified by Main and Solomon (1990) as indicative of disorganization. This prompted Teti and Gelfand (1997) to suggest that these children be more parsimoniously termed "disorganized," in keeping with Main and Solomon's (1986, 1990) original conceptual formulations about disorganization as reflecting an inability to marshal a coherent, logical strategy coupled with behavioral indices of fear, confusion, and/or dissociation. Such a change in terminology would also be welcome because of my discomfort with the label "anxious depressed," a term that has the flavor of a psychiatric diagnosis. These children singularly lacked a coherent means for accessing their attachment figures, showing striking parallels in some cases with disorganized infants by the presence of freezing/stilling and other D-like indices. It is argued that attachment classificatory systems can be most useful if they do not stray from Bowlby's (1969) and Ainsworth's (Ainsworth et al., 1978) original formulations regarding the secure base construct as the principal underlying framework for classifying children. Stated differently, attachment classification systems should describe attachment behavior and not become proxies for psychiatric diagnostic systems. If they do, they run the risk of overspecifying the very construct they purport to measure, and in turn jeopardizing the viability of that construct if the system cannot be empirically supported (see Cook & Campbell, 1979, for a discussion of this issue).

The significance of constructing this behaviorally disorganized composite group of anxious depressed, insecure–other, and defended/coercive children was evident in comparisons between this group and the more typical or "organized" PAA classifications (Teti et al., 1995). Indeed, this group was clearly the most maladapted of all attachment groupings for both maternal and child indicators of functioning. Nine of the 11 children in this group were children of clinically depressed mothers and comprised 29% of all children of clinically depressed mothers. In separate comparisons, mothers in this composite group reported significantly higher levels of parenting stress and were rated by "blind" observers during 10-minute observations of feeding and free play as significantly less behaviorally competent than were mothers of secure, defended, and coercive children.

Thus, these findings identified preschoolers with incoherent behavioral strategies and their mothers to be the most at-risk of all attachment groups in this variable risk sample. Although "classic" signs of disorganization, using Main and Solomon's (1990) criteria, were not present in every child in this group, *all* children were lacking a single, coherent behavioral strategy in the strange situation procedure. For simplicity and clarity, such children will heretofore be referred to as *behaviorally disorganized*.

MENTAL VERSUS BEHAVIORAL DISORGANIZATION: REVISITING MAIN AND SOLOMON

This still leaves us with somewhat of a conundrum in conceptualizing controlling children. On the one hand, they are viewed within the framework of Cassidy–Marvin as disorganized, with two studies establishing strong longitudinal links between controlling patterns at age 6 years and disorganization in infancy (Main & Cassidy, 1988; Wartner et al., 1994). On the other hand, Crittenden (1992) views the caregiving and punitive patterns as reflecting face valid, organized strategies for maintaining access to an attachment figure and considers them to be more maladaptive variants of her defended and coercive categories, respectively.

Additional evidence from Main et al. (1985), and more recently from Solomon et al. (1995) and George and Solomon (1998), on 6-year-olds may offer a way out of this dilemma. In these studies, controlling children's *mental* representations of attachment, as assessed from their responses to hypothetical parent–child separations and to family photographs, were qualitatively distinct from those of secure, insecure–avoidant, and insecure–ambivalent children. Main et al. (1985) found secure children's verbal responses to be characterized by flexibility, openness, fluency, and ease of access to affect and memory, which was reflective of the balanced, open style of emotion regulation and coping that typifies secure infants in the strange situation procedure. Secure children responded with interest and positive (but not overbright) emotion to a family photograph. Insecure–

avoidant children, by contrast, presented an avoidant pattern in their verbal responses to the vignettes, showing discomfort when discussing emotions in response to hypothetical parent–child separations and actively
avoiding family photographs. Insecure–disorganized–controlling children
were highly dysfluent in their responses and provided distressed and/or
irrational responses to the parent–child separation vignettes. When presented with a family photograph, these children frequently manifested
depression and some behavioral disorganization (e.g., one child became
quiet for 12 seconds while bending over the photograph, reminiscent of a
"stilling" response that characterizes some disorganized infants). Comparisons in this study involving the insecure–ambivalent classification were not
performed because only 2 children among the 40 assessed at age 6 were so
classified.

Solomon et al. (1995) and George and Solomon (1998) provided an
essential replication of these findings in their study, reviewed earlier, of
attachment representations in 69 six-year-olds. Although this study combined behaviorally disorganized (insecure–other, in Main and Cassidy's
[1988] system) children with controlling children, it is important to note
that *all* such children had *mental* representations of attachment that
reflected underlying themes of fear, confusion, chaos, and disorganization.
In addition, George and Solomon (1988) reported from semistructured
interviews with mothers that mothers of controlling children, regardless of
whether the children has been classified as punitive or caregiving,
reported feeling helpless and out of control in their relationships with their
children (in contrast to mothers of children with more typical, organized
attachments). This study also provided evidence suggesting that the punitive and caregiving classifications have qualitatively distinct caregiving
antecedents. Mothers of punitive children described their relationships
with their children as confrontational, combative, and adversarial, with
continual attempts by both mother and child to take control of the relationship. By contrast, mothers of caregiving children appeared to be disinvest-
ed in their relationships with their children, expressing the desire to withdraw, flee, or disappear from them.

From these findings and those from Teti and his colleagues on behaviorally disorganized preschoolers, it is proposed that controlling and
behaviorally disorganized preschoolers and young school-age children represent two different levels of disorganization. At the behavioral level, and
following Crittenden's (1992) formulations, controlling children can be
considered organized, based on the existence of behavior patterns that are
coherent, strategic means for managing their relationships with their caregivers. Perhaps beginning as behaviorally disorganized in infancy, these
children have learned over time that their caregivers are best accessed via

role reversing, reparative nurturance, and overbrightness, or by a harsh use of embarrassment and punishment that is used strategically to meet these children's attachment needs. Controlling behavior patterns have been viewed as developing in response to unpredictable, potentially frightening caregiving environments (Main & Cassidy, 1988; Main & Hesse, 1990). At the behavioral level, controlling patterns might thus be considered strategic, learned response patterns that develop over time in response to parental insufficiency. George and Solomon (1998) have proposed that punitive behavior patterns evolve in response to maternal confrontation and hostility, whereas caregiving patterns develop as a reparative response to maternal withdrawal. These behavior patterns may thus be adaptive in the short run, but may be be maladaptive over the longer term or in other contexts (see Jacobvitz & Hazen, Chapter 5, this volume). In either case, however, caregiving and punitive strategies are viewed here as more adaptive than is the absence of a coherent behavioral strategy. Controlling children remain disorganized at the representational level, however, as empirically demonstrated by Main et al. (1985), Solomon et al. (1995), and George and Solomon (1988).

Behavioral disorganization in the preschool and early school-age years would by default also be expected to be disorganized at the representational level, a premise again receiving support from Solomon et al. (1995). Behavioral disorganization in the preschool years would be an expected product of long-term chronically and severely impaired parenting, like the behaviorally disorganized preschoolers of persistently debilitated and depressed mothers in Gelfand and Teti's maternal depression project. One can only speculate as to the nature and quality of the caregiving environments to which behaviorally disorganized children are exposed over the long term. What seems clear, however, is that such children have not been able to develop a compensatory strategy (e.g., a caregiving or punitive pattern), either because of their own developmental limitations and/or perhaps because their caregiving environments are sufficiently and chronically unpredictable, frightening, and overwhelming that the development of a compensatory strategy was not possible. These children are expected to manifest greater levels of relational difficulties with parents and to be at greater risk more generally than are controlling children, because the former have been unable to develop a coherent means of coping with caregiver dysfunction. Until now, this hypothesis has not been systematically tested, although the findings of Cicchetti and Barnett (1991) are consistent with it. Cicchetti and Barnett found greater proportions of children with a mixture of avoidance and resistance (indicative of behavioral disorganization) in their abused group relative to nonabused controls but no group differences in the proportions of controlling children.

A COMPARISON OF SECURE, CONTROLLING, AND BEHAVIORALLY DISORGANIZED CHILDREN

This hypothesis is tested here in a preschool sample examined in collaboration with Donna Gelfand (see Teti et al., 1995; Gelfand, Teti, Seiner, & Jameson, 1996). Secure, controlling, and behaviorally disorganized preschoolers of depressed and nondepressed mothers are compared with respect to mother–child interaction; maternal reports of depressive symptoms, negative life events, and their children's fussy-difficultness; and children's performance on the Bayley Mental Developmental Index (MDI; Bayley, 1969). If behaviorally disorganized preschoolers reflect higher levels of parent–child dysfunction than do controlling children, we expected to find more frequent differences between secure and behaviorally disorganized children than between secure and controlling children. We also expected differences to emerge between the behaviorally disorganized and the controlling groups, with the latter showing more favorable functioning.

A principal aim of the Gelfand–Teti project was to examine the effects of clinical maternal depression on the socioemotional and intellectual functioning of infants and preschoolers. All depressed mothers who were recruited were in therapy for depression, with a DSM-III-R diagnosis of either major depression, dysthymia, or adjustment disorder with depression as a major feature, and were referred to the project by their therapists. Nondepressed mothers were recruited from similar neighborhoods as the depressed mothers through the help of the Utah Department of Health. All mothers had infants in the first year of life (M age = 7.16 months of age) at recruitment, and both questionnaire and observational data were obtained from mothers and their children at four time points in this longitudinal study: Time 1 (recruitment), Time 2 (approximately 13 months after recruitment), Time 3 (approximately 20 months after recruitment), and Time 4 (approximately 32 months after recruitment).

The present analyses are concerned with questionnaire and mother–child observational data obtained at Times 1, 2, and 3. The preschool attachment data reported here were obtained from strange situation videorecordings made in the university laboratory at Time 2, using Crittenden's PAA for all children 21 months of age and older (n = 54) Children under 21 months of age were separately assessed using the Ainsworth's traditional classification system and Main and Solomon's (1990) criteria for classifying disorganization in infancy, and will not be discussed here. Questionnaire data analyzed include mothers' reports of depressive symptoms from the Beck Depression Inventory (Beck, Ward, Mendelson, Mock, & Erbaugh, 1961), negative major life events (from an adaptation of the Life Experiences Survey; Sarason, Johnson, & Siegel, 1978); and child's fussy-difficultness (from the Infant Characteristics Questionnaire; Bates, Freeland, & Lounsbury, 1979). Observational measures included home-based ratings of maternal and child behavior during 10-minute observations of feeding and free play with toys. Raters blind to all other maternal–child data rated mothers on four 5-point Likert-type scales adapted from Zoll, Lyons-Ruth, and Connell (1984): *sensitivity* (ability to read and respond appropriately to child signals), *warmth* (quality of affection expressed toward child), *flatness of affect* (amount of impassive, expressionless affect expressed toward child), and *disengagement* (disconnection from child as gleaned from body positioning, pacing, or control of interaction). These four behaviors as a group possessed high internal reliability (see Teti et al., 1995), and after adjusting ratings as necessary so that higher scores reflected more optimal behavior, these four scales were summed into a composite measure, *maternal behavioral competence*, to be used in analyses. Children's behavior in interactions with mother were rated on two variables derived from the Infant Behavior Record of the Bayley Scales of Infant Development (Bayley, 1969), *interest in and involvement with mother* (higher scores mean more interest/involvement during interactions), and *general emotional tone* (lower scores mean higher levels of fussy, negative behavior during interactions). Finally, the Bayley MDI (Bayley, 1969), administered at Time 2, is also analyzed here. The reader is referred to Teti et al. (1995) and Gelfand et al. (1996) for a detailed description of the full project.

Three PAA-derived attachment groups of children and their mothers were of interest here: Secure (Group B, $n = 14$), controlling (a combined group of caregiving [defended subgroup A3, $n = 6$] and punitive [coercive subgroup C3, $n = 6$] children, combined $n = 12$), and behaviorally disorganized children (a subsample consisting of 9 anxious depressed children, 1 insecure–other child, and 1 defended/coercive child, combined $n = 11$). With the exception of the Bayley MDI, which was analyzed at Time 2 only, the means of all dependent variables across Times 1, 2, and 3 were used. One-way analyses of variance were conducted with planned contrasts (nonorthogonal) that compared secure with controlling, secure with behaviorally disorganized, and controlling with behaviorally disorganized children. Because these analyses were considered exploratory and hypothesis generating, no special control of Type I error was taken, although such control would of course be essential in subsequent attempts by others to replicate or extend these findings.

Omnibus F values for each analysis were significant, and Table 8.4 summarizes the results of the planned contrasts. No significant differences emerged between secure and controlling children, with the exception of the Bayley MDI scores, which favored secure children over controlling children. However, *all* comparisons between secure and behaviorally disorganized children were significant. Mothers of behaviorally disorganized chil-

TABLE 8.4. Comparisons among Secure, Controlling, and Behaviorally Disorganized Preschoolers of Depressed and Nondepressed Mothers

	Variable means						
	Maternal			Child			
Attachment group	Severity of maternal depression	Negative life events	Behavioral competence	Fussy–difficultness	General emotional tone	Interest in and involvement with mother	Bayley MDI
Secure (PAA group B, $n = 14$)	13.6 (9.1)[a]	3.0 (2.2)[a]	33.4 (3.6)[a]	27.2 (7.8)[a]	7.9 (0.7)[a]	7.1 (1.0)[a]	111.6 (17.8)[a]
Controlling [Caregiving (PAA subgroup A3, $n = 6$) + punitive (PAA subgroup C3, $n = 6$); total $n = 12$]	13.4 (8.9)[a]	4.8 (2.7)[a]	31.5 (3.4)[a]	30.1 (7.0)[ab]	7.3 (0.9)[ab]	7.2 (1.1)[a]	98.4 (11.2)[b]
Behaviorally disorganized [PAA anxious/depressed ($n = 9$), insecure–other ($n = 1$), and defended/coercive ($n = 1$); Total $n = 11$]	21.1 (9.8)[b]	5.6 (2.2)[b]	27.5 (4.6)[b]	36.0 (5.0)[b]	6.8 (0.8)[b]	5.9 (0.7)[b]	93.6 (12.3)[b]

Note. Values in parentheses are standard deviations. Groups without superscripts in common are significantly different, $p < .05$. All group means presented were averaged across Times 1, 2, and 3 of the project, except the Bayley MDI (Time 2 only). See text for further variable description.

dren reported more depressive symptoms, more negative life events, and saw their children as fussier than did mothers of secure children. Furthermore, "blind" observers of mother–child interaction rated mothers of behaviorally disorganized children as significantly less competent than mothers of secure children, and behaviorally disorganized children as showing less interest in, and responsivity to, their mothers, and more negative emotion, than secure children. Behaviorally disorganized children also received poorer scores on the Bayley MDI than did secure children. The behaviorally disorganized group also differed significantly from the controlling group on several variables, including maternal depressive symptoms, negative life events, maternal behavioral competence, and children's interest in, and responsivity to, the mother. All differences indicated poorer functioning in the behaviorally disorganized group.

COMPARING SECURE, CAREGIVING, AND PUNITIVE CHILDREN

A final set of comparisons was conducted among the secure, caregiving, and punitive groups to explore whether caregiving or punitive children could be differentially distinguished from secure children on the same dependent variable set. These analyses, presented in Table 8.5 suffered from low statistical power due to small cell sizes in the caregiving ($n = 6$) and punitive ($n = 6$) groups, and Table 8.5 thus indicates any difference for which $p < .10$. Noteworthy among these findings is the paucity of differences between the secure (Group B) and caregiving (subgroup A3) group, with only one comparison marginally significant, involving negative life events, favoring the secure group ($p < .10$). By contrast, the punitive group (subgroup C3) differed from the secure group on child fussy-difficultness ($p < .10$), children's general emotional tone during interactions with mothers ($p < .05$), and on Bayley MDI scores ($p < .05$). In all cases, worse functioning was associated with the punitive group. Finally, punitive children received poorer scores during interactions with mothers on general emotional tone ($p < .10$) and interest in and involvement with the mother ($p < .10$) than did caregiving children. Although these results are exploratory and require replication, they suggest that punitive children look worse to observers than do caregiving children, which is not necessarily surprising given that punitive children, by definition, are more aggressive and oppositional in their interactions with their caregivers and perhaps to nonfamilial adults. It would be premature to conclude, however, that the punitive attachment classification confers a higher risk status on children than does the caregiving classification in light of George and Solomon's (1988) findings that both punitive and caregiving children were disorganized at the

TABLE 8.5. Comparison among Secure, Caregiving, and Punitive Attachment Groups

	Variable means						
	Maternal				Child		
Attachment group	Severity of maternal depression	Negative life events	Behavioral competence	Fussy–difficultness	General emotional tone	Interest in and involvement with mother	Bayley MDI
Secure (PAA group B, $n = 14$)	13.6 (9.1)[a]	3.0 (2.2)[a]	33.4 (3.5)[a]	27.2 (7.8)[a]	7.9 (0.7)[a]	7.1 (1.0)[ab]	111.6 (17.8)[a]
Caregiving (PAA subgroup A3, $n = 6$)	9.7 (6.4)[a]	5.6 (3.7)[b]	32.3 (3.7)[a]	27.0 (4.9)[ab]	7.8 (0.9)[a]	7.7 (1.2)[a]	100.5 (8.3)[ab]
Punitive (PAA subgroup C3, $n = 6$)	18.0 (10.2)[a]	3.9 (0.9)[ab]	30.8 (3.3)[a]	33.9 (7.9)[b]	6.8 (0.4)[b]	6.6 (0.7)[b]	96.3 (14.0)[b]

Note. Values in parentheses are standard deviations. Groups without superscripts in common are different, $p < .10$ or lower. All group means presented were averaged across Times 1, 2, and 3 of the project, except the Bayley MDI (Time 2 only). See text for further variable description.

level of representation. Determining if caregiving versus punitive children have different caregiving antecedents, and examining the developmental sequelae of such classifications, are viewed here as critically important to the field.

CONCLUSIONS AND FUTURE DIRECTIONS

This chapter has attempted to clarify disparate findings regarding the construct of disorganization in the preschool years and to provide the beginnings of an integrative framework that might guide future research on the conceptualization and measurement of disorganization during these periods. It has been argued that controlling patterns of behavior in the preschool period represent strategic, behaviorally organized, albeit maladaptive means of achieving and maintaining access to attachment figures. Given their empirical links with disorganization in infancy, these patterns have been hypothesized to develop in compensatory fashion as a learned response to potentially frightening caregiving behavior (Crittenden, 1992; George & Solomon, 1999; Main & Cassidy, 1988; Main & Hesse, 1990; Solomon & George, 1996). These patterns may assist children over the short run in coping more effectively with serious parental insufficiency, which would help explain the similarity between the controlling and secure groups in the present analyses, and the equivocal findings in earlier reports regarding the degree to which such children are at higher risk than children who are placed into the standard attachment groups. Such compensatory behavior patterns, however, belie these children's representations of attachment, which are earmarked by fear, confusion, and/or inhibition (Main et al., 1985; Solomon et al., 1995, George & Solomon, 1998). Thus, although controlling children evince organized, albeit compensatory strategies at the behavioral level, they remain disorganized representationally. What long-term disadvantages this representational status confers on controlling children in their relationships with their attachment figures and other emergent attachment figures later in life is unclear.

The premise that caregiving and punitive preschoolers and early school-age children deploy coherent, organized attachment behavior patterns calls for more systematic attempts to understand how these two groups differ in terms of the manner in which the caregiver, the infant, and the social environment contribute jointly to different controlling patterns in the preschool years. This perspective is consistent with George and Solomon (1999), who recently noted an evolving emphasis in attachment research that incorporates not only maternal sensitivity but also infant, familial, and social–contextual influences on attachment security. George and Solomon (1999) are particularly concerned with such influences, as they impact on the quality of care provided to young children. Although both punitive and caregiving patterns are viewed as strategic means of gaining and maintaining access to caregivers (Crittenden, 1992; George & Solomon, 1998, 1999), of particular interest is whether, or how, infant temperamental styles and mothers' social environments might contribute to individual differences in maternal caregiving, and in turn, to differences in attachment quality. Are hostile, confrontational caregiving, and, in turn, punitive behavior patterns in preschoolers, more likely to develop in response to infants who are temperamentally prone to distress and negative affect, and/or in the context of a hostile family environment? In what ways might infant temperamental difficulty and/or lack of emotional or instrumental support from fathers contribute to a mother's desire to withdraw and escape from her relationship with her child? Exploring such questions would require extensive, systematic investigation of the caregiver, child, and family interactions in the home, over successive time points, in the pioneer spirit of Ainsworth et al.'s (1978) validation of the infant classification system.

Subsequent research should address the extent to which there are any long-term differential consequences of caregiving versus punitive attachment strategies. In light of the present analyses, it would be of particular interest to explore whether punitive children are more predisposed toward higher levels of externalizing symptoms in home and school contexts over the long term than are caregiving children, and to assess whether caregiving children might be more predisposed toward manifesting internalizing symptomatology. Treating caregiving and punitive children as distinct entities, as Solomon et al. (1995) and George and Solomon (1998) have begun to do, may yield important insights about how these attachment strategies impact on the child over the long term.

Finally, it has been proposed that children who lack clear-cut, coherent strategies for accessing attachment figures, termed "behaviorally disorganized" herein, may be at substantially higher risk for relational and behavioral problems than are controlling children and should be treated as a distinct group rather than combined with controlling children. Indeed, that behavioral disorganization exists at all beyond infancy raises questions about etiology and developmental significance. What differentiates the caregiving environments of disorganized infants who are able to develop compensatory controlling patterns by the preschool years from those of children who start off as disorganized in infancy but remain unable to develop compensatory, organized behavioral strategies vis-à-vis their caregivers beyond infancy? It is proposed that behaviorally disorganized children are exposed to significantly worse caregiving environments (e.g., caregiving that is persistently chaotic, unpredictable, and frightening) than are children who develop controlling strategies, rendering impossible the development of a compensatory controlling strategy. Testing this hypothesis, it is argued, is a worthy goal of attachment research.

REFERENCES

Ainsworth, M. D. S., Blehar, M. C., Waters, E., & Wall, S. (1978). *Patterns of attachment: A psychological study of the Strange Situation.* Hillsdale, NJ: Erlbaum.

Bates, J. E., Freeland, C. A., & Lounsbury, M. L. (1979). Measurement of infant difficultness. *Child Development, 50,* 794–803.

Bayley, N. (1969). *Manual for the Bayley Scales of Infant Development.* San Antonio, TX: Psychological Corporation.

Beck, A. T., Ward, C. H., Mendelson, M., Mock, J., & Erbaugh, J. (1961). An inventory for measuring depression. *Archives of General Psychiatry, 4,* 561–571.

Bowlby, J. (1969). *Attachment and loss: Vol. 1. Attachment.* New York: Basic Books.

Bretherton, I., Ridgeway, D., & Cassidy, J. (1990). Assessing internal working models of the attachment relationship: An attachment story completion task for 3-year-olds. In M. T. Greenberg, D. Cicchetti, & E. M. Cummings (Eds.), *Attachment in the preschool years: Theory, research, and intervention* (pp. 273–308). Chicago: University of Chicago Press.

Carlson, V., Cicchetti, D., Barnett, D., & Braunwald, K. (1989). Disorganized/disoriented attachment relationships in maltreated infants. *Developmental Psychology, 25,* 525–531.

Cassidy, J. (1988). Child–mother attachment and the self in six-year-olds. *Child Development, 59,* 121–134.

Cassidy, J., Marvin, R. S., & the Working Group of the John D. and Catherine T. MacArthur Foundation on the Transition from Infancy to Early Childhood. (1987/1990/1991/1992). *Attachment organization in three- and four-year olds: Coding guidelines.* Unpublished manuscript, University of Virginia, Charlottesville.

Cicchetti, D., & Barnett, D. (1991). Attachment organization in maltreated preschoolers. *Development and Psychopathology, 3,* 397–411.

Cohn, D. A. (1990). Child–mother attachment of six-year-olds and social competence at school. *Child Development, 61,* 152–162.

Cook, T. D., & Campbell, D. T. (1979). *Quasi-experimentation: Design and analysis issues for field settings.* Chicago: Rand McNally College.

Crittenden, P. M. (1992). Quality of attachment in the preschool years. *Development and Psychopathology, 4,* 209–241.

Crittenden, P. M. (1995). *Coding Manual: Classification of quality of attachment for preschool-aged children.* Miami, FL: Family Relations Institute.

DeMulder, E. K., & Radke-Yarrow, M. (1991). Attachment with affectively ill and well mothers: Concurrent behavioral correlates. *Development and Psychopathology, 3,* 227–242.

Easterbrooks, M. A., Davidson, C. E., & Chazan, R. (1993). Psychosocial risk, attachment, and behavior problems among school-aged children. *Development and Psychopathology, 5,* 389–402.

Gelfand, D. M., Teti, D. M., Seiner, S. A., & Jameson, P. B. (1996). Helping mothers fight depression: Evaluation of a home-based intervention program for depressed mothers and their infants. *Journal of Clinical Child Psychology, 25,* 406–422.

George, C., & Solomon, J. (1998, July). *Attachment disorganization at age six: Differences in doll play between punitive and caregiving children.* Paper presented at the meeting of the International Society for the Study of Behavioural Development, Bern, Switzerland.

George, C., & Solomon, J. (1999). Attachment and caregiving: The caregiving behavioral system. In J. Cassidy & P. R. Shaver (Eds.), *Handbook of attachment: Theory, research, and clinical application* (pp. 649–670). New York: Guilford Press.

Greenberg, M. T., Speltz, M. L., DeKlyen, M., & Endriga, M. C. (1991). Attachment security in preschoolers with and without externalizing behavior problems: A replication. *Development and Psychopathology, 3,* 413–430.

Klagsbrun, M., & Bowlby, J. (1976). Responses to separation from parents: A clinical test for young children. *British Journal of Projective Psychology and Personality Study, 21,* 7–27.

Lyons-Ruth, K., Connell, D. B., Grunebaum, H., & Botein, S. (1990). Infants at social risk: Maternal depression and family support services as mediators of infant development and security of attachment. *Child Development, 61,* 85–98.

Main, M., & Cassidy, J. (1988). Categories of response to reunion with the parent at age 6: Predictable from infant attachment classifications and stable over a 1-month period. *Developmental Psychology, 24,* 415–426.

Main, M., & Hesse, E. (1990). Parents' unresolved traumatic experiences are related to infant disorganized attachment status: Is frightened and/or frightening parental behavior the linking mechanism? In M. T. Greenberg, D. Cicchetti, & E. M. Cummings (Eds.), *Attachment in the preschool years: Theory, research, and intervention* (pp. 161–182). Chicago: University of Chicago Press.

Main, M., Kaplan, N., & Cassidy, J. (1985). Security in infancy, childhood, and adulthood: A move to the level of representation. In I. Bretherton & E. Waters (Eds.), Growing points of attachment theory and research. *Monographs of the Society for Research in Child Development, 50*(1–2, Serial No. 209), 66–104.

Main, M., & Solomon, J. (1986). Discovery of a new, insecure–disorganized/disoriented attachment pattern. In M. Yogman & T. B. Brazelton (Eds.), *Affective development in infancy* (pp. 95–124). Norwood, NJ: Ablex.

Main, M., & Solomon, J. (1990). Procedures for identifying infants as disorganized/disoriented during the Ainsworth Strange Situation. In M. T. Greenberg, D. Cicchetti, & E. M. Cummings (Eds.), *Attachment in the preschool years: Theory, research, and intervention* (pp. 121–160). Chicago: University of Chicago Press.

Manassis, K., Bradley, S., Goldberg, S., Hood, J., & Swinson, R. P. (1994). Attachment in mothers with anxiety disorders and their children. *Journal of the American Academy of Child and Adolescent Psychiatry, 33,* 1106–1113.

Moss, E., Parent, S., Gosselin, C., Rousseau, D., & St-Laurent, D. (1996). Attachment and teacher-reported behavior problems during the preschool and early school-age period. *Development and Psychopathology, 8,* 511–525.

Posada, G., Waters, E., Cassidy, J., & Marvin, R. S. (in press). Q-sort observations of secure-base behavior at home are not strongly related to security classification based on separation and reunion behavior in the laboratory at age 3 years. In E. Waters, B. E. Vaughn, G. Posada, & D. Teti (Eds.), *Patterns of secure-base behavior: Q-sort perspectives on attachment and caregiving in infancy and childhood.* Hillsdale, NJ: Erlbaum.

Rodning, C., Beckwith, L., & Howard, J. (1991). Quality of attachment and home environments in children prenatally exposed to PCP and cocaine. *Development and Psychopathology, 3,* 351–366.

Sarason, I. G., Johnson, J. H., & Siegel, J. M. (1978). Assessing the impact of life changes: Development of the Life Experiences Survey. *Journal of Consulting and Clinical Psychology, 46,* 932–946.

Schuengel, C. (1997). *Attachment, loss, and parental behavior: A study on intergenerational transmission.* Unpublished dissertation, Leiden University, Leiden, The Netherlands.

Shouldice, A., & Stevenson-Hinde, J. (1992). Coping with security distress: The Separation Anxiety Test and attachment classification at 4.5 years. *Journal of Child Psychology and Psychiatry, 33,* 331–348.

Solomon, J., & George, C. (1996). Defining the caregiving system: Toward a theory of caregiving. *Infant Mental Health Journal, 17,* 183–197.

Solomon, J., George, C., & De Jong, A. (1995). Children classified as controlling at age six: Evidence of disorganized representational strategies and aggression at home and at school. *Development and Psychopathology, 7,* 447–463.

Speltz, M. L., Greenberg, M. T., & DeKlyen, M. (1990). Attachment in preschoolers with disruptive behavior: A comparison of clinic-referred and nonproblem children. *Development and Psychopathology, 2,* 31–46.

Spieker, S. J., & Booth, C. (1988). Maternal antecedents of attachment quality. In J. Belsky & T. Nezworski (Eds.), *Clinical implications of attachment* (pp. 300–323). Hillsdale, NJ: Erlbaum.

Stevenson-Hinde, J., & Shouldice, A. (1995). Maternal interactions and self-reports related to attachment classifications at 4.5 years. *Child Development, 66,* 583–596.

Teti, D. M., & Gelfand, D. M. (1997). The Preschool Assessment of Attachment: Construct validity in a sample of depressed and nondepressed families. *Development and Psychopathology, 9,* 517–536.

Teti, D. M., Gelfand, D. M., Messinger, D. S., & Isabella, R. (1995). Maternal depression and the quality of early attachment: An examination of infants, preschoolers, and their mothers. *Developmental Psychology, 31,* 364–376.

Wartner, U. G., Grossmann, K., Fremmer-Bombik, E., & Suess, G. (1994). Attachment patterns at age six in south Germany: Predictability from infancy and implications for preschool behavior. *Child Development, 65,* 1014–1027.

Waters, E. (1995). Appendix A: The Attachment Q-set (version 3.0). In E. Waters, B. E. Vaughn, G. Posada, & K. Kondo-Ikemura (Eds.), Caregiving, cultural, and cognitive perspectives on secure-base behavior and working models: New growing points of attachment theory and research. *Monographs of the Society for Research in Child Development, 60*(Nos. 2–3, Serial No. 244), 234–246.

Zoll, D. A., Lyons-Ruth, K., & Connell, D. (1984, August). *Infants at psychiatric risk: Maternal behavior, depression, and family history.* Paper presented at the 92nd Annual Convention of the American Psychological Association, Toronto.

CHAPTER 9

The Effects on Attachment of Overnight Visitation in Divorced and Separated Families

A Longitudinal Follow-Up

JUDITH SOLOMON
CAROL GEORGE

The study of separation from the caregiver is a cornerstone of attachment theory; however, attachment research has yet to explore whether early experiences of separation from caregivers in the context of marital separation and divorce influence the development of infant attachment. Several years ago we began the first study of its kind designed to address this question. The results of our baseline analyses of infant attachment revealed a very high rate of attachment disorganization among 1-year-olds who participated in regular overnight visitation schedules with the father (Solomon & George, in press-b). In this chapter, we report key findings from our longitudinal follow-up of these infants in toddlerhood and examine the implications of our findings for understanding attachment disorganization more generally.

BACKGROUND

It is increasingly common for visitation arrangements for infants and toddlers in separated families to involve regular overnight stays with the nonresidential parent, usually the father, of one to several nights duration. This practice has gained favor with some parents and the courts as a way to ensure the infant's frequent and continuing contact with both parents. Surveys from California and Wisconsin indicate that over one-third of children age 2 or younger in separated/divorced families participate in overnight visitation with a second parent (Maccoby, Depner, & Mnookin, 1988; Seltzer [Wisconsin Parent Survey], personal communication, May 1992). Although many jurisdictions directly favor schedules that include overnights, this practice runs counter to the advice of some traditional child development and mental health practitioners (Goldstein, Freud, & Solnit, 1973; Hodges, 1986; Skafte, 1985). Concerns continue to be expressed by court personnel (e.g., Kings County Family Court Services, 1989; Spokane County Bar Association, 1996), as well as by many parents and mental health practitioners. Serious objections to this practice are usually based on classic studies of long-term separations of very young children from their mothers (Bowlby, 1969/1982, 1973; Heinicke & Westheimer, 1965; Robertson & Robertson, 1989). In the context of divorce and separation, concerns have been expressed about both acute effects of the stress of repeated separations of the infant from his or her primary caregiver and possible long-term effects on the infant's attachment security with mother.

In order to explore the effects of overnight visitation on infant–parent attachment and to determine what risk and buffering factors may exist in these families, we embarked upon a study of infants, age 12 to 18 months, in separated/divorced and maritally intact families. In the separated/divorced couples, the parents' relationship typically had dissolved by the time the infant was 4 months of age; however, some relationships dissolved much earlier. The key attachment-related issue for infants, therefore, was not one of loss of the father, but of developing primary relationships to both parents in the midst of repeated separations and the emotional aftermath of marital disruption. For their part, parents were faced with the enormous challenge of sustaining an adequate coparenting relationship, often with an individual whom they had little reason to trust either as a parent or as a supportive adult partner.

Our findings from the baseline period played a central role in focusing our questions about the sequelae of attachment when we saw the children again, approximately 1 year later, at age 2½. We found at baseline significantly more disorganized/unclassifiable infant–mother attachments than secure and avoidant attachments among infants who had experienced overnight visitation schedules (the overnight group) as compared both to infants who saw their fathers regularly but did not have overnights (the no-overnight group) and infants from intact families (the married group). About two-thirds of the attachments in the overnight group were judged disorganized/unclassifiable, in comparison to one-third such classifications in the married group sample.[1] Although we had anticipated that overnight visitation might be associated with greater insecurity in infant–mother attachment, we had not predicted that disorganized attachments would predominate. Based on findings available when we initiated the study on the effects of early day care (Bargolow & Vaughn, 1987; Belsky, 1986; Blehar, 1974), we had expected that overnight visitation effects, if any, would be revealed in the form of higher avoidance of the mother in laboratory reunions.[2]

In order to understand our findings, we returned to the now-classic observations of young children who have undergone prolonged separations (Bowlby, 1973/1980; Heinicke & Westheimer, 1965; Robertson & Robertson, 1989). These observations seemed to make sense of our puzzling findings because they suggested links between the experience of prolonged separation and the display of disorganized attachment behavior. In these classic studies, prolonged separation was observed to be associated with detachment from the mother, a phenomenon that has since been linked to avoidant attachment (Main, 1981). Our reexamination of the earlier observations revealed, however, that separated children's behavior was far more extreme and incoherent than either avoidance or resistance and fit more easily into Main and Solomon's (1990) classification criteria for attachment disorganization. Other behaviors reported in these early observations, such as sudden or out-of-context provocative behavior or hostility directed toward the mother were also observed in our sample. When these behaviors were not mixed with other signs of disorganization of disorientation they resulted, in our study, in the designation of the relationship as "unclassifiable" (see Solomon & George, Chapter 1, this volume, for a more detailed discussion). Thus, the parallels between disorganized and unclassifiable behavior in our sample, and the observations of children following more extended separations, suggested that the unexpected numbers of such classifications in our overnight visitation group reflected something about the children's reaction to repeated overnight separations from the mother.

The Conditions of Overnight Separation in Divorcing Families

Bowlby (1969/1982, 1973) and Rutter (1972) emphasized that the conditions of separation and reunion—including the quality of care during separation and the mother's behavior following reunion—would determine both acute and long-term effects of major separation. This context-sensitive view was supported in our baseline data. With regard to risk and protective factors, we found that no particular aspect of overnight visitation arrangements predicted organization or disorganization of attachment. Disorganization in the overnight group was, however, significantly associated with high parental conflict, low parental communication about the baby, and lower psychological protection of the infant by the mother in the visitation context. Mothers who received low ratings for psychological protection described themselves in interviews as unable to demand visitation arrangements that they felt were more suitable to the baby and as failing to provide comfort and reassurance to the infant when he or she was obviously distressed before and after visitation. In contrast, mothers in the overnight group whose infants were classified as having an organized attachment strategy (A, B, or C) described themselves as active and confident in providing psychological protection in the visitation context.

Thus, some infants experienced overnight visitation under fairly tranquil and supportive circumstances. Their parents were able to respond flexibly to their attachment signals and needs, for example, by providing increased reassurance at departures and reunion, or by changing the schedule when infants seemed distressed by separations or were ill. In contrast, the majority of infants in the overnight group were more likely to experience their mothers as oblivious, helpless to reassure them, or alarming at precisely those moments when their attachment system was likely to be most strongly activated, that is, during separations and reunions. In addition, it was particularly during transitions between mother's and father's care that parents interacted with each other. At these times, they were likely to become angry with one another, anxious, or rigid and remote. Sometimes parents' anxiety or anger was redirected toward the infant.

We have hypothesized that the caregiving of some of the mothers in the overnight group became disorganized or disabled by their belief that they could not protect their infant from the stresses of separation or care by a father whom they believed to be insensitive. Although we had no adequate way to evaluate independently the fathers' caregiving in this study, we have evidence (from parents' interviews and substantial clinical experience with families such as these) that the mother's mistrust of the father, although often founded on accurate perception, was fueled or exacerbated by the divorce and visitation context. Especially notable aspects of this context included lack of communication between the parents, entrenched and mutually generated hostility, and hypervigilance that arose from entirely expectable maternal separation anxiety and the infant's own behavior.

Our interviews with mothers suggested that many mothers of disorganized or unclassifiable infants might have been quite adequate caregivers under other circumstances. This impression was supported in our analyses of the relation between mothers' representations of themselves as a "secure base" (an evaluation of caregiving representations that takes into consideration a wide variety of commonplace and stressful situations) and their psychological protection scores (Solomon & George, in press-a). Both ratings were made from the same, hour-long interview about the mother–child relationship, but the psychological protection measure was based only on the mother's comments about visitation itself. These measures showed only a moderate positive correlation within the divorce group as a whole. Furthermore, while both scales were found to contribute independently to infant attachment security, psychological protection scores made a larger contribution. Thus, the quality of the mother's caregiving in the context of visitation was not simply an extension of the quality of her general caregiving, and her behavior in the visitation context may be more crucial in determining attachment security for infants in the overnight group.

We have suggested elsewhere that the mother's scores on psychological protection reflect her psychological resolution of the challenges to caregiving presented by the divorce and overnight situation (Solomon & George, in press-c). It appears that, under these circumstances, few mothers are able to reorient and reorganize their caregiving strategies at the representational and behavioral levels so as to provide adequate care to the infant. This use of the resolution construct was suggested by, and parallels, Pianta and Marvin's use of the term "resolution" as applied to studies of mothers with neurologically compromised infants (Pianta, Marvin, Britner, & Borowitz, 1996; Pianta, Marvin, & Morog, Chapter 14, this volume; see also Barnett et al., Chapter 7, this volume). Similar to our view of divorce, these researchers have reported that the mother's failure to resolve the assault to caregiving posed by infant disability also threatens the child's attachment security.

Hypotheses for the Follow-Up Assessment

The follow-up phase of the study was designed to evaluate the stability and sequelae of the differences we had observed in mother–infant attachment at baseline. A well-validated classification system for attachment is not available for children ages approximately 20–36 months of age (Solomon & George, 1999); thus, a strict comparison between baseline and follow-up classifications is not possible at this time. Attachment researchers have been successful, however, in demonstrating *coherence* in development, that is, in finding systematic relations between the quality of infant attachment and both concurrent and later differences in mother–child interaction in other salient developmental tasks of early childhood (Sroufe, 1979). Across a variety of problem-solving and cooperative tasks, securely attached infants or children have been found to be more autonomous (enthusiastic and persistent) and more cooperative with their mothers than insecurely attached children. Correlatively, the mothers of securely attached infants or children are also judged to provide superior support and guidance in these tasks compared to mothers of insecurely attached children (Achermann, Dinneen, & Stevenson-Hinde, 1991; DeMulder & Radke-Yarrow, 1991; Erickson, Sroufe, & Egeland, 1985; Matas, Arend, & Sroufe, 1978; Moss, Parent, Gosselin, Rousseau, & St-Laurent, 1996; Moss, Rousseau, Parent, St-Laurent, & Saintonge, 1998; Stevenson-Hinde & Shouldice, 1995). Furthermore, studies have shown that mothers of disorganized infants and children generally fail to maintain reciprocal, affectively attuned, task-appropriate communication and behavior as compared with mothers of organized infants and children (Easterbrooks, Biesecker, & Lyons-Ruth, 1997; Jacobvitz & Hazen, Chapter 5, this volume; Moss et al., 1996, 1998; Moss, St-Laurent, & Parent, Chapter 6, this volume).

Based on this body of literature, we expected to find that organized dyads—those classified into one of the organized attachment groups (A, B, or C)—performed better in problem-solving and clean-up tasks at follow-up than disorganized dyads. Although we recognized that attachment relationships might be less stable in divorcing than intact families, given the absence of prior research in this area, we made no specific predictions about the overall effect of family group. We did, however, predict a statistical interaction between attachment organization and family group on behavior in the follow-up tasks. This prediction was based on our hypothesis that, in the overnight dyads, the disorganized and/or unclassifiable classifications reflected the deleterious effects of the visitation context on mother–child interaction. We also had particular questions regarding differences between children who had been judged disorganized and those who had been judged "unclassifiable" in the overnight group. Infants were assigned to the unclassifiable group when their attachment behavior was judged "incoherent" or contradictory, and yet did not correspond to the guidelines for the disorganized classification. We wondered whether it was this unclassifiable subgroup, rather than the more "conventionally" disorganized subgroup, whose attachment behavior reflected difficult separation experiences rather than more pervasive problems in the mother–child relationship. For this reason, unclassifiable cases were treated as a separate classification group from both the organized and disorganized groups in the analyses.

METHODS

Sample

The subjects in this study were mothers and toddlers who had participated approximately 1 year earlier in the baseline assessments for this study.

Eighty-five percent of the baseline sample returned for the follow-up. The majority of families that did not return had moved out of the area. The total follow-up sample size was 126, although not all data were available and/or codable for all subjects for all variables. Forty of the returning dyads had been members of the *baseline overnight group;* that is, the parents were separated or divorced, and the children were participating in overnight visitation schedules with the father 1 year earlier; 42 dyads had been members of the *baseline no-overnight group*; that is, at baseline, the infants saw their fathers regularly but did not stay overnight with them; and 44 were members of the *baseline married group.* Children averaged 29 months of age at the time of follow-up. The sex distribution of the toddlers was the same as it was at baseline: 55% of the toddlers were boys.

Demographic and other background characteristics of the sample as well as recruitment procedures are described fully in Solomon and George (in press-a). In brief, the mothers in our sample were generally mature (approximately 30 years of age) and represented a wide range of ethnicities, education levels, and incomes. Although the groups were well matched on many variables, married mothers were somewhat better educated, reported higher incomes, and were less likely to work full time at baseline. None of the variables on which groups differed was found to be related to attachment classification.

Group membership had changed somewhat by the time of the follow-up assessment. The overnight and married comparison groups were generally stable. Five of the baseline overnight dyads had gotten married or had changed to no-overnight schedules. Five of the married couples were separated or divorced and had established visitation arrangements for the toddler (overnight and no-overnight). There was a great deal more change in the baseline no-overnight group. Twenty-one (48%) families changed groups: 18 families (41%) moved to an overnight plan, and 3 couples (7%) started living together (i.e., were eligible for the married group). The sample sizes of the follow-up family groups, therefore, were as follows: overnight (55); no-overnight (29); married (42).

Procedures

Baseline procedures, including attachment classification procedures, are described fully in Solomon and George (in press-a, in press-b). At follow-up, mother and child attended a single session in our laboratory playroom, where they were videotaped in a set of activities lasting about 1½ hours. The session consisted primarily of two interactive tasks. The first was a problem-solving task in which the focus was on the child's autonomy (e.g., enthusiasm, persistence in problem solving) and the quality of the mother's support. The second was a cleanup task in which we observed how the mother gained the child's cooperation and the quality of the child's cooperation with her.

The problem-solving task, or "puzzle box" was adapted from a task developed by Matas et al. (1978). The puzzle box was a large plexiglas box (approximately 4 feet wide × 2 feet high × 2 feet deep) through which extended a long Plexiglas lever (approximately 6 feet long). A small box containing a few M & M candies was attached to one end of the lever; this could only be reached by the child through the top of the box. In order to accomplish this task, the lever had to be held in place with a heavy block at the far end (the end opposite the candy box). The physical and cognitive requirements of this task were such that the mother's participation and support were necessary for successful completion. No limit was placed on the duration of this task. The cleanup task required sorting and shelving a large variety of toys. Six minutes was the amount of time allotted for this task. Mothers were instructed in both tasks to give the child an opportunity to do the task on his or her own and then to provide whatever assistance the child seemed to need.

A brief separation and reunion occurred before each task. Prior to the problem-solving task, the mother left the room while the child remained for 3 minutes with a friendly adult, as in the strange situation. Children generally seemed unperturbed by this separation. Prior to cleanup, the child was left alone in the room for 5 minutes before the mother's return. Not surprisingly, more toddlers seemed distressed and angry during this separation. Eight minutes elapsed from the end of the second separation to the beginning of cleanup, during which time mother and child were free to interact as they wished.

Prior to the laboratory session, mothers completed a set of questionnaires about themselves, their toddlers, and their relationship with the child's father, similar to those they had completed at baseline. Mothers were also interviewed briefly about current visitation arrangements and their feelings about them. These data are not included in the present report.

Measures

Problem Solving

The quality of mother's support for the child's autonomous exploration in the problem-solving situation was rated using a scale adapted from Sroufe, Matas, and Rosenberg (1983), called *Supportive Presence*. This is a 7-point scale, with the odd points anchored by definitions. Raters carefully considered the mother's attentiveness, affective involvement, self-assurance, and the quality and timing of her cues in arriving at a rating. The child's *Task Orientation* was rated on a 7-point scale also adapted from the work of Sroufe et al. (1983). High scores were given to children who were enthusiastic, persistent, and comfortable with incorporating mother's suggestions. Low scores were given to children who seemed actively to avoid the task. Both ratings were made from videotape by trained coders who were blind to all other information about the families and the hypotheses of the study. The interrater correlations on a randomly selected and independently rated subsample ($n = 17$) was .84 for Supportive Presence and .93 for Task Orientation.

Cleanup

Mothers' behavior during the cleanup task was rated on a 7-point *Authoritativeness* scale developed for this study. Raters carefully considered the quality of the mother's involvement and support, the extent to which she provided structure and leadership, and the sensitivity of her interventions with the child. Children were rated on a 7-point scale for *Self-control*, a scale also developed for this study. High scores were given to children who showed initiative in cleanup in the context of an overall partnership with the parent, in which cleanup was a mutual goal. The lowest scores were given to children who were completely uncooperative with the parent. To receive the lowest scores, negativity or resistance had to be clearly directed toward the parent and unresolved by the end of the session. Cleanup ratings were completed by a different team of raters from those who worked on the problem-solving task and who were blind to all other information about the families and the hypotheses of the study. Interrater correlations on a randomly selected and independently rated subsample ($n = 25$) was .94 for Supportive Presence and .91 for Task Orientation.

RESULTS

Hypotheses related to mother–child interaction in the follow-up tasks were examined using mothers' and children's scores on each task as dependent variables in separate analyses of variance (ANOVAs) or analyses of covariance (ANCOVAs) with attachment status (organized, disorganized, unclassifiable) as one factor and family group as the second. Due to our interest in examining differences between disorganized and unclassifiable children, and the fact that unclassifiable cases were rare in the no-overnight ($n = 4$) and married family groups ($n = 6$), these family groups were combined into a single comparison family group. Preliminary two-way ANOVAs had shown that there were no significant differences between them on the relevant dimensions (no effects of family group and no interactions between attachment organization and family for any of the dependent variables).

Problem-Solving Task

Table 9.1 shows the means for maternal and child behavior in the problem-solving task, grouped according to baseline family group (overnight vs. comparison) and attachment organization (organized, disorganized, unclassifiable). As predicted, a two-way ANOVA showed a significant overall effect of attachment organization on maternal supportive presence, $F = 5.37$, $df = 2,115$, $p = .006$, and no effect was found for family group. That is, mothers of infants with organized attachments were rated as more supportive than mothers of infants with disorganized and unclassifiable attachments. There was also, as predicted, a significant interaction between attachment and family group, $F = 5.90$, $df = 2,115$, $p = .004$. Follow-up analyses of simple main effects showed that this interaction was due to differences in the behavior of mothers of unclassifiable infants across family groups, $F(\text{unclassifiable}) = 9.71$, $df = 1,19$; $p = .002$, with unclassifiable mothers providing more adequate support in the overnight families than in the comparison families. Paired comparisons of attachment groups within the overnight families showed that mothers of both organized and unclassifiable infants were significantly more supportive than mothers of disorganized infants ($p < .05$, step-down multiple stage F test correction) and were not significantly different from one another. In contrast, in the

TABLE 9.1. Mothers' and Children's Behavior in the Problem-Solving Task as Related to Baseline Family Group and Attachment Status

Attachment group	Overnight (baseline)			Comparison (baseline no-overnight and married)		
	N	Mean	SD	N	Mean	SD
Mothers' supportive presence						
Organized (A, B, C)	12	3.50	(1.04)	50	3.99	(1.38)
Disorganized (D)	13	2.65	(1.13)	21	2.98	(1.08)
Unclassifiable (U)	10	4.40	(.87)	10	2.70	(1.18)
Children's task orientation[a]						
Organized (A, B, C)	12	5.41	(1.30)	50	4.37	(1.50)
Disorganized (D)	13	4.08	(1.01)	21	3.78	(1.59)
Unclassifiable (U)	10	4.44	(1.90)	10	4.86	(1.45)

[a]Age at follow-up as covariate. $F(\text{age}) = 5.65$; $df = 1,115$; $p = .02$. Means in table are adjusted for age at follow-up.

comparison dyads, mothers of unclassifiable infants were comparable to mothers of disorganized infants. This is consistent with our hypothesis that at least some proportion of attachment relationships were unclassifiable due to the infant's response to overnight separation from the mother under adverse conditions. Again, although we have hypothesized that mothers of such children are unavailable, unresponsive, or even aversive during separation and reunions, they are not necessarily so in general.

Preliminary analyses showed a low but significant correlation between the child's age at follow-up assessment and task orientation ($r = .24$, $n = 116$, $p = .008$); this variable was included, therefore, as a covariate in the statistical analyses. Results of the ANCOVA analysis, shown in Table 9.1, revealed a significant main effect for attachment organization, $F = 3.93$, $df = 2,115$, $p = .02$; no significant effect of family group, and, in contrast to the maternal data, no significant interaction between factors. Follow-up paired comparisons of the attachment groups using the step-down multiple stage F-test correction showed that disorganized toddlers were significantly lower ($p < .05$) in task enthusiasm and persistence than toddlers in either the organized or unclassifiable groups. Thus, although the comparison group mothers of unclassifiable children received very low ratings for supportive presence, this apparently did not have an impact on their children's performance.

Cleanup

As shown in Table 9.2, mother and child behavior in the cleanup task were in the expected directions—mothers of children who were organized at baseline were judged to be more authoritative than mothers whose children were judged disorganized; children who had been classified into one of the organized attachment categories were rated higher in self-control than children who had been classified as disorganized. The main effects for attachment organization, however, fell short of statistical significance in the two-way ANOVAs (F(authoritativeness) = 2.68, $df = 2$, 109, $p = .07$; F(self-control) = 2.05, $df = 2,109$, $p = .13$). There was no main effect for family group on behavior and no significant interactions between factors.

Patterning in Children's Responses across Tasks

The weaker findings in the cleanup task in comparison to the problem-solving task might be attributed to the fact that cleanup is a somewhat less developmentally appropriate task than problem solving in the third year of life. The cleanup task certainly was not as enjoyable for mother or child as the puzzle box, as indicated by the overall lower scores received by children and mothers in cleanup as compared with problem solving. Nevertheless,

TABLE 9.2. Mothers' and Children's Behavior in Cleanup Task as Related to Baseline Family Group and Attachment Status

Attachment group	Overnight (baseline)			Comparison (baseline no-overnight and married)		
	N	Mean	SD	N	Mean	SD
Mothers' authoritativeness						
Organized (A, B, C)	12	3.17	(1.47)	47	3.21	(1.65)
Disorganized (D)	13	2.39	(1.77)	19	2.16	(1.83)
Unclassifiable (U)	9	2.44	(1.86)	10	3.70	(1.84)
Children's self-regulation						
Organized (A, B, C)	12	2.92	(1.37)	50	3.21	(1.56)
Disorganized (D)	13	2.23	(1.52)	21	2.89	(1.97)
Unclassifiable (U)	10	2.28	(1.60)	10	3.30	(1.89)

we had expected a positive correlation in performance across both tasks. This was not borne out in across-task correlations ($r_{mothers}$ = .07, n = 106, p = .44; $r_{children}$ = .06, n = 106, p = .21).

This raised a question as to whether it might be more appropriate to think of the laboratory session as a whole than as a set of different tasks. There was a 5-minute separation between problem solving and cleanup, during which the child was entirely alone in the room, followed by a reunion. As we mentioned earlier, no construct-validated attachment classification system exists for 2½-year-olds (Solomon & George, 1999); however, we wondered whether we could infer something about attachment security by comparing the child's interaction with the mother before and after the separation.

Following prolonged separations, observers have noted that young children who have otherwise returned to normal may "break down" to anger, anxiety, and distress when presented with reminders of the separation (Bowlby, 1973; Heinicke & Westheimer, 1965, Robertson & Robertson, 1971). By analogy, we hypothesized that children who have experienced repeated overnight separations from the mother might be more likely than other children to show a marked decline or "breakdown" in the quality of their interactions with the mother following the brief laboratory separation to which we had subjected them.

It was also possible that postseparation breakdown was related to attachment organization. Indeed, at the most general level, both disorganized and unclassifiable attachments are characterized by a breakdown of an underlying organized attachment strategy (Main & Solomon, 1986,

1990). In addition, Suomi (1991) has reported that "peer-reared" rhesus monkeys, although otherwise comparable in social behavior to mother-reared monkeys, show far greater behavioral and physiological indices of distress when later separated from their social groups. Thus, "insecurity" resulting from inadequate early attachment relationships became evident only under conditions of marked separation-related stress. Given the evidence that attachment disorganization is associated with a very high level of insecurity and that such children have difficulty in regulating affect and physiological functioning following separation (Spangler & Grossmann, 1993; Spangler, & Grossmann, Chapter 4, this volume), it seems plausible that these children might show evidence of continuing negative affect toward the mother that would be manifested as lack of self-control in the cleanup task.

In order to evaluate these two hypotheses, we defined two distinct patterns from among children who had performed well in the problem solving task. A "breakdown" pattern was defined as adequate performance in problem-solving (a score of 4 or higher on problem-solving task orientation), followed by an extremely low score on self-control (a score of 1 or 2). It will be remembered that low self-control scores explicitly were designed to represent a failure on the part of the child to engage in a cooperative partnership with the parent in the cleanup context. Children who received very low scores were, by definition, very wild, angry, or miserable by the end of the cleanup period (usually, so were their mothers by that time). A second pattern, identified as "no breakdown," comprised children whose performance began high (task orientation > 4) and continued, relatively, in this vein (self-regulation > 2).

The breakdown variable was entered as one factor in a hierarchical loglinear analysis, along with the child's follow-up family group (overnight, comparison) and attachment organization group (organized, disorganized, unclassifiable). Main effects of each factor and higher-order interactions were eliminated in a backward-stepping procedure until only those effects that provided the best possible model of the data remained. The final best-fitting model consisted of both two-way interactions: breakdown × follow-up group (likelihood ratio χ^2 = 4.65, df = 1, p = .03) and breakdown × attachment organization (likelihood ratio χ^2 = 8.07, df = 2, p = .017). Thus, both hypotheses were confirmed. The data corresponding to each interaction are shown in Table 9.3.

Considering the interaction between follow-up family group and breakdowns, children who were participating in overnight visitation schedules were twice as likely to show a breakdown in interaction with mother as children in the comparison group. Postseparation breakdowns were characteristic of about half (51%) of the follow-up overnight children who scored 4 or above in the problem-solving task, but were shown by only 27%

TABLE 9.3a. Breakdown in Children's Performance across Tasks as related to Follow-Up Family Group

| | Overnight (follow-up) | | Comparison (follow-up no-overnight and married) | | |
	n	(%)	n	(%)	Total
Breakdown	19	(51%)	10	(27%)	29
No-breakdown	18	(49%)	27	(73%)	45
Total	37		37		74

Note. Likelihood ratio χ^2 = 4.65, *df* = 1, *p* = .03).

TABLE 9.3b. Breakdown in Children's Performance across Tasks as Related to Baseline Attachment Group

| | Organized (A, B, C) | | Disorganized (D) | | Unclassifiable (U) | | |
	n	(%)	n	(%)	n	(%)	Total
Breakdown	11	(26%)	9	(60%)	9	(56%)	29
No-breakdown	32	(71%)	6	(40%)	7	(44%)	45
Total	43		15		16		74

Note. Likelihood ratio χ^2 = 8.076, *df* = 2, *p* = .017.

of the comparison children. Turning to the relation between breakdowns and attachment organization, 60% and 56%, respectively, of disorganized and unclassifiable toddlers who performed well in problem solving broke down in the cleanup task. In contrast, only 26% of the organized children broke down.

DISCUSSION

The results of this study partially confirmed our hypotheses about the continuity of infant–mother relationships in separated/divorced and maritally intact families, and provided important additional information about the effects of overnight visitation arrangements in early childhood. Mothers of children who 1 year earlier had been judged to have an organized attachment with mother (Groups A, B, or C) provided significantly more sensitive and appropriate support for their child's autonomous exploration in a problem-solving task than mothers whose children were earlier judged to have a disorganized attachment. Similarly, children who 1 year earlier had been judged to have an organized attachment also were judged to show more persistent and enthusiastic problem-solving behavior than children in the disorganized group. This predicted pattern of differences between the organized and disorganized attachment groups also emerged for mothers' authoritativeness and children's self-control in the cleanup task, but just missed conventional levels of significance. These findings are consistent with previous studies of mother–child interaction outside the strange situation that have shown that disorganized attachment status is associated with pervasively poor mother–child interaction and communication (Easterbrooks, Biesecker, & Lyons-Ruth, 1997; Jacobvitz & Hazen, Chapter 5, this volume; Moss et al., in press; Moss et al. Chapter 6, this volume; Stevenson-Hinde & Shouldice, 1995).

A striking feature of mother–toddler interaction in the disorganized dyads was its lack of coordination at the level of behavior, affect, and attention. This was most often evident in the failure of mother and child to respond contingently to one another. For example, the toddler might start to lose interest in the puzzle box and the mother would be unable to recapture the child's attention or persuade him or her to return to it. In other instances, the child might carry on very well with the puzzle box or the cleanup, but the parent would become markedly withdrawn or unhelpful. Thus, while communication flowed predictably and reasonably effectively within organized dyads, communication in the disorganized dyads was itself "disorganized." This use of the term is very different than what is referred to as disorganized attachment behavior, but it aptly describes the interactive quality that was observed in these dyads.

In the case of maternal supportive presence in problem solving, the overall prediction from baseline attachment organization to later performance in the tasks was modified by an expected statistical interaction between attachment and family group. Within the baseline overnight group (i.e., children who participated in overnight visitation arrangements at baseline), mothers whose children had earlier been judged to be unclassifiable in attachment received ratings that were comparable to those received by mothers of children with organized attachment classifications and higher than those earned by mothers of disorganized infants. In the baseline comparison families (no-overnight or married at baseline), mothers of unclassifiable children performed at the same low level as the mothers of "conventionally" disorganized infants. This supports our view that a number of baseline classifications in the overnight group reflected the effects on attachment behavior of the infant's adverse experience of repeated overnight separations from the mother rather than more pervasive difficulties in the mother–infant relationship.

Baseline family group did not interact statistically, however, with infant attachment classifications in the case of the child's problem-solving orientation or mothers' or children's cleanup behavior in toddlerhood. In part, this may reflect the overriding effects of the tasks themselves. The majority of toddlers were highly motivated to solve the intriguing puzzle box and often persisted with little or no maternal support. Possibly, the use of a series of problems, paralleling more closely Matas et al.'s (1978) procedures, would have yielded better discrimination between groups of toddlers. In contrast, the cleanup task, which was not intrinsically compelling and tapped the later-maturing capacity for self-control on the part of the child (Kopp, 1982, 1987), was associated with poorer performance across attachment and family groups.

Exploratory analyses indicated, however, that mother–child interaction in cleanup was in part a function of the child's *current* separation experiences: Children who were participating in overnight visitation with father at follow-up were significantly more likely to show a marked deterioration in performance across tasks than children who were not. Such children approached problem solving with gusto and enthusiasm but during cleanup were resistant, angry, and refused to participate in a working partnership with their mothers. The critical event, we believe, was not the cleanup task itself but the fact that the cleanup was immediately preceded by a 5-minute separation of mother and child in the laboratory. This "breakdown" phenomenon strongly suggests that the overnight experience had sensitized children to separations and reunions with the mother. In other words, "breakdown" was observed in these toddlers in response to stress following strong activation of attachment. Although replication of this phenomenon is necessary, it is consistent with separation-related findings in other contexts. For example, observers of young children who have experienced prolonged separations noted a resurgence of out-of-context aggression and separation anxiety in the presence of individuals or other cues associated with the separation many weeks following separation, after a return to apparently normal behavior (Bowlby, 1973; Heinicke & Westheimer, 1965; Robertson & Robertson, 1971). Similarly, as noted earlier, Suomi (1991) reported for rhesus macaques that long-term negative effects of deviant rearing regimes were evident only when monkeys were briefly separated from their social group, but not in the usual course of social interaction.

Breakdowns in behavior across follow-up tasks may also shed light on a key feature of the baseline findings—the very high numbers of disorganized and unclassifiable attachments that were found at baseline in overnight visitation families (Solomon & George, in press-b). Among children who were participating in overnight visitation schedules at the time of follow-up, those who had been classified as disorganized or unclassifiable 1 year earlier were significantly more likely to break down in performance in the follow-up tasks than children who had been placed into one of the organized attachment classification groups. Organization of attachment at baseline was unrelated to breakdowns, however, among children who had never participated in overnight visiting schedules. This finding provides another source of evidence that adverse separation experiences can influence infant attachment strategies, causing them to break down or become disorganized.

In contrast to the findings for maternal support discussed previously, it is noteworthy that both disorganized and unclassifiable children in the overnight group were likely to break down in the follow-up assessment. One reason for this may be overlap in the classification criteria. Many overnight children were judged to be unclassifiable in the strange situation because of the display of sudden, out-of context aggression or defiance toward the mother. In essence, anger toward the mother broke through or overwhelmed attachment behavior or avoidance, paralleling the eruption of anger and defiance that was observed in the cleanup task. A number of other overnight children were placed in the disorganized group proper, on the basis of behavior that fit the Main and Solomon guidelines for "sequential contradictory behavior patterns," such as low distress in separation followed by inconsolable behavior upon reunion, the reverse pattern (distress in separation followed by avoidance of the mother on reunion), or full, bright greetings to the mother followed by marked avoidance. These patterns are contradictory without seeming inherently conflicted and may signal the "breaking through" of distress and separation anxiety rather than the fear or apprehension of the mother that is believed to lie at the core of other indices of disorganization (see Main & Hesse, 1990, for a discussion of fear of mother as source of disorganization, and Solomon & George, Chapter 1, this volume, for additional discussion of this issue). Thus, depending upon the specifics of the child's behavior, that is, whether anger or distress was expressed in an out-of-context or contradictory way, a child might be assigned to either the unclassifiable or disorganized group. Further study may reveal that sequential contradictory patterns are associated with different etiologies than the other disorganization indices. On the other hand, as noted earlier, there appears to be considerable overlap in the behavior of children who have experienced prolonged separations from the mother and the indices for disorganization specified in the Main and Solomon system. Thus, it may be a mistake to try to infer etiology in any one case solely on the basis of the specific behaviors displayed by the child (see also Barnett et al., Chapter 7, this volume; Teti, Chapter 8, this volume).

METHODOLOGICAL, THEORETICAL, AND CLINICAL IMPLICATIONS

There is a persistent tension in attachment research and theory about the relation between and the developmental impact of, specific attachment-related assaults on the one hand, and more enduring features of the child-rearing environment on the other. In his early writing, Bowlby emphasized the effects of particular events such as prolonged separation or early loss, although at the same time, he was clearly aware that the impact of events was itself a function of the relational context in which the events occurred and other conditions, such as the child's level of cognitive development. In *Separation*, the second volume of his Attachment trilogy (1973), Bowlby defined "security" by its negation, as it were, that is, as the absence of "fear, apprehension, or alarm" (p. 182). By focusing on middle-class families under generally stable circumstances, Ainsworth's research paradigm (Ainsworth, Blehar, Waters, & Wall, 1978) provided an operational definition of security (confidence in the availability and responsiveness of the attachment figure), resulting in a theoretical and empirical shift away from the study of major assaults or trauma to the attachment system. Indeed, researchers typically exclude from their samples any infants who have recently undergone major separations or families currently in crisis in recognition of the disruptive effects such events may have on the assessment of the "underlying" infant–parent attachment relationship. The questions addressed in this longitudinal investigation of visitation and divorce required us to ignore this methodological rule of thumb, although we did exclude children who had participated in overnights for a month or less.

Against this historical background, the interpretation of our findings is obviously problematic. Were the disorganized and unclassifiable children in this study less secure about the mother's *psychological* availability, either in general, or in the context of separation and reunion? Or were they simply more frightened or anxious about separation itself and, consequently, very angry at their mothers and emotionally more fragile? And, how do we define and operationalize these constructs independently from one another? These are critical issues for researchers who are attempting to evaluate the effects of the all-too-common experiences of separation and loss in the lives of very young children, and there are no definitive answers available at this time.

In this study, we attempted to provide at least preliminary answers to these questions by observing mother–child interaction outside the context of separation and reunion, and by comparing interaction before and after separations. On the basis of this kind of empirical triangulation, we tentatively conclude that overnight visitations schedules can disorganize the child's attachment strategies, but that such disorganization does not necessarily pervade or reflect the overall quality of the mother–child relationship. Whereas there is now considerable research demonstrating poor developmental outcomes for children in normative or other kinds of high-risk samples who are classified as insecure–disorganized (see Lyons-Ruth & Jacobvitz, 1999, for recent reviews of this literature), based on our findings, the same prognosis should not necessarily apply to disorganized and unclassifiable children who are participating in overnight visitation schedules. Possibly, over the long term, and to the extent that their mothers are adequately sensitive, these children will be no different from their organized counterparts in a variety of problem-solving or social contexts. We would predict, however, that they will continue to be more emotionally vulnerable or brittle in the context of separation, both in contrived laboratory situations and outside the laboratory as well. This is consistent with our findings about the breakdown in communication and cooperation in these dyads following a laboratory separation, and with our clinical experience with toddlers in quite similar family circumstances. In the latter context, we have noticed that these toddlers are unwilling to be separated from their primary caregivers, even when the surroundings are familiar, and have greater than expected difficulty with other transitions, such as departing from the clinical playroom. This difficulty is sometimes exhibited as protest, resistance, and anger at departure. Once departure is seen as inevitable, however, the majority of these toddlers are unable to depart with the parent in a leisurely and pleasant manner. Instead, they avert their face from the playroom or therapist and literally run away. Whether there are long-term consequences of this separation-related vulnerability is a matter for future investigation.

ACKNOWLEDGMENTS

This research was funded by a grant to Judith Solomon from the Bureau of Maternal and Child Health Research Program (No. MCJ-060616). An earlier version of this chapter was presented at the biennial meetings of the Society for Research in Child Development, Washington, DC, April 1997.

NOTES

1. Unusually high numbers of disorganized classifications and insecure classifications in general are a common feature of normative samples in our region (San Francisco Bay Area). These have now been reported in several samples and for different age/classification systems (infants, preschoolers, and kindergartners) in studies conducted by independent laboratories, using a variety of experienced coders

(Main, personal communication, 1994; Silverman, 1990; Solomon, George, & Silverman, in press; Solomon, George, & DeJong, 1995).

2. More recent studies relevant to separation effects have reported conflicting findings. The NICHD Early Child Care Research Network (1997) found no relation overall between attachment classification and early child care. Sagi, van IJzendoorn, Aviezer, Donnell, and Mayseless (1994) reported that Israeli kibbutz infants who regularly sleep away from the mother are more likely to be classified resistant than secure.

REFERENCES

Achermann, J., Dinneen, E., & Stevenson-Hinde, J. (1991). Cleaning up at 2.5 years. *British Journal of Developmental Psychology, 9*, 365–376.

Ainsworth, M., Blehar, M., Waters, E., & Wall, S. (1978). *Patterns of attachment: A psychological study of the Strange Situation.* Hillsdale, NJ: Erlbaum.

Bargalow, P., & Vaughn, B. (1987). Effects of maternal absence due to employment on the quality of infant–mother attachment in a low-risk sample. *Child Development, 58*, 945–954.

Belsky, J. (1986). Infant day-care: A cause for concern? *Zero to Three, 6*,1–6.

Blehar, M. (1974). Anxious attachment and defensive reactions associated with day care. *Child Development, 45*, 683–692.

Bowlby, J. (1969/1982). *Attachment and loss: Vol. 1. Attachment.* New York: Basic Books.

Bowlby, J. (1973). *Attachment and loss: Vol. 2. Separation.* New York: Basic Books.

Bowlby, J. (1980). *Attachment and loss: Vol. 3. Loss.* New York: Basic Books.

DeMulder, E. K., & Radke-Yarrow, M. (1991). Attachment with affectively ill and well mothers: Concurrent behavioral correlates. *Development and Psychopathology, 3*, 227–242

Easterbrooks, A. M., Biesecker, G., & Lyons-Ruth, K. (1997). *Infancy predictors of emotional availability in middle childhood: The role of attachment and maternal depression.* Manuscript submitted for publication.

Erickson, M. F., Sroufe, L. A., & Egeland, B. (1985). The relationship between quality of attachment and behavior problems in preschool in a high-risk sample. In I. Bretherton & E. Waters (Eds.), Growing points of attachment theory and research. *Monographs of the Society for Research in Child Development, 50*(1–2, Serial No. 209), 147–166.

Goldstein, J., Freud, A., & Solnit, A. (1973). *Beyond the best interests of the child.* New York: Free Press.

Heinicke, C. M., & Westheimer, I. (1965). *Brief separations.* New York: International Universities Press.

Hodges, W. F. (1986). *Interventions for children of divorce: Custody, access, and psychotherapy.* New York: Wiley.

Kings County Family Court Services. (1989). *Access guidelines.* Seattle, WA: Kings County Family Court Services.

Kopp, C. B. (1982). Antecedents of self-regulation: A developmental perspective. *Developmental Psychology, 18*, 199–214.

Kopp, C. B. (1987). The growth of self-regulation: Caregivers and children. In N. Eisenberg (Ed.), *Contemporary topics in developmental psychology* (pp. 41–56). New York: Wiley.

Lyons-Ruth, K., & Jacobvitz, D. (1999). Attachment disorganization: Unresolved loss, relational violence, and lapses in behavioral and attentional strategies. In J. Cassidy & P. Shaver (Eds.), *Handbook of attachment: Theory, research, and clinical applications* (pp. 520–554). New York: Guilford Press.

Maccoby, E., Depner, C. E., & Mnookin, R. H. (1988). Custody of children following divorce. In M. Hetherington & J. Aresteh (Eds.), *Impact of divorce, single parenting, and stepparenting on children* (pp. 91–116). Hillsdale, NJ: Erlbaum.

Main, M. (1981). Avoidance in the service of attachment: A working paper. In K. Immelman, G. Barlow, L. Petrinovich, & M. Main (Eds.), *Behavioral development: The Bielefeld interdisciplinary project* (pp. 651–693). New York: Cambridge University Press.

Main, M., & Hesse, E. (1990). Parent's unresolved traumatic experiences are related to infant disorganized attachment status: Is frightened and/or frightening behavior the linking mechanism? In M. Greenberg, D. Cicchetti, & M. Cummings (Eds.), *Attachment in the preschool years* (pp. 161–182). Chicago: University of Chicago Press.

Main, M., & Solomon, J. (1986). Discovery of an insecure–disorganized attachment pattern: Procedures, findings, and theoretical implications. In T. B. Brazelton & M. Yogman (Eds.), *Affective development in infancy* (pp. 95–124). New York: Academic Press.

Main, M., & Solomon, J. (1990). Procedures for identifying infants as disorganized/disoriented during the Ainsworth Strange Situation. In M. Greenberg, D. Cicchetti, & M. Cummings (Eds.), *Attachment in the preschool years* (pp. 121–160). Chicago: University of Chicago Press.

Matas, L., Arend, R. A., & Sroufe, L. A. (1978). Continuity of adaptation in the second year: The relationship between the quality of attachment and later competence. *Child Development, 49,* 547–556.

Moss, E., Parent, S., Gosselin, C., Rousseau, D., & St-Laurent, D. (1996). Attachment and teacher-reported behavior problems during the preschool and early school-age period. *Development and Psychopathology, 8,* 511–525.

Moss, E., Rousseau, D., Parent, S., St-Laurent, D., & Saintonge, J. (1998). Attachment at school-age: Maternal reported stress, mother–child interaction, and behavior problems. *Child Development, 69,* 1390–1405.

NICHD Early Child Care Research Network. (1997). The effects of infant child care on infant–mother attachment security: Results of the NICHD study of early child care. *Child Development, 68,* 860–879.

Pianta, R. C., Marvin, R., Britner, P., & Borowitz, K. (1996). Mothers' resolution of their children's diagnoses: Organized patterns of caregiving representations. *Infant Mental Health Journal, 17,* 239–256.

Robertson, J., & Robertson, J. (1989). *Separation and the very young child.* London: Free Association Books.

Rutter, M. (1972). Maternal deprivation reassessed. *Journal of Psychosomatic Research, 16,* 241–250.

Sagi, A., van IJzendoorn, M. H., Aviezer, O., Donnell, F., & Mayseless, O. (1994).

Sleeping out of home in a kibbutz communal arrangement: It makes a difference for infant–mother attachment. *Child Development, 65,* 992–1004.

Silverman, N. (1990). *Attachment security, maternal behavior, and preschool competence at age three.* Unpublished doctoral dissertation, Boston, University, Boston, MA.

Skafte, D. (1985). *Child custody evaluations.* Beverly Hills, CA: Sage.

Solomon, J., & George, C. (1999). The measurement of attachment security in infancy and early childhood. In J. Cassidy & P. Shaver (Eds.), *Handbook of attachment: Theory, research, and clinical applications* (pp. 287–316). New York: Guilford Press.

Solomon, J., & George, C. (in press-a). The caregiving system in mothers of infants: A comparison of divorcing and married mothers. *Attachment and Human Development, 2.*

Solomon, J., & George, C. (in press-b). The development of attachment in separated and divorced families: Effects of overnight visitation, parent, and couple variables. *Attachment and Human Development, 1.*

Solomon, J., & George, C. (in press-c). Toward an integrated theory of maternal caregiving. In J. Osofsky & H. Fitzgerald (Eds.), *WAIMH handbook of infant mental health.* New York: Wiley.

Solomon, J., George, C., & De Jong, A. (1995). Children classified as controlling at age six: Evidence of disorganized representational strategies and aggression at home and at school. *Development and Psychopathology, 7*(3), 447–464.

Solomon, J., George, C., & Silverman, N. (in press). Maternal caregiving Q-sort: Describing age-related changes in mother–infant interaction. In E. Waters, B. Vaughn, & D. Teti (Eds.), *Patterns of attachment behavior: Q-sort perspectives in secure base behavior and caregiving in infancy and childhood.* Hillsdale, NJ: Erlbaum.

Spangler, G., & Grossmann, K. E. (1993). Biobehavioral organization in securely and insecurely attached infants. *Child Development, 64,* 1439–1450.

Spokane County Bar Association. (1996). *Child-centered residential schedules.* Spokane, WA: Spokane County Superior Court.

Sroufe, L. A. (1979). The coherence of individual development. *American Psychologist, 43,* 834–841.

Sroufe, L. A., Matas, L., & Rosenberg, D. M. (1983). *Manual for scoring mother and child variables in tool-use task: Applicable for 2-year-old children.* Unpublished manuscript, University of Minnesota, Minneapolis.

Stevenson-Hinde, J., & Shouldice, A. (1995). Maternal interactions and self-reports related to attachment classifications at 4.5 years. *Child Development, 66,* 583–596.

Suomi, S. J. (1991). Early stress and adult emotional reactivity in rhesus monkeys. *In Ciba Foundation Symposium 156: The childhood environment and adult disease* (pp. 171–188). Chichester, UK: Wiley.

CHAPTER 10

Explaining Disorganized Attachment

Clues from Research on Mild-to-Moderately Undernourished Children in Chile

EVERETT WATERS
MARTA VALENZUELA

One of John Bowlby's primary goals in developing modern attachment theory was to preserve Sigmund Freud's genuine insights about close relationships. In order to accomplish this, Bowlby replaced Freud's view of attachment as a bond based on mental energy with the concept of attachment as a secure base relationship organized by a behavioral control system. The hallmarks of an infant's secure base behavior are (1) exploration away from the caregiver; (2) monitoring the caregiver's accessibility during exploration; (3) increased alertness to, or proximity to, the caregiver under circumstances that would impede monitoring or access; (4) preferential proximity and contact seeking in the face of uncertainty or threat; and (5) finding comfort in proximity and contact. In contrast to psychoanalytic and social learning views of the infant as clingy and demanding, Bowlby envisioned an active inquisitive infant, intent on exploration and mastery, and all the more able to pursue these goals for its confidence in an attachment figure's availability, responsiveness, and competence. When these behaviors are employed in an organized way and with respect to just one or a few caregivers across time and across situations, they are referred to as the secure base phenomenon.

Control systems theory enabled Bowlby to explain the complexity, environmental and situational sensitivity, developmental adaptiveness, and apparently purposefulness of secure base behavior without invoking unverifiable psychological constructs or endowing the infant with unlikely cognitive sophistication. Control systems models are also a useful way of formalizing ideas about the organization of the secure base phenomenon (Bischof, 1975; Bretherton, 1985; Waters, 1981). They also anchor Bowlby's and Mary Ainsworth's concept of attachment security. Secure attachment is closely linked to the notion of a well-configured, well-functioning control system. Although researchers have shown little interest in parametric analysis of secure base functioning, this framework has served as a useful conceptual tool and guide to assessment for over 30 years.

It is somewhat surprising, therefore, that the control systems perspective does not anticipate or suggest a second powerful device that has served attachment theory and research for just as long as control systems theory has. This is the notion of patterns of attachment. The control system model emphasizes the skilled nature of secure base behavior. Within this perspective, attachment security is just a matter of some infants being more skillful at secure base behavior than others. A continuum, nothing more.

In fact, the situation appears more complex. As Ainsworth pointed out, there is a wide range of individual differences in secure base behavior. Not only are some infants more skilled than others, but also there is quite a bit of diversity in the secure base behavior of the more skilled infants and even more among those whose secure base behavior seems less skilled. This is particularly evident under the stress of separation and reunion in the standard strange situation, and particularly during reunion episodes. Secure infants are characterized by comfortable exploration in mother's presence, reduced exploration when she leaves, positive greeting or proximity seeking when she returns, effective comforting by contact if needed, and return to preseparation levels of exploration. Within this framework, some secure infants favor independent exploration, whereas others some prefer interactive play. Some cry during separation, others do not. And reunion behavior ranges from active distance interaction to close contact. These patterns tend to be stable across time and are entirely consistent with the organization and adaptive function of the secure base concept.

The most surprising aspect of infant attachment behavior is that ineffective secure base behavior in the strange situation finds two very different expressions. Avoidant infants show little greeting or proximity seeking in reunion episodes. They may in fact abort active approaches, actively avert gaze, or ignore the mother's call. They may also show flashes of anger in their expression or cries. Mary Main (1981) has suggested that, at low levels, this behavior heightens maternal attachment behavior. And indeed, mothers often chide avoidant infants saying, "Oh, you're angry" or "Don't be angry," and seeking to engage them or pick them up.

Resistant (ambivalent) infants are extremely distressed by separation and yet approach behavior is weak or entirely absent when mother returns. In addition, they find little comfort in contact and are often angered if mother tries to comfort them with a toy. They are sometimes termed "ambivalent" in reference to the fact that they mix weak contact maintaining with strong protest if mother puts them on the floor. Exploratory behavior rarely recovers to preseparation levels during the reunion episodes.

The avoidant and the resistant patterns are not merely attenuated secure base behavior; they are entirely paradoxical. Both reflect distress at separation and, from the point of view of the secure base phenomenon, self-defeating behavior upon reunion. Separation is the source of the infant's distress.[1] And when mother returns and greets them from the door, the solution to their problem is at hand. They need only take it. But they do not. The question is why?

Each of these patterns has a certain coherence or logic to it. This has led some to suggest that they are strategic (Main, 1990) even adaptive in human evolution (Belsky, 1999). In addition, they are clearly discrete; that is, they are not arbitrary divisions on a spectrum. They are also very consistent and have a wide range of competence-related correlates (Colin, 1996). And perhaps most surprisingly, the secure, avoidant, and resistant patterns have proven to be useful prototypes for describing patterns of attachment in adults (Main & Solomon, 1986).

The primary attachment classifications (secure, avoidant, and resistant) and their subgroups were discovered early, and relatively few new groups have been added. The first was the B4 subgroup of secure infants. These infants are extremely distressed by separation but, unlike resistant infants, they show active proximity seeking and contact maintaining. Most importantly, they are comforted by contact and return to effective play as long as they are permitted to stay close to the mother or on her lap. This pattern was first noticed in Sylvia Bell's (1970) dissertation research and has become quite familiar in subsequent research. The disorganized pattern described by Main and Solomon (1986) has been the only widely accepted addition to this catalogue.

Although secure, avoidant, and resistant attachment patterns are familiar, it would be too much to say that we fully understand them. Understanding an attachment pattern involves three steps: identification, validation, and explanation. Identification is a matter of establishing that the pattern exists: coding it reliably and determining that the pattern happens frequently enough to be considered significant, that it shows stability and change consistent with attachment theory. Validation is the process of demonstrating that the pattern reflects individual differences in secure base behavior, not temperament, developmental quotient (DQ), or some other behavioral or psychological construct. Validation research typically involves examining predicted correlates such as maternal sensitivity or maternal state of mind with respect to attachment, secure base behavior at home, and affective, behavioral and cognitive correlates in naturalistic and standardized settings. It also involves examining alternative interpretations by independently assessing temperament, IQ, and so forth. Finally, explanation is the process of developing and testing hypotheses about the mechanisms underlying an attachment pattern. Ideally, these would involve detailed understanding of links between an underlying attachment control system and attachment classification.

This could be accomplished in any of several ways. For secure patterns, this could involve mapping classification criteria into a specific control systems model and arguing persuasively that the conditions leading to secure attachment also play a role in the development of this particular control system. This would also be relevant to explaining an insecure pattern. Alternatively, or in addition, one could develop a persuasive argument that specific failures in a control system would account for (i.e., predict) the behavior associated with the insecure pattern. For example, all control systems models include appraisal and effector components. Appraisal components integrate information about the environment, caregiver behavior, infant state, and so forth, and output information about the infant's "felt security." In response to this information, effector components select and integrate proximity seeking and other secure base behaviors until output from the appraisal system returns to acceptable limits. Failures in either system would interfere with the kind of active response and return to play that is the hallmark of secure attachment.

And finally, it would be a step toward explaining an insecure pattern if we could make the case that experiences specifically associated with its development or with activation of characteristic behaviors would in fact interfere with an underlying control system in specific ways. Each of these involves close argument and empirical support. These, in turn, depend on developing specific hypotheses about the components and organization of the attachment control system and on establishing behavioral facts that can be used to distinguish between alternative control systems models and various hypotheses about the development and activation of the behaviors associated with an attachment pattern.

Each of the primary attachment classifications is now well justified and validated. With the publication of this volume, we believe, much the same can be said of the disorganized pattern. The task now is to move from validation to explanation. Unfortunately, attachment theorists rarely achieve or even attempt the kind of analytic explanation of attachment patterns discussed above. Instead, we most often settle for hypotheses that make only informal reference to mechanisms or that invoke mechanisms without the expectation that they will, or can be, rigorously tested against empirical data.

Despite the limitations of current theory and methods, it is worth defining analytical explanation in terms of control systems models as a standard against which to measure other approaches to explaining attachment patterns. This is the kind of explanation Bowlby had in mind when he proposed the control systems model and defining it as a goal is an important step toward keeping the control systems concept and the secure base phenomenon at the heart of attachment theory. Focusing on analytic explanation also ensures that we do not settle for identification and validation alone. These are important but they do not take us to the level of mechanisms that ultimately is necessary truly to explain attachment patterns and realize Bowlby's goal of an effective prevention and therapy.

This chapter reports data that can stimulate hypotheses about the development and activation of the disorganized attachment pattern and help sort out alternative interpretations. This takes us beyond identification and validation, and brings us a step closer to the kind of explanation outlined earlier. Our data are from samples of well-nourished and mild-to-moderately undernourished children living on the outskirts of Santiago, Chile. The primary goal of the study was to examine links between maternal sensitivity and the children's nutritional status. In the course of the research, the children were seen in the strange situation at 18 and 28 months of age. Especially at the younger age, a surprisingly large number of the subjects could not be assigned to any of the traditional attachment classifications. Instead, they were extremely inconsistent, showing behavior characteristic of one classification in the first reunion and then a very different pattern in the next. Because these data were connected prior to the widespread use of the disorganized classification, and prior to the emergence of systems for scoring the strange situation beyond infancy, these infants were classified "atypical." As described below, this corresponds to at least a subset of the infants who would today be classified Disorganized. This chapter reports that atypical attachment is strongly associated with nutritional status and that rates of atypical attachment diminished markedly with age. These surprising findings suggest interesting and testable hypotheses about the nature of disorganized attachment and provide information that can be used to evaluate existing hypotheses. They also have implications for our perspective on the development of secure attachment.

ATTACHMENT STABILITY AND CHANGE

Stability of infant–mother attachment between 18 and 20 months has been examined in a wide range of samples. Overall, studies on stability of attachment have found secure–anxious classification in the strange situation to be stable in middle-class samples when no major changes were experienced by the families between the two assessments. Several researchers have demonstrated the long-term stability of attachment. Connell (1976), using a discriminant analysis classification procedure, found 80% stability between attachment classification at 12 months and later classification at 18 months. Similarly, Waters (1978) using classifications made by trained coders, reported 96% stability at 12 and 18 months. Main and Weston (1981) reported 80% stability of attachment toward the mother at 12 and 20 months in all major classifications, including an "unclassifiable" group. In a follow-up study designed to assess continuity of organization of attachment behaviors beyond infancy, Main, Kaplan and Cassidy (1985) also reported significant stability of attachment in children assessed in the strange situation at 12 months, and later assessed at 6 years, in a modified procedure to assess attachment at this age.[2]

These data have been important in establishing the reliability of strange situation assessments and have played a part in the adoption of this assessment for a wide range of research on the early social and emotional development of children. Data on changes in attachment classification over a 6-month period in relation to changes in family circumstances and stressful life events have also contributed to our confidence in the strange situation and to our understanding of the individual differences it measures. In particular, Thompson, Lamb, and Estes (1982) have shown that strange situation classifications can change markedly when mothers of 1-year-olds are returning to work after spending the child's first year at home. Reported stability by these authors is 53% for overall classification of children seen at 13 and 20 months old. Vaughn, Egeland, Sroufe, and Waters (1979) have also reported substantial change in strange situation classification from 12 to 18 months in a low socioeconomic status sample. Most importantly, they were able to relate patterns of change to stressful life events mothers experienced between the two assessments. Mothers of infants who were anxiously attached at both assessments reported the highest number of stressful events. Those whose infants had been secure and changed to anxious reported fewer stressful events. Fewer still were reported by mothers whose infants improved from anxious to secure. Fewest occurrence of stressful life events of all were reported by mothers of stable, secure children.

These data have been important for several reasons. First, Bowlby's attachment theory is a theory of the infant's responsiveness to salient environmental cues and to patterns of maternal care. It stipulates that infant–mother attachment develops from interaction and requires that relationships be responsive to changes in infants experience. In addition, infant attachment relationship has come to be viewed as being modified by changes in the caregiver or the infant for mutual accommodation in a predictable manner. This responsiveness to life events, along with data indicating that attachment relationships with mother and father are not highly correlated, have contributed to provide decisive evidence against a temperament interpretation of strange situation classifications (Sroufe, 1985).

A noteworthy feature in the stability studies to date has been a tendency for change to involve attachment classification moves from anxious to secure, rather than at random, in studies that have not involved specific stressors between test and retest assessments. This phenomenon may be understood in terms of the organism's self-righting tendencies in development (Sameroff & Chandler, 1975), the infant's active role in eliciting care (Main, 1981) and in the increasing influence of infant behavior on the caregiver with age (Bell & Harper, 1977).

The present analysis of attachment stability was undertaken within the context of a study examining relations between maternal sensitivity, child nutrition, and attachment security of low-income, mild-to-moderately chronically undernourished children at 18 months (Valenzuela, 1990, 1997). This research has already demonstrated links between insensitive maternal care, poor infant nutrition, and high rates of insecure attachment.

The present longitudinal data were collected for several reasons. First, strange situation stability data in our low income control group were obtained for comparison with data from low income samples in North America (e.g., Vaughn et al., 1979). Similar stability results in Chile would be one of several types of evidence supporting our use of the strange situation in this culture. Second, these data were also collected in order to evaluate the stability of the relationships between the nutritional and the attachment variables described by Valenzuela (1990) at 18 months. Finally, stability data were collected because our initial assessment at 18 months indicated that there was a very high rate of atypical attachments (51%, which also included 32% of an anxious–avoidant–resistant pattern) in our chronically undernourished sample. These are rare in middle-class, nonclinical samples, and they have not been closely studied. Retest data are a potentially valuable source information about atypical strange situation classifications and about their relationships to other attachment patterns.

SUBJECTS

The subjects for this project were 34 nutritionally healthy children (> 90% of expected weight for age) and 37 mild-to-moderately undernourished children (70–85% of expected weight for age) and their mothers. Both samples were recruited through neighborhood community health clinics in an impoverished neighborhood of Santiago, Chile. There were no statistically significant differences between the two different nutritional groups in family income, mother's age or education, father's age, education or type of occupation, family size, or number of children. All children were last born, full-term, and normal birth weight.

The families lived in a treeless, impoverished community of approximately 15,000 on the outskirts of Santiago, a city of approximately 5 million. In general, the unpaved streets were clean, and violent crimes (as opposed to property crimes) were rare. However, crowding, health problems, underemployment, family conflict, and male alcohol abuse were significant problems in this community. The families lived in one- to two-room concrete block structures with earthen floors. All of the homes had clean indoor water and basic electricity. The number of children ranged from one to four per family. All of the fathers earned subsistence incomes as laborers, peddlers, or in subsidized employment (e.g., cleaning parks or construction sites) in Santiago. All but one of the mothers was at home full time; one mother, employed as a peddler, took her child with her each day. Mothers' earnings for work performed at home were intermittent and minimal.

The community was served by a system of community health centers that provided basic health care (including birth control) consultation, services, and referrals. Each center was staffed by physicians, nurses, nutritionists, and social workers. The present study was conducted in three centers that specialized in child health care and nutrition. Each provided well-baby care and distributed free supplies of powered milk for children under 6 years old. All of the subjects lived within walking distance of one of these centers.

With the exception of two of the dyads, all subjects came from intact families. Between the first and the second assessment, no major changes in family composition occurred, no mothers started working outside the home, no new child care arrangements were made, and no child had started day care or experienced illness requiring hospitalization. Only 7% of the families seen in the second assessment changed residence between assessments. Fourteen (16.5%) mother–infant dyads were not seen in the second assessment. These families changed residence outside the city or moved within the city limits but did not notify the Community Health Clinic of a change of address.

ASSESSMENT PROCEDURES

All mother–infant dyads were initially seen in the strange situation procedure at a mean age of 18 months (range = 17–21 months). The second assessment was conducted at a mean age of 28 months (range = 24–32 months). The strange situation is a standardized, well-validated procedure to assess quality of infant–mother attachment. It consists of eight 3-minute episodes, including two separations and two reunions with mother. The Ainsworth et al. (1978) procedures were used without modification at both ages and were recorded on videotape.

Behavior in the strange situation is only scoreable if the child has both the locomotor and cognitive competence necessary to recognize the novelty of the situation, to note and recall the mother's absence and return, and (in principle) to activate secure base behavior during reunions. In home-reared middle-class infants, these are well consolidated in virtually all healthy 1-year-olds. Because we could not assume that 12-month-olds reared in extreme poverty would display fully developed secure base behavior, our initial assessments were conducted at 18 months.

Children were classified into Ainsworth's major (A, B, or C) attachment categories according to the scoring system outlined by Ainsworth et al. (1978). Although this system is best validated for infants 12–18 months of age, it seemed more appropriate for the present sample than adaptations designed for older children (e.g., Cassidy & Marvin, 1992). First of all the Ainsworth procedure is not irrelevant to children as old as 28 months. Bosso, Corter, and Abramovitch (in press) report a strong association between Ainsworth strange situation classifications and Q-sort observations of secure base behavior at home in a sample of 18- to 32-month-olds (mean age = 26.3 months). Moreover, the Ainsworth scoring criteria seemed entirely adequate to the task in this sample. We saw few indications that the content or organization of the subjects' secure base behavior involved the kinds of developmental and strategic shifts cited in the Cassidy and Marvin (1992) system. For example, there was little indication that avoidance was more subtle than in infant samples (Cassidy & Marvin, 1992, p. 15). There was also little indication that resistant behavior was accompanied by or had been replaced by controlling behavior (p. 56). Nor did verbal behavior play a prominent role in the infants' secure base behavior (pp. 35, 42). The relevance of the Ainsworth scoring system at both 18 and 28 months is also supported by the fact that agreement between independent coders was high and approximately equal at both ages.

Even within the Ainsworth scoring system, a substantial number of subjects could not be assigned standard classifications. These were infants, especially in the mild-to-moderately undernourished sample, whose behavior was easily scored within episodes but was inconsistent across episodes. Their behavior was (1) typical of one insecure group (A or C) in the first reunion and then a distinctively different (C or A) pattern in the second; (2) typical of one insecure group (A or C) in the first moments of a reunion episode; followed by a change to a distinctively different (C or A) insecure pattern during the remainder of the episode, or (3) alternated between A- and C-type responses throughout the final reunion episode. To avoid the risk of overinterpreting unexpected behavior in these cross-cultural and very deprived samples, we designated these subjects "insecure–atypical" rather than disorganized. We also used this designation because we noted few of the "odd" behaviors that are today associated with the disorganized attachment pattern. Nonetheless, most of these "atypical" children would meet Main and Solomon's (1990) criteria for the "D" classification by virtue of "sequential display of contradictory behavior patterns."[3]

Both authors independently scored the 18- and 28-month strange situations. The follow-up strange situations were scored approximately 1 year after the 18-month sessions. In addition, the two sets of videotapes were not identified by name or identical subject numbers. Agreement was 88.2% for the 18-month data and 83.7% for the 28-month data. Disagreements led to review of the videotapes, and final classification was- decided by the more experienced rater. Nutritional status was not readily apparent from the video records at either age.

RESULTS

All of the subjects retained the same nutritional status for the duration of the study.

Nutritionally Healthy Sample

The 18- and 28-month classifications for the low-income, normally developing children are presented in Table 10.1. Fifty percent (17/34) of the adequately nourished infants were classified secure at the 18 months and 67.6% (23/34) were classified secure at 28 months (n.s.). Overall, 21/34 (61.8%) of the children received the same secure vs. insecure classification at both ages (kappa = .24, $p < .17$). Using four categories (A, B, C, Atypical), 21/34 (61.8%) of the children received the same received the same classification at both ages (kappa = .3 7, $p < .01$). As in previous research (e.g., Ainsworth, Blehar, Waters & Wall, 1978; Waters, 1978; Egeland & Farber, 1984), secure classifications were more stable than insecure classifications.

Among secure infants, 14/17 (82.4%) received the same classification at both ages. Only 8/17 (47.1%) insecure infants received the same classification at both ages. These rates of secure versus insecure attachment and stability versus change are comparable to data from a large North American sample of low socioeconomic status families (Vaughn et al., 1979).

TABLE 10.1. Attachment Classification at 18 and 28 Months
in the Well-Nourished Group

18-month attachment classifications	28-month attachment classifications				
	Avoidant	Secure	Resistant	Atypical	Total
Avoidant	4	2	0	0	6
Secure	1	14	1	1	17
Resistant	0	3	3	0	6
Atypical	1	4	0	0	5
Total	6	23	4	1	34

Mild-to-Moderately Undernourished Sample

The 18- and 28-month classifications for the mild-to-moderately undernourished sample are presented in Table 10.2. Only 8.1% (3/37) of the
children in this sample were classified secure at 18 months, and 27% (10/
37) were classified secure at 28 months ($p < .04$). These rates are significantly lower than in the socioeconomically matched adequately nourished
sample at both 18 months ($p < .01$) and 28 months ($p < .01$).

Overall, 24/37 (64.9%) of the mild-to-moderately undernourished
children received the same secure versus insecure classification at both
ages (kappa = –.14, $p < .56$). This is comparable to stability of secure versus
insecure classifications in the nutritionally healthy sample ($p < .99$). Using
four categories (A, B, C, Atypical), only 12/37 (32.4%) of the moderately
undernourished subjects received the same classification (A, B, C, Atypical) at both ages (kappa = 13, $p < .15$).

This is significantly less than the stability of four-group classifications
in the adequately nourished sample ($kappa_1$ vs. $kappa_2$, $p < .01$).

None (0/3) of the children classified secure at 18 months received the

TABLE 10.2. Attachment Classifications at 18 and 28 Months
in the Mild-to-Moderately Undenourished Group

18-month attachment classifications	28-month attachment classifications				
	Avoidant	Secure	Resistant	Atypical	Total
Avoidant	4	1	0	1	6
Secure	2	0	1	0	3
Resistant	0	1	4	2	7
Atypical	5	8	4	4	21
Total	11	10	9	7	37

same classification at 28 months. This is significantly less than the 82.4% stability of insecure attachment in the adequately nourished sample ($p <$ .01).[4] In contrast, 24/34 (70.6%) children classified insecure at 18 months were also classified insecure at 28 months. This is significantly greater than the 47.1% stability of insecure attachment in the adequately nourished sample ($p < .05$).

In brief, adequately nourished children were more likely than mild-to-moderately undernourished children to be securely attached. They were more likely to receive the same four-group attachment classification across age. As discussed below, this was largely due to the high rate and instability of atypical attachment in the mild-to-moderately undernourished sample.

Atypical Attachment

Atypical attachment was more common among mild-to-moderately under-nourished children at both ages (56.8% (21/37) vs. 14.7% (5/34), $p < .01$ at 18-months, and 18.9% (7/37) vs. 2.9% (1/34), $p < .04$ at 28 months). In addition, the proportion of insecure infants classified atypical declined across age in both samples. This effect was especially marked in the mild-to-moderately undernourished sample (91.9% (21/34) of the insecure classifications at 18 months versus 25.9% (7/27) of the 28-month insecure classifications, $p < .01$).

This explains the fact that the stability of secure versus insecure classifications was similar across samples, while four-group classifications were less stable in the mild-to-moderately undernourished sample.

Finally, it is worth noting that the fate of atypical attachment was different in the two samples. In the adequately nourished sample, 4/5 (80%) of the atypical 18-month-olds were secure at 28 months. In the mild-to-moderately undernourished sample, only 8/21 (38.1%) became secure. The remainder (9/21) were classified avoidant or resistant and 4/21 remained Atypical.

DISCUSSION

A substantial number of children in this study showed an atypical attachment pattern in the strange situation. This involved inconsistent patterns of avoidant and resistant behavior across reunion episodes, changing from avoidance to resistance (or vice versa) within reunion episodes, and occasionally alternating between avoidance and resistance throughout the final reunion episode. Under the traditional strange situation classification system these infants would most often be informally classified A/C and simply be scored as insecure for most data analyses. If it were necessary to force an A or C classification, most coders would give greater weight to behavior in the second reunion.

Main and Solomon's (1986, 1990) recognition of disorganized responses to separation and reunion has focused attention on the possibility that there may a logic to such behavior. A wide range of studies reviewed and included in this volume have shown that the disorganized attachment pattern can be scored reliably, has good discriminant validity vis-à-vis temperament constructs, and has a wide range of important correlates in maternal behavior and competence-related outcomes. The task now is to move from identification and validation to explanation.

Although the children in our samples did not show the full range of behaviors associated with the disorganized attachment pattern, they uniformly displayed sequences of contradictory behaviors. The hallmark of their strange situation behavior was inconsistent patterns of avoidant and resistant behavior within and across reunion episodes. We described these infants as "atypical" rather than disorganized, because our data were initially scored before the Main and Solomon (1986) scoring system was fully validated. In addition, we wanted to avoid overinterpreting the behavior of children from a cultural and socioeconomic context quite unlike those in which the traditional Ainsworth classifications and the Main and Solomon scoring system were developed. Nonetheless, most of the atypical children in our sample would today be classified disorganized.

Interestingly, there was little evidence of misdirected or incomplete behaviors, stereotypies, freezing, confusion or disorganized behavior, or apprehension regarding the parent. This suggests that there may be distinct subgroups of disorganized attachment, perhaps associated with different etiologies (Spangler, Fremmer-Bombik, & Grossmann, 1996). This said, it is useful to examine alternative explanations for the behavior we observed and the relevance of these explanations to the broader concept of disorganized attachment. As mentioned earlier, attachment theory and research have not yet reached the point of explaining attachment patterns in terms of specific control systems models and their operating characteristics. It is not too early, however, to move beyond identification and validation to consider the types of mechanisms that might explain disorganized attachment. Indeed, this is a good time to start asking what the answer may be like.

Infant Characteristics and Atypical Attachment

Because both of our samples were drawn from the same neighborhoods, the high rate of Atypical attachment in the mild-to-moderately undernourished children cannot be explained in terms of greater socioeconomic disadvantage. It is possible, however, that poor nutrition itself contributed to this effect. For example, poor nutritional status might contribute directly to high and stable rates of insecure attachment by interfering with a child's tolerance of stress and thus with the ability to organize coherent separation and reunion responses. This would be consistent with Spangler and Grossmann (1996 and Chapter 4, this volume) interpretation of disorganized attachment. This emphasis on the ability to produce organized behavior under stress articulates well with Main and Solomon's emphasis on conflict and approach–avoidance as motivational factors in Disorganized attachment. For as Sroufe and Waters (1976) have noted, increasing ability to maintain organized behavior under stress (i.e., greater stress tolerance) is a hallmark of early socioemotional development.

What is missing from such explanations is specific reference to the effects of stress on a secure base control system; that is, if stress and conflict are truly explanatory, we should be able to detail how stress impacts on a specific control systems model to produce exactly the behavior associated with disorganized attachment. In principle, stress could interfere with the input, integrative, or output functions of an attachment control system; that is, it could interfere with (1) a child's perception of separation and reunion situations, (2) access to representations of past experience, (3) appraisal processes, and/or (4) selection, activation, and coordination of secure base responses.

Developing testable hypotheses at this level of analysis is important to achieving the goals Bowlby had in mind for the control systems model. Indeed, without this kind of analysis, explanations in terms of stress and conflict are largely post hoc. It is not enough to explain atypical or disorganized attachment in terms of stress. We have to ask why we see disorganization in some aspects of behavior and not in others, and why these patterns of attachment are associated with some stressful contexts and rearing environments and not others. As in other areas of psychology, stress and coping can easily explain too much and reduce explanation to the empty notion that all good (and bad) things go together. The best protection against this is to ask stress and coping theorists to outline the mechanisms through which stress and coping could produce all of the behaviors that need to be explained, without producing behaviors that in fact are not observed.

Hypotheses about the mechanisms underlying the effects of stress and coping can be addressed indirectly through correlational data and close examination of secure base behavior at home and in the strange situation. They can also be addressed via experimental analyses of secure and Disorganized children's perceptions, appraisals, and secure base responses to well defined circumstances and patterns of maternal behavior. Although stress is most often treated as a unitary construct, it is in fact a very complex phenomenon with wide individual differences in its eliciting conditions and modes of expression (Nachmias, Gunnar, Mangelsdorf, Parritz, & Buss, 1996). For these reasons, measures of psychobiological variables such as stress related hormones may prove useful for manipulation checks and as dependent variables in some of this research.

Caregiver Behavior and Atypical Attachment

The association between poor nutrition and atypical attachment is also consistent with the hypothesis that a third variable contributes independently to poor nutrition and insecure attachment. The obvious candidate is inadequate maternal behavior. As mentioned earlier, the mothers in this sample were poorly educated, underemployed, impoverished, and had little hope that their circumstances would improve. Under these circumstances, chronically detached and depressed mothers might well have provided both inadequate nutrition and inadequate secure base behavior.[5]

As with stress and coping constructs, reference to maternal behavior easily explains too much and too easily leads us toward the hypothesis that all good (and bad) things go together. Again, the best defense is specificity. Insofar as possible, parental behavior as explanations of disorganized attachment should specify exactly what aspect of parental behavior is involved and how its interaction with an attachment control system would produce observed behaviors without also producing behaviors that are not observed. Unfortunately, this is easier to achieve conceptually than empirically. All of the factors that influence parental behavior can create correlations across a wide range of caregiving responses. Thus, it is difficult to isolate specific components of parental care in empirical research, especially because much that is important in parental care cannot ethically be manipulated. Faced with these same constraints, Bowlby's strategy was to seek conceptual clarity in control systems theory and hope that this would reveal the best possibilities for empirical analysis.

The best known explanation of disorganized attachment is Main and Hesse's (1990) "frightened and/or frightening maternal behavior" hypothesis. They note that the hallmarks of disorganized attachment are competition among, or inhibition of, attachment behaviors, especially just as they are being initiated (p. 173). They also note that freezing and apprehensive behavior are part of the disorganized attachment pattern. Thus, Main and Hesse (1991) suggest that initiation and then inhibition of an attachment behavior sequence by fear is central to the disorganized attachment pattern.[6]

Following Bowlby, Main and Hesse suggest that the infant's fear reflects something in its actual experience. Obvious examples include physical abuse and extreme behaviors associated with parental psychosis.

They also suggest that a parent suffering from unresolved mourning may still be frightened by the loss and, as a result, may display anxiety, unusual vocal patterns and speech content, unusual movements, and lapses of cognitive monitoring that an infant or young child might find frightening. The clarity and testability of this explanation is enhanced by the fact that Main and Hesse explicitly cast it in terms of Bowlby's attachment control systems construct. This proves a useful framework within which to contrast the cognitive and motivational state of avoidant and resistant infants with that of disorganized infants at various points in separation and reunion episodes. Their analysis emphasizes that, for the disorganized infant, the mother herself, not the situation, is the source of distress. The control systems framework clarifies how this limits the child's response options and sets the stage for sustained high levels of stress. This, they suggest, leads to behavioral inhibition and disorganization.

This analysis has much to recommend it. It is relatively detailed and closely mapped into Bowlby's control systems model. As a result, it suggests a wide range of testable hypotheses. Nonetheless, we have several reservations that could be addressed empirically. First, it is not clear that lapses of monitoring, behavioral dysfluencies, and related behavior would stand out among the imperfections, interruptions, and intrusions that come with even the most sensitive maternal care in a real environment. Nor is it clear that they would be perceived as frightening if they were. These issues can certainly be addressed in naturalistic observations and in experimental studies of infants' reactions to simulated lapses, dysfluencies, and so on.

A second concern is that Main and Hesse's analysis does not anticipate heterogeneity among disorganized infants; that is, it does not anticipate that in a study such as ours, children would show sequential incongruities but not misdirected or interrupted behavior, stereotypies, freezing, or apprehension. It is possible that the "frightening and/or frightened maternal behavior" hypothesis can be elaborated to accommodate this concern. This might be facilitated by a taxonomic search to identify subgroups of disorganized infants and children. It would be useful if this included data on ordinary secure base behavior from naturalistic settings, as well as emergency behavior from contexts such as the strange situation.

Finally, the "frightening and/or frightened maternal behavior" hypothesis does not anticipate the significant decline in atypical attachment observed in the present study. Although one could speculate that with maturation infants are increasingly able to maintain organized behavior in the face of frightening and/or frightened maternal behavior. However, this implies that disorganized behavior would be rare after early childhood, which it is not, especially in clinical samples (van IJzendoorn, Schuengel, & Bakermans-Kranenburg, 1999).

Caregiver Behavior and Attachment Organization

Bowlby suggested that the attachment behavior control system is part of our primate evolutionary endowment. This, and his references to imprinting, has led many to think of the attachment control system as a fully organized blueprint genetically mapped in the human brain, ready to emerge fully organized when activated by appropriate maternal behavior. Although there is some support for this view in Bowlby's writings, he consistently emphasized the role of experience over time and contexts in attachment development. As Waters, Kondo-Ikemura, Posada, and Richters (1991) point out, our primate endowment is less likely to be a fully organized blueprint than a set of biases in our learning abilities that make it easy to integrate control system components through experience with an organized pattern of caregiver behavior. This is what Bowlby was referring to when he stated that attachment development depends on experience of species-typical parental care. Indeed, an organized and organizing environment is critical to the development of every physiological perceptual and complex behavior control system. Building upon organization in the environment reduces the amount of information that has to be encoded genetically and also allows developing systems to adapt to prevailing conditions.

This perspective suggests an alternative view of parental behavior and disorganized attachment patterns. If the attachment control system depends on organized and organizing patterns of secure base support, it follows that it will not be properly organized if such support is absent, disorganized, or markedly discrepant from the caregiving environment that our primate heritage takes for granted. This would lead to dysfluent and perhaps even disorganized attachment behavior in both ordinary and emergency situations.

Naturalistic observations have consistently demonstrated links between maternal sensitivity and infant secure base behavior (Ainsworth et al., 1978; Pederson, Moran, Sitko, Campbell, Ghesquire, & Acton, 1990; Kondo-Ikemura & Waters, 1995; Posada, Jacobs, Carbonell, Alzate, & Bustamante, 1999). However, most of this work has used broad measures of maternal sensitivity and infant security. Attachment researchers have not yet examined in detail the roles of specific caregiver behaviors in the emergence and integration of specific secure base control systems components. One of the key issues is whether integration of control systems components depends on specific facets of care (e.g., physical contact, comforting, response to social referencing) or on the aggregate effect of sensitivity across modalities.

Another concerns the role that infants' own behavior and maternal responses play in establishing and consolidating dominant secure base responses; that is, what makes a particular response or pattern of response more "available" and thus more likely to be activated in a particular situation? And what keeps alternative responses from being activated and competing with the dominant response? Clearly, the answer is experience, but what kind of experience? And which components of the secure base control system are involved? Unfortunately, we understand little about the development of integration within and across input, appraisal response selection, and output components of the attachment control system. One of the first issues to address here is how inconsistent care differs from the lack of care. Another is the relative contributions of (1) mixed signals in the caregiving environrunent (e.g., Main, 1981; Main & Hesse, 1990) and (2) problems within the secure base control system to disorganized attachment patterns. Until such issues are examined in detail, understanding of secure, insecure, and disorganized attachment patterns are necessarily speculative and not very specific.

Many of the mothers in our Chilean samples were chronically disengaged and many would have met the criteria for clinical depression. Disengagement and depression were particularly evident in the mothers of the mild-to-moderately undernourished children. It seems likely that they also provided poorly organized secure base support.

Although poorly organized secure base support could affect almost any aspect of a developing attachment control system, the inconsistency across episodes observed in our sample and the simultaneous display of incompatible behaviors, incomplete and interrupted behaviors, and "odd" movements that define the D classification suggest that the problem is primarily one of response selection. One of the functions of the attachment control system is to integrate information about the physical situation, the mother, and the child's expectations, the attachment control system, and to pass the result to components that select an appropriate response. We suggest that some of the hallmarks of disorganized attachment result when the control systems components responsible for this integration fail to pass along a signal that is strong enough and or selective enough to activate and maintain a single predominant response. Under various circumstances, this could produce a wide range of outputs, ranging from no response to interrupted responses, activation of more than one response, and alternating responses. Moreover, the inability to produce or maintain an adaptive response could prove very stressful.

This analysis has two important implications. The first is that the primary factor in disorganized attachment may prove to be response selection rather than fear or apprehension regarding the mother. The second is that fear or apprehension regarding the mother is not a necessary condition for disorganization. The inability to select and maintain an organized (be it secure or insecure) response can itself be a cause of fear and apprehension; that is, fear and "apprehension" may be the *result* rather than the cause of behavioral disorganization.

This response selection hypothesis is consistent with many of the observations cited in support of the "frightened and or frightening matemal behavior" hypothesis. For example, both abusive and psychologically disturbed caregivers are likely to provide poor secure base support. The same may be said of caregivers whose unresolved mouming distracts them or undermines motivation necessary to provide organized and organizing secure base support. In addition, it anticipates that as a child gets older, he or she may be more able to detect weak or inconsistent organization in the caregiver's behavior. It may also be more able to actively elicit organized care. Depending on why the caregiver's behavior was deficient in the first place, this might lead to secure attachment in some cases and to well-configured insecure attachment patterns in others. If the caregiver is seriously disturbed, or the caregiving environment is inconsistent with organized and organizing secure base support, the disorganized attachment pattern would persist. In contrast, the "frightened and or frightening matemal behavior" hypothesis suggests that both the caregiver's problems and the child's experience of aversive secure base support are relatively enduring. Consequently, it predicts that disorganized attachment will typically endure. Our results indicate that this is not always the case. The mothers in our sample were, after all, far more disadvantaged that disturbed. And as a result, they may have been able to provide more organized and organizing secure base support when, after infancy, their children could present stronger or clearer demands for secure base support.

One Pattern of Disorganized Attachment or Several?

Diversity among children with disorganized attachment is a difficult problem for any theory. Most can be adapted post hoc to account for specific examples of diversity. But few can predict patterns of diversity in advance. In all likelihood, some of the diversity among disorganized attachment patterns win be due to the fact that more than one variable is in play; that is, children will inevitably have different experiences and develop different expectations from even similar experiences. In addition, there will always be wide individual differences in cognitive, behavioral, and physiological coping mechanisms, and in thresholds for distress. There are also many different ways that the structure or function of a secure base control system might lead to disorganized behavior. Some of these might be examined via computer simulation.

The present study illustrates the diversity of disorganized attachment patterns. It also provides interesting findings that can be used to test the power of hypotheses about the mechanisms underlying disorganized attachment. If we cannot yet predict the ways in which disorganized attachment will be diverse, we can at least discover and carefully describe them.

Thus, taxonomic research on the ordinary and emergency secure base behavior of disorganized infants and children deserves high priority in attachment research. We hope the results will suggest useful hypotheses about the origins of this diversity and about the nature of disorganized attachment. In turn, this may contribute to our understanding of avoidant, resistant, and secure attachment patterns.

ACKNOWLEDGMENTS

The data for this study were collected as part of a longitudinal study of nutrition and socioemotional development. This project was designed and directed by Marta Valenzuela with the generous support of the Nestle Foundation.

NOTES

1. Heart rate telemetry indicates that even avoidant infants, whose low level of overt distress is sometimes mistaken for lack of concern, find separation stressful (Spangler & Grossmann, 1993; Sroufe & Waters, 1977.

2. This is not to say that attachment security exhibits trait-like stability regardless of circumstances. As Vaughn, Egeland, Sroufe, and Waters (1979) and Waters, Kondo-Ikemura, Posada, and Richters (1991) indicate, Bowlby's theory predicts both that attachment security tends to be consistent across time in ordinary rearing environments and open to revision in light of experience. As a result, it can change if caregiving changes across time (e.g., Vaughn et al., 1979; Belsky, Campbell Cohn, & Moore, 1996).

3. As mentioned earlier, we noticed few behaviors in the 28-month strange situations that seemed inconsistent with standard Ainsworth et al. (1978) classification criteria. Indeed, Bosso, Abramovitch, and Corter (in press) have demonstrated the validity of these criteria in a sample of 2- to 3-year-olds by comparing them to direct observations of secure base at home with the Attachment Q-set (Waters & Deane, 1985). Virtually all of the subjects classified secure, avoidant, and resistant at the 28-month follow-up would have received corresponding classifications in the Cassidy and Marvin (1992) revised classification system for 30- to 54-month-olds. The majority of the "atypical" infants would have been classified insecure–other. Because most of the inconsistency in their behavior was across rather than within episodes, few would have met the criteria for insecure–controlling–disorganized. In addition, inconsistency across episodes would also have precluded our reporting underlying ("forced") classifications for most of the Atypical subjects.

4. Although the difference between the stability of secure (0/3) and insecure classifications (24/34) in this sample is significantly greater than 0 ($p < .01$), we cannot accurately estimate the stability of secure attachment from only three cases.

5. As mentioned earlier, free infant nutritional supplements were provided by the community health centers.

6. They allow, however, that disorganized attachment behavior might arise as well from neurological impairment or confusion due to inconsistent signals from the caregiver.

REFERENCES

Ainsworth, M., Blehar, M., Waters, E., & Wall, S. (1978). *Patterns of attachment.* Hillsdale, NJ: Erlbaum.

Bell, R. A., & Harper, L. (1977). *Child effects on adults.* Hillsdale, NJ: Erlbaum.

Bell, S. (1970). The development of the concept of the object as related to infant–mother attachment. *Child Development, 41,* 291–311.

Belsky, J. (1999). Modern evolutionary theory and patterns of attachment. In J. Cassidy & P. Shaver (Eds.), *Handbook of attachment: Theory, research, and clinical applications* (pp. 141–161). New York: Guilford Press.

Belsky, J., Campbell, S., Cohn, J., & Moore, G. (1996). Instability of attachment security. *Developmental Psychology 32,* 921–924.

Bischof, N. (1975). A systems approach toward the functional connections of attachment and fear. *Child Development, 46,* 801–817.

Bosso, O. R., Corter, C., & Abramovitch, R. (in press). Attachment behavior at home, sibling behavior, and Strange Situation classifications of 2- and 3-year olds. In. E. Waters, B. Vaughn, G. Posada, & D. Teti (Eds.), *Patterns of secure base behavior: Q-sort perspectives on attachment and caregiving at in infancy and childhood.* Mahwah, NJ: Erlbaum.

Bretherton, I. (1985). Attachment theory: Retrospect and prospect. In I. Bretherton & E. Waters (Eds.), Growing points of attachment theory and research. *Monographs of the Society for Research in Child Development, 50*(1–2, Serial No. 209), 3–35.

Cassidy, J., & Marvin, R. (1992). *Attachment organization in preschool children: Procedures and coding manual.* Unpublished manuscript, Department of Psychology, University of Maryland, College Park.

Colin, V. (1996). *Human attachment.* Philadelphia: Temple University Press

Connell, D. (1976). *Individual differences in attachment: An investigation into stability, implications and relationships to structure of early language development.* Unpublished doctoral dissertation, Syracuse University, Syracuse, NY.

Egeland, B., & Farber, E. (1984). Infant–mother attachment: Factors related to its development and changes over time. *Child Development, 55,* 753–771.

Kondo-Ikemura, K., & Waters, E. (1995). Maternal behavior and infant security in Old World monkeys: Conceptual issues and a methodological bridge between human and non-human primate research. In E. Waters, B. Vaughn, G. Posada, & K. Kondo-Ikemura (Eds.), Caregiving, Cultural, and Cognitive Perspectives on Secure Base Behavior and Working Models. *Monographs of the Society for Research in Child Development, 60,* 97–110.

Main, M. (1981). Avoidance in the service of attachment: A working paper. In K. Immehnann, G. W. Barlow, L. Petrinovich, & M. Main (Eds.), *Behavioral development: The Bielefeld interdisciplinary project* (pp. 651–693). New York: Cambridge University Press.

Main, M. (1990). Cross-cultural studies of attachment organization: Recent studies, changing methodologies, and the concept of conditional strategies. *Human Development, 33,* 48–61.

Main, M., & Hesse, E. (1990). Parents' unresolved traumatic experiences are related to infant disorganized attachment status: Is frightened/frightening parental behavior the linking mechanism? In M. Greenberg, D. Cicchetti, & M. Cummings (Eds.), *Attachment in the Preschool Years,* pp. 161–182. Chicago: University of Chicago Press.

Main, M., Kaplan, N., & Cassidy, J. (1985). Security in infancy, childhood and adulthood. A move to the level of representation. In I. Bretherton & E. Waters (Eds.), Growing points of attachment theory and research. *Monographs of the Society for Research in Child Development, 50*(1–2, Serial No. 209), 66–104.

Main, M., & Solomon, J. (1986). Discovery of a new, insecure–disorganized/disoriented attachment pattern. In T. B. Brazelton & M. Yogman (Eds), *Affective development in infancy* (pp. 95–124). Norwood, NJ: Ablex.

Main, M., & Solomon, J. (1990). Procedures for identifying disorganized/disoriented infants during the Ainsworth Strange Situation. In M. Greenberg, D. Cicchetti, & M. Cummings (Eds), *Attachment in the preschool years* (pp. 121–160). Chicago: University of Chicago Press.

Main, M., & Weston, D. (1981). The quality of the toddler's relationship to mother and to father: related to conflict behaviour and the readiness to establish new relationships. *Child Development, 52,* 932–940.

Nachmias, M., Gunnar, M., Mangelsdorf, S., Parritz, R., & Buss, K. (1996). Behavioral inhibition and stress reactivity: The moderating role of attachment security. *Child Development, 67*(2), 508–522.

Pederson, D. R., Moran, G., Sitko, C., Campbell K., Ghesquire, K., & Acton, H. (1990). Maternal sensitivity and the security of infant–mother attachment. *Child Development, 61,* 1974–1983.

Posada, G., Jacobs, A., Carbonell, O., Alzate, G., & Bustamante, M. (in press). Maternal caregiving and child secure base behavior in two naturalistic contexts: Emergency and everyday, *Developmental Psychology.*

Sameroff, A. J., & Chandler, M. J. (1975). Reproductive risk and the continuum of caretaking casualty. In F. D. Horowitz, M. Hetherington, S. Scarr-Salapatek, & E. G. Siegel (Eds.), *Review of child development research* (Vol. 4). Chicago: University of Chicago Press.

Spangler, G., & Grossmann, K. E. (1993). Biobehavioral organization in securely and insecurely attached infants. *Child Development, 64,* 1439–1450.

Sroufe, L. A. (1985). Attachment classification from the perspective of infant–caregiver relationships and infant temperament. *Child Development, 56,* 1–14.

Sroufe, L. A., & Waters, E. (1977).. Heart rate as a convergent measure in clinical and developmental research. *Meffill-Palmer Quarterly, 23,* 3–27.

Thompson, I., Lamb, M., & Estes, D. (1982). Stability of infant–mother attachment and its relationship to changing life circumstances in an unselected middle-class sample. *Child Development, 53,* 144–148.

Valenzuela, M. (1990). Attachment in chronically underweight young children. *Child Development, 61,* 1984–1996.

Valenzuela, M. (1997). Maternal sensitivity in a developing society: The context of urban poverty and infant chronic undernutrition. *Developmental Psychology, 33,* 845–855.

van IJzendoorn, M., Schuengel, C., & Bakermans-Kranenburg, M. (1999). Disorganized attachment in early childhood: Meta-analysis of precursors, concomitants, and sequelae. *Development and Psychopathology, 11,* 225–249.

Vaughn, B., Egeland, B., Sroufe, L. A., & Waters, E. (1979). Individual differences in infant-mother attachment at twelve and eighteen months: Stability and change in families under stress. *Child Development, 50,* 971–975.

Waters, E. (1978). The reliability and stability of individual differences in infant–mother attachment. *Child Development, 49,* 483–494.

Waters, E. (1981). Traits, behavioral systems, and relationships: Three models of infant–mother attachment. In K. Immelman, G. W. Barlow, L. Petrinovich, & M. Main (Eds.), *Behavioral development* (pp. 621–650). Cambridge, UK: Cambridge University Press.

Waters, E., & Deane, K. (1985). Defining and assessing individual differences in attachment relationships: Q-methodology and the organization of behavior in infancy and early childhood. In I. Bretherton & E. Waters (Eds.), Growing points of attachment theory and research. *Monographs of the Society for Research in Child Development, 50*(1–2. Serial No. 209), 41–65.

Waters, E., Kondo-Ikemura, K., Posada, G., & Richters, J. (1991). Learning to love: Mechanisms and milestones. In M. Gunner & A. Sroufe (Eds.), *Minnesota Symposia on Child Development: Vol. 23. Self Processes and Development* (pp. 217–255). Hillsdale, NJ: Erlbaum.

PART 4

Adult and Clinical Applications

Disorganization of Attachment as a Model for Understanding Dissociative Psychopathology

GIOVANNI LIOTTI

The possibility that an individual constructs, very early in his or her life, multiple, segregated, or dissociated models of the self and of a particular attachment figure was first discussed by John Bowlby (1973, p. 205). The theme of multiple internal working models (IWMs) of self and of a single attachment figure has been developed by Mary Main (1991) in a seminal paper that emphasizes the relationship between multiple models of attachment and deficits in metacognitive development. Recent research on disorganization/disorientation of attachment behavior (henceforth called attachment disorganization for the sake of brevity) promises to illustrate in detail how multiple, reciprocally incompatible, and segregated (dissociated) IWMs of self and of the attachment figure are constructed, and how they may interfere with the integrative functions of memory, consciousness, and identity (Liotti, 1992a, 1995; Main, 1995; Main & Morgan, 1996).

This chapter aims to follow on Bowlby's idea that the consequences of an early construction of a multiple working model[1] may provide important keys for the understanding of adult psychopathology (Bowlby, 1973, p. 205). As to the types of psychopathology most amenable to a preliminary study in terms of multiple IWMs of attachment, it is immediately clear that the dissociative disorders, with their tendency toward a clinically evident multiple representation of the self, constitute the best candidate (Liotti,

1992a, 1995).[2] Bowlby approached the topic of dissociation and dissociative identity disorders when he further developed his 1973 idea of the relationships between multiple models and psychopathology (see Bowlby, 1980, Chap. 4, and especially pp. 56–61; see also Bowlby, 1988, Chap. 6). On the other hand, disorganization of attachment, among the different types of early attachments, provides the clearest hints at the interpersonal dynamics that may lead to the construction of multiple IWMs (Liotti, 1992a; Main, 1991; Main & Hesse, 1992; Main & Morgan, 1996). Looking at the early construction of multiple IWMs, it does not matter greatly whether one chooses to classify infant attachment behavior in the A–C category range (Crittenden, 1995) or using the additional D category (Main & Solomon, 1990; Main, 1995). Both the A–C (avoidant/ambivalent) and the D (disorganized/disoriented) categories portray equally well the basic idea of an early construction of incompatible, simultaneous representations of the self and of a single other person.

Thus, this chapter elaborates on the theme of attachment disorganization as an antecedent of dissociative processes and focuses on the role of early disorganized attachment in the etiology of the dissociative disorders.[3] This leads us to reconsider the prevailing view of dissociation as *primarily* a defense against trauma (see, e.g., Putnam, 1995, p. 585). The construction of multiple, dissociated working models of self and the attachment figure in the context of early disorganized attachment prompts us to regard dissociation not exclusively or essentially as a mental device protecting against the experience of painful emotions, but also, and perhaps more basically, as the sign and substance of a primary breakdown in the intersubjective processes (Stolorow & Atwood, 1992) that normally generate an integrated and coherent sense of self.

It should be emphasized, here at the beginning, that the model of dissociation expounded in this chapter—although based not only on clinical experience and clinical speculations, but also on the interrelated results of a few empirical studies—is mainly the outcome of an exercise in theory building. Its underpinnings are reasonable hypotheses related to empirical and controlled observations rather than definitely proved assertions. The theory, however, like many clinical theories emerging from the field of attachment studies, is formulated in such a way as to be empirically testable, and, indeed, it is in the process of being tested. Those research findings that are the outcome of the first attempts at testing the theory are briefly discussed in a later section of this chapter. My hope that the theory will soon be subjected to more stringent tests is my main reason for writing this chapter.

In order to examine the possible relationships between disorganized attachment and dissociation, a clear definition of the concept of dissociation is mandatory. Let us, then, briefly review how the concept was originally defined, about a century ago, by Pierre Janet. This definition still conveys most clearly, according to many students of the theme (Davies & Frawley, 1994, p. 31; Hilgard, 1986, pp. 5–13; van der Hart & Horst, 1989; van der Kolk & van der Hart, 1989), what is meant by dissociation.

JANET'S CONCEPT OF DISSOCIATION

According to Janet (1889/1973, 1907/1965), the essential aim of the working of the mind is adaptation to the environment rather than defense against inner unacceptable impulses. Adaptation to the environment is achieved through the "personal synthesis" of meaning structures (see also van der Kolk & van der Hart, 1989). The personal synthesis of generalized meanings, at its highest level, involves the sense of self. Dissociation,[4] according to Janet's original formulation of the concept, is the failure of the personal synthesis, brought about not only by psychological trauma, but also by other conditions (e.g., vehement emotions, temperamental variables, debilitating illnesses). Even when the dissociative processes are set into motion by trauma—as is often the case when dissociation reaches pathological proportions—they are not an active defense of the mind against the psychological consequences of the traumatic event, but rather, directly, those very consequences. One aspect of the psychological consequences of trauma is the breakdown of the adaptive mental processes leading to the maintenance of an integrated sense of self. Another, related aspect is that the memory of the traumatic event assumes a subconscious status not as the result of defensive mechanisms (as Freud's theory postulated), but because it never reaches a full representation in consciousness. To become fully conscious of an event is synonymous with being able to "tell the story" of that event.[5] Telling the story of an event in a coherent way corresponds to the higher possible success of the personal synthesis, which is exactly the mechanism with which trauma interferes. In this respect, Janet's view of the higher possible level of consciousness (*fonction du réel*) seems in keeping with the recent theory of consciousness formulated by Edelman (1989), according to which higher level consciousness implies the integration, mediated by language, of memories of the social self and the social non-self (see also van der Kolk & van der Hart, 1989, p. 1534).

It has been asserted that Janet's view of the working of the mind is based, as a root metaphor, on the second law of thermodynamics, while Freud's view is based on the first law (Semerari, 1995). According to Freud, conscious mental work is based on a specific mental energy, which, if not discharged in consciously regulated action, may remain segregated in the unconscious system. If the mental energy being bound to a defensively repressed memory is warded off from the conscious system, it cannot be discharged and must be transformed into an unconscious piece of mental work—for instance, transformed into a conversion symptom, or into a dream (hence, the metaphorical similarity with the first law of thermodynamics, which asserts the conservation and transformation of energy). For Janet, on the contrary, the working of the mind is (like life itself; see Lorenz, 1981) a form of negentropy, an effort to create order and meaning in opposition to the entropic tendencies of the multiple, chaotic information streams continuously impinging on the sense organs. The failure of this mental, conscious work of meaning making, of extracting order and unity out of chaotic, multifarious information, leaves whatever types of information that escape personal synthesis (such as traumatic information) in the disordered status of subconscious processing.

The emphasis that Janet and Freud placed on these different root metaphors of the working of the mind—the first and the second law of thermodynamics—may lie at the ground of a difficulty still facing students of dissociation. On the one hand, Janet's concept of dissociation as a basic breakdown, in the face of traumatic events, of the integrative, meaning-making functions of consciousness and memory is of great clinical appeal. On the other hand, it is difficult to bring Janet's basic ideas to bear on the three issues that, since Freud, are indispensable to any modern dynamic approach to psychopathology but were not of any great concern to the great French psychopathologist: personality development since early periods of life, interpersonal influences, and the often unconscious dynamics of the motivational processes. I argue in the following paragraphs that disorganized attachment in infancy provides us with a useful model for the study of dissociation throughout the lifespan that could solve this difficulty and place Janet's concept of dissociation within the context of personality development mediated by interpersonal influences and motivated by unconscious motivational systems. In order to approach this goal, I begin with a summary of the observable similarities, the clinical observations and the research findings that authorize the hypothesis that suggests a link between dissociative states and disorganized attachment.

PHENOMENOLOGICAL RESEMBLANCE BETWEEN DISSOCIATIVE STATES AND DISORGANIZED ATTACHMENT

Main and Morgan (1996) discussed the phenotypic resemblance between dissociative states on the one hand, and, on the other, (1) disorganized infant attachment behavior observed in the strange situation; and (2) lapses in the monitoring of reasoning or discourse observed in adults during the discussion of traumatic experiences as an aspect of the Adult

Attachment Interview. Examples of these similarities are trance-like or dazed expressions, simultaneous or sequential display of contradictory behavioral systems, and sudden disoriented and disorienting changes in posture and in action patterns.

Phenotypic resemblance between two phenomena does not imply that the same basic process is at work in producing them. However, the phenotypic resemblance between disorganized attachment and dissociation allows for the hypothesis that Janet's concept of a failure in the personal synthesis may be applied equally to dissociated mental processes in adult patients, to disorganized infant behavior in the strange situation, and to lapses in the metacognitive monitoring of reasoning and discourse during the Adult Attachment Interview.

In order to support this hypothesis, we should be able to identify similarities not only between the outward behavior of dissociative patients and children's disorganized attachment behavior, but also between the types of cognitive processes accompanying these behaviors. In terms of contemporary cognitive psychology, what Janet described as "personal synthesis" may be expressed as implying the successful, coherent integration of explicit (semantic and episodic) and implicit memories (for a discussion of implicit memory in relation to attachment, see Amini et al., 1996). Let us, then, consider whether it is possible to identify similarities between disorganized attachment and dissociative states with regard to a defect in the integrative functions of memory.

The implicit memories of the repetitive patterns of attachment–caregiving interactions are supposed to be integrated gradually, in the child's meaning structures, with the developing processes of semantic knowledge, giving rise to those memory structures that Bowlby (1969/1982, 1973, 1980) called internal working models (IWMs) of the attachment relationship. The IWM corresponding to disorganized attachment, I argue below, is very likely multiple and incoherent, while that of secure attachment is held to be integrated and coherent (Liotti, 1992a, 1995, in press; Main, 1991; Main & Morgan, 1996). This means that a failure of the integrative functions of memory characterizes disorganized attachment. Disorganized infants and children are unable to synthesize their overall experience of the interaction with the caregiver into a cohesive memory structure. Their memory of past interactions with the caregiver is composed of separate meaning structures that cannot be reciprocally integrated. A similar defect in the integrative functions of memory characterizes, by definition, pathological dissociation (see, e.g., Putnam, 1995). Thus, there is not only a formal resemblance between disorganized attachment behavior and dissociative behavior but also the hypothesized cognitive–emotional processes underpinning these two classes of behavior may be held to be similar.

RESEARCH FINDINGS AND CLINICAL OBSERVATIONS

Empirical evidence that supports the hypothesis of a relationship between disorganized attachment in infancy and pathological dissociation in adult life is gradually accumulating.

Disorganized attachment is much more frequent (up to 83% of the infants studied) in high-risk samples of parent–child dyads—in which the child is at risk of parental maltreatment or the parent is suffering from unresolved losses, major depression, substance abuse, and the effects of divorce—than in low-risk samples (for references, see Carlson & Sroufe, 1995; Main, 1995; Main & Morgan, 1996). The family situation of infants at risk for developing disorganized attachment is therefore similar to that described by most adult patients whose history of traumatic family interactions is causally linked to their dissociative symptoms by most clinicians and researchers. These findings do not disconfirm, and therefore authorize, the hypothesis that disorganized attachment is the *first step* in a developmental pathway leading, perhaps through a long sequence of dramatic or violent family interactions from infancy onward, to pathological dissociation in adult life.

Another finding that supports the hypothesis of a developmental continuity between disorganized attachment in infancy and adult dissociation has been provided by a study on adult dissociative and nondissociative psychiatric patients (Liotti, Intreccialagli, & Cecere, 1991). The rationale of this study is based on the well-documented finding that an index of unresolved loss significantly differentiates the caregivers of children disorganized in their attachment from the caregivers of other insecurely or securely attached children (Ainsworth & Eichberg, 1991; Main & Hesse, 1990; van IJzendoorn, 1995). Therefore, if disorganized attachment is linked to adult dissociation, dissociative patients should have had more often than nondissociative psychiatric patients the experience of being cared for, in infancy, by a caregiver suffering from an unresolved loss. Liotti et al. (1991) asked 46 patients showing dissociative phenomena (the "cases") and 109 patients free from dissociative experiences (the "controls") the following question: "Did your mother lose through death, in the 2 years before your birth or in the 2 years following it, one of her parents, a sibling, a child, or her husband (your father)?" While about 62% of the cases answered this question in the affirmative, only 13% of the controls did so. The statistical difference is highly significant.

In support of the hypothesized link between disorganized attachment in infancy and dissociative tendencies in adulthood, Coe, Daleenberg, Aransky, and Reto (1995) recently found that a fearful attachment style in adulthood (which is believed to arise from early experience of disorganized attachment) is significantly related in a nonclinical population to a greater likelihood of dissociative experiences (depersonalization). Anderson and Alexander (1996) also found that fearful attachment was significantly correlated with dissociation in a sample of adult survivors of childhood sexual abuse, while abuse variables (such as age of onset, coercion, nature of the abuse, and even centrality of the relationship between the perpetrator and the victim) did not significantly predict dissociation. It should be noted that these two studies (Coe et al., 1995; Anderson & Alexander, 1996) used a semistructured interview for the assessment of adult attachment styles (Bartholomew & Horowitz, 1991) that has not yet been shown to be related to infant classification in the strange situation. Therefore, these results may be taken to support only tentatively the hypothesis of a relationship between dissociation and disorganization of early attachment.

The preliminary results of a recent longitudinal study also tend to support the hypothesis of a link between early disorganization of attachment and later dissociative processes. Carlson (1997) reports a significant association between disorganized attachment status with mother in infancy (assessed in the strange situation) and dissociative tendencies in middle childhood and adolescence (assessed by teachers). Teachers, in Carlson's study, rated their pupils according to a dissociative scale including such items as the following: confused, seems to be in a fog, accident prone, explosive unpredictable behavior, stares blankly, strange behavior. Infant disorganized attachment, in Carlson's study, was also related at ages 17 and 19 to overall history and self-report of dissociative episodes as measured by the Dissociative Experience Scale (DES; Bernstein & Putnam, 1986).

Hesse and van IJzendoorn (in press) examined the relation between (1) participants' propensities toward absorption, as assessed by Tellegen's Absorption Scale (Tellegen & Atkinson, 1974); and (2) the anamnestic data of participants' parents who experienced the loss by death of a close relative within the 2 years preceding or following the birth of the participant. They report a significant relation between the two variables: experience of loss in the parent and absorption in the child. Since absorption is an aspect of dissociative tendencies (Putnam, 1995)—and the parent's experience of a serious loss near the birth of the child increases the risk for the child to develop a disorganized pattern of attachment toward that parent—this study could also be considered to lend support to the hypothesis discussed in this chapter. It is intriguing, however, that Hesse and van IJzendoorn were unable to find in their sample the expected significant relationship between parents' experience of loss near the birth of the child and infant disorganization of attachment in the strange situation. This relationship has been consistently found in at least six samples (Ainsworth & Eichberg, 1991; Benoit & Parker, 1994; Carlson, 1990; Main & Hesse, 1990; Radojevic, 1992; Ward & Carlson, 1995), while it was absent in only one sample other than that studied by Hesse and van IJzendoorn (Kolar, Vondra, Friday, & Valley, 1993). A possible explanation of Hesse and van IJzendoorn's finding is that, while the experience of loss in the parents facilitates the propensity toward absorption in the growing child, a *clinically evident* disorganization of the child's attachment is not a *necessary* mediating factor. In other words, the mental state of the parent who is suffering from an unresolved loss may influence the child's mental state, so that dissociative tendencies are facilitated even when the overt behavior of the child in the strange situation is not such as to allow a clear-cut classification within the disorganized subgroup. Children may be able to develop an organized attachment strategy toward an "unresolved" parent even when they begin to suffer from mild dissociative tendencies. If these dissociative tendencies in response to the attachment figure's more seriously unresolved mental status grow beyond a certain limit, overt disorganization of the child's attachment behavior will become evident. This explanation, it should be noted, is in keeping with Janet's view of success in the personal synthesis as a matter of degree within a continuous process of meaning making rather than as an all-or-none phenomenon.

Clinical studies of dissociative patients in psychotherapy do not disconfirm, and intuitively support, the idea that disorganized attachment may be linked to dissociation. The typical transferential responses of dissociative patients in psychotherapy closely resemble the attachment behavior of the disorganized child in its chaotic mixture of approach–avoidance behaviors toward the attachment figure (Davies & Frawley, 1994; Lichtenberg, Lachmann & Fosshage, 1992, pp. 164–168; Liotti, 1993, 1995, in press; Lowenstein, 1993; Putnam, 1995, p. 600). In the course of psychotherapy, whenever the attachment system of patients suffering from dissociative disorders becomes activated and directed toward the therapist, dissociative experiences (blank spells, amnesia, trance-like states), resembling the disoriented states of children whose attachment is classified in the disorganized category (Main, 1995; Main & Solomon, 1990) may occur in the course of the psychotherapeutic dialogue (Liotti, 1993, 1995). Moreover, during the psychotherapeutic dialogues, patients suffering from dissociative disorders seem to construe their own behavior and the therapist's according to multiple and incoherent representational models. These models, I argue, closely resemble the multiple IWMs hypothesized as typical of disorganized attachment (Liotti, 1995).

THE MEANING STRUCTURES
OF DISORGANIZED ATTACHMENT

The IWM of the attachment relationship is originally constructed at about the end of the first year of life by synthesizing repetitive implicit memories of the interaction between the infant and the caregiver (Amini et al., 1996). Later on, these "implicit memories of attachment interactions that have been generalized" (cf. the concept of RIG, Representations of Interactions that have been Generalized, in Stern, 1985) develop into semantic memories that can be expressed verbally.

The meaning of the semantic memories composing the IWM of secure attachment may be expressed in the expectation of being effectively cared for when in trouble and in the positive appraisal of one's feelings and emotions. The meanings emerging from the IWM of avoidant attachment convey the expectation of being disapproved of or rejected if one expresses the need for care, and of negative appraisal of one's emotions of attachment. Ambivalent attachment is reflected in doubts and uncertainty concerning whether and when help will be forthcoming (see, e.g., Carlson & Sroufe, 1995; George & Solomon, 1996; Main, 1995). The meaning structures emerging from the IWM of disorganized attachment, I now argue, are more complex and dramatic. Moreover, they are likely to be multiple, contradictory, and reciprocally dissociated (Liotti, 1992a, 1995, in press; Main, 1991, 1995; Main & Hesse, 1992; Main & Morgan, 1996).

The implicit memories of the early interactions leading to disorganization of attachment, being very likely based on frightened and/or frightening parental reactions to the approaching child (Main, 1995; Main & Hesse, 1990, 1992; Main & Morgan, 1996), contain the experience of fear in the child and the memory of frightened and/or aggressive expressions in the parent. Together with these, there will also be, however, memories of comfort both in the child and in the parent. Notwithstanding the barrier of fear and/or aggression in the parent, the disorganized child will eventually be able, in most instances, to achieve proximity (otherwise, he or she could not survive). The contact with little children is comforting for most adults, however distressed they might have been before the contact (for a discussion of the comforting emotions mediated in the parent by the activation of the caregiving system, see Solomon & George, 1996). Once the parent is calmer and momentarily more affectionate, the disorganized child will experience some degree of comfort in his or her arms.

The meaning structures emerging from implicit memories in which emotions of fear, aggression, and comfort dramatically follow each other (both in the self and in the perceived behavior of the attachment figure) are necessarily multiple (Liotti, 1992a, 1995, in press; Main & Hesse, 1990, 1992; Main & Morgan, 1996). Disorganized children may construe—simultaneously and with equal likelihood—what they have repeatedly experienced in their attachment interactions as: (1) their being responsible for the fear and/or aggression they perceive in the attachment figure when they approach him or her; (2) the attachment figure being the cause of their extreme experience of fear (they record the experience of being frightened by the expression of fear they notice in the attitudes of the attachment figure); (3) the attachment figure being able to comfort them; (4) their being able to comfort the attachment figure; (5) both themselves and the attachment figure being the victims of some unseen, inexplicable outside danger.

In other words, disorganized children will extract from their implicit memories of attachment interactions at least three reciprocally incompatible, basic meanings for the representation of the self, and three for the representation of the attachment figure. Children may variously combine these three meanings in the representation of the attachment interaction, so that they use more than three, and at least five, incompatible themes to *try* to give sense and structure to the autobiographical memories of the attachment relationships. The first of the three meaning structures has to do with the experience of being frightened and helpless (self and/or the attachment figure as "victim"); the second, with the experience of being the cause of the other's fear and helplessness (the "persecutor"); the third, with the experience of being comforting to the frightened other (the "rescuer").[6] Thus, the relationship of disorganized attachment implies a *simultaneous*—or almost simultaneous—construction of the child's self as victim of a "persecuting" (i.e., fear-inducing) attachment figure; as the "persecutor" of a helpless, frightened attachment figure; as a victim of impending dangers from which the attachment figure is the rescuer; and as the "rescuer" of the vulnerable attachment figure. Moreover, both the self and the attachment figure may be construed as helpless victims of an inexplicable, invisible external threat. Being so strongly contradictory and reciprocally incompatible, these constructions of self-with-others are likely to hamper seriously the mental synthesis of a unitary sense of self. If, in the course of further development, one of these representations displaces the others in the organization of conscious experience, the displaced representations of self-with-others will come to constitute, in Janet's terminology, an early example of dissociated mental states.

The hypothesis of multiple, incompatible, and thereby unintegrated (i.e., reciprocally dissociated) representations of self-with-others stemming from early relationships of disorganized attachment is supported by an increasing number of longitudinal studies. Children judged disorganized in their attachment relationships during infancy often show role-reversing ("controlling") attitudes toward the attachment figure at age 6, being either punitive toward the parent or inappropriately solicitous and caregiving (Main & Cassidy, 1988; Wartner, Grossmann, Fremmer-Bombik, & Suess, 1994). These either punitive or solicitous interpersonal strategies may correspond to the original representations of the self as the "persecutor" and the "rescuer" of the parent. Thanks to this selection of a representational and behavioral controlling strategy (that empowers the child at the expense of disowning any representation of the self as helpless and needing comfort), some degree of mental and behavioral coherence is achieved. When, however, the child's attachment system is strongly activated (e.g., by presenting the child with family photographs or with the pictures of the Hansburg's Separation Anxiety Test), this coherence is quickly destroyed. Bizarre, irrational, catastrophic, or self-destructive ideational contents are then elicited, while disoriented or disorganized responses are likely to come to substitute for the former seemingly organized controlling strategy (George, 1996; Main, 1995; Main, Kaplan, & Cassidy, 1985; Main & Morgan,1996).

This pattern of response in children who had been disorganized in their infant attachment—shifting from an organized, controlling strategy to disorganization in the context of a strong activation of the attachment system—is in keeping with the idea of a multiple, dissociated IWM of attachment underpinning the seemingly unitary representation of the self as "controlling." This idea is also supported by two recent studies (Jacobsen, Edelstein, & Hoffmann 1994; Solomon, George, & De Jong, 1995) showing that children classified as controlling at age 6 are characterized by a disorganization of representational processes "consistent with models of segregated or unintegrated systems of representation" (Solomon et al., 1995, p. 460). The general pattern of these segregated (i.e., dissociated) representational processes—as it emerges from an overall consideration of the previously quoted studies—suggests the simultaneous presence of the three poles of the "drama triangle" (Karpman, 1968): Self as *rescuer* (evidenced by controlling–caregiving strategies), self as *victim* (evidenced by themes of catastrophes and helplessness characterizing the incoherent narratives these children produce during tests of separation anxiety), and self as *persecutor* (evidenced by self-descriptions as particularly "evil," and by the description both parents and teachers provide of these children as unable to control their supposedly malignant aggressiveness; Cassidy, 1988; Hesse & Main, in press; Lyons-Ruth, 1996; Solomon et al., 1995).

This pattern of three incompatible, dramatic representations of the self, and of three corresponding, equally incompatible representations of the attachment figure, bears close resemblance to the multiple representations of self and others that characterizes dissociative disorders. Such a pattern of multiple, segregated, incompatible representations of self and others along the poles of the drama triangle (rescuer, persecutor, and victim) is suggested by the existence of three major types of alter personalities in the dissociative identity disorder: The three more common types of alter personalities—as assessed by Ross (1989) in his careful study of multiple personalities in contemporary samples of dissociative patients—are a helpless child personality that often is the one who preserves the clearer memory of episodes of abuse (the "victim"); a hostile personality that aims to

inflict suffering or death either to the primary personality or to other people (the "persecutor"); and a benevolent, helping personality that strives to
protect the primary personality from the painful memories of the abuse
and from difficult or potentially traumatic aspects of everyday life (the "rescuer"). Aside from the problems posed by multiple personalities (a diagnosis that may be overemphasized by many students of dissociation), the multiplicity of dissociated representations of self and others emerges in the
treatment of dissociative patients in the form of multiple transferences, as
the multiplicity has been repeatedly described by clinicians (Davies &
Frawley, 1994: Liotti, 1995; Putnam, 1995, p. 600). During the therapeutic
dialogues, these patients shift, sometimes very quickly, from (1) construing
the therapist as the idealized rescuer of an impotent, victimized self to (2)
seeing him or her as a persecutor who is expected to repeat the abusive or
seriously neglecting behavior of an early parental figure, to (3) construing
both the therapist and the self as helpless victims of overwhelming
dramatic and ill-defined situations, to (4) regarding the therapist as the
potential victim of the malignant, "persecutor" self, to (5) perceiving the
therapist as vulnerable and needing the comfort and reassurance the
omnipotent "rescuer" self is held able to provide. Davies and Frawley
(1994)—who do *not* use a model based on disorganized attachment in their
careful study of the psychotherapy of adult survivors of childhood sexual
abuse—have reached conclusions highly compatible with the model discussed in this chapter. They describe eight main transference–countertransference positions in the treatment of these dissociative patients: In
these positions, according to Davies and Frawley's terminology, therapists
and patients shift between the roles of the unseeing parent and the
neglected child, of the sadistic abuser and the helpless victim, of the idealized, omnipotent rescuer and the entitled child, and of the seducer and the
seduced. These shifts make it possible, according to Davies and Frawley, to
detect eight basic transference–countertransference positions that follow
each other during the psychotherapeutic process and are pathognomonic
of this particular class of dissociative patients.

On the basis of the model outlined here, which postulates a phenomenological and etiological continuity between disorganized attachment and
dissociation, we may consider in a new light the important and complex
topic of the relationship between trauma and dissociation.[7]

DISSOCIATION, TRAUMA, AND ATTACHMENT

Attachment theory postulates that the attachment system is activated whenever a human being is exposed to a fearful or traumatic event. Pain, fear,
and humiliation—the unavoidable consequences of any traumatic event—

innately motivate human beings to search for the protective proximity of an attachment figure "from the cradle to the grave" (Bowlby, 1979, p. 129). The IWM constructed on the basis of early attachments, however, modulates how this search for protective proximity will be performed later in life and may even inhibit it. While the IWMs of secure attachment allows for the efficient search for, and the likely attaining of, comfort and reassurance after a traumatic event, those corresponding to insecure attachments variously hamper it. The expectations of being rejected or kept at a distance (avoidant attachment), of being inefficiently or clumsily comforted (ambivalent attachment), of being frightened by the attachment figures or of being frightening to them (fearful and disorganized attachment), hinder the search for protective proximity to other human beings after having experienced a traumatic event. Therefore, we may expect that the secure IWM of attachment will constitute a protective factor against the likelihood of developing acute and chronic posttraumatic stress disorders after the experience of trauma. In contrast, the IWMs of insecure attachment will likely constitute vulnerability factors for the acute and chronic posttraumatic stress disorders (see Yehuda & MacFarlane, 1995, for a discussion of the problem of vulnerability to posttraumatic stress disorder).

The IWM of disorganized attachment not only hinders the search for help and comfort when a child faces the emotional consequences of trauma but also it actively increases at least one of those consequences, namely, the experience of fear. The child's expectation of being frightened further by the attachment figures when approaching them in fear and pain, or of being frightening to them, creates an inescapable, paradoxical loop of ever-increasing fear (Main & Hesse, 1990) that may conceivably be understood as a major risk factor for reacting to trauma with dissociation. On the phenotypic level of the cognitive processes implied in it, the interpersonal situation corresponding to disorganized attachment closely resembles the confusion technique used by Milton Erickson (1964) to induce hypnotic trances. In both interpersonal situations, an altered state of consciousness (dissociation) appears in an inescapable situation in which there is no possibility of choosing between contradictory meanings implied by the ongoing interpersonal transactions (Liotti, 1992b, 1993). In the hypnotic technique, the contradictory meanings are deliberately created by the hypnotherapist, while in the disorganized attachment relationship, they are created by the child's inborn need for protective proximity coupled with the fugue-inducing frightened–frightening behavior of the attachment figure (Main & Hesse, 1990).

Thus, the IWM of disorganized attachment may be a major risk factor for reacting with dissociation to any type of trauma, because it reactivates in the inner representations of self-with-the-attachment-figure that are mobilized by the traumatic experience a paradoxical loop of frightening and contradictory meanings. If, moreover, the traumatic events are created by a mal-treating parent to whom the child is previously bound by a disorganized pattern of attachment, the paradox of being forced by inborn needs (the attachment behavioral system) to rely for protection on the very source of danger is greatly strengthened. We may conceivably expect that extreme degrees of dissociation will be the outcome of such an interpersonal situation, not because of primarily defensive purposes, but just because there is no possible *organized* way of construing such a situation. In these circumstances, to think of dissociation as a defense would be analogous to thinking of bone fractures as defensive reactions to physical traumas.

The hypothesis that dissociation is related to the activities of the attachment system may explain the intriguing empirical finding that children's memory does *not* respond with dissociation to catastrophic life events (tornadoes, fires, airplane crashes, kidnapping) taking place outside their family network of affectional bonds, while adults' memory more often does (Spiegel & Cardena, 1991; Kotre, 1995, p. 137). Children do suffer from the emotional consequences of such overwhelming extrafamily events, but their memory's integrative functions seem unaffected. *Thus, emotional suffering induced by acute catastrophic events, when these events do not take place within the context of family relationships, is not linked to dissociation of memory functions in children.* This finding has been explained by the hypothesis that only chronic exposure to trauma as it may happen in the relationship with a repeatedly maltreating parent may lead to the use of dissociative defenses impairing children's memory and consciousness. Adults, for unexplained reasons, are held to be prone to use dissociative defenses after a single exposure to catastrophic events.

An alternative explanation is reached if one considers the hypothesis expounded, among others, by Horowitz (1986) that the *meaning* of trauma, rather than its intensity or frequency, impedes its integration into conscious memory structures. "The essence of psychological trauma is the loss of faith that there is order and continuity in life," and this loss of faith occurs "when one loses the sense of having a safe place to retreat within or outside oneself to deal with frightening emotions " (van der Kolk, 1987, p. 31). For this reason, those who regard psychological trauma as implying the disruption of meaning structures state also that an event is traumatic only insofar as it brings over "the sudden, uncontrollable disruption of affiliative bonds" (van der Kolk, 1987, p. xii). If this hypothesis is true, then we may explain in the following way the lower probability that children will dissociate in response to traumas when the trauma takes place outside their family. Children's cognitive processing of emotional information before the adolescent phase of cognitive development that Piaget has called "formal operations" is concerned with meanings concretely bound to their actual relationships, mediated by the attachment system. Only after adolescence does the cognitive apparatus operate in an hypothetical–

deductive fashion on such abstract meaning structures as "God," "World," "Reality," or "Destiny," which subsume, among other semantic structures, also the original IWM of attachment. Therefore, for children, trauma is able to produce dissociation only insofar as it is able to interfere with the synthesis of meaning structures concretely related to parents and family members, while in adults, trauma may also dissociate meaning structures related to abstract concepts such as "God," "World," "Destiny," or "Reality." Children, in the face of traumas inflicted by attachment figures, may have dissociative experiences while asking themselves, consciously or otherwise, "Why has Daddy (or Mummy, or Brother) done this to me?" Adults, on the contrary, may also be prone to dissociation in the effort to extract meaning from impersonal traumatic events (e.g., natural catastrophes) by asking themselves, "Why has Destiny (or God, Reality, the World) done this to me?" This cognitive explanation of the differential dissociating effect of acute extrafamilial traumas in children and adults should not induce us to overlook the interpersonal–emotional dynamics, related to the attachment system, that are recursively intertwined with the cognitive processing of traumatic experiences (see note 2). Children who are the victim of acute traumas taking place outside the family can turn to attachment figures for emotional comfort and for empathic help in the cognitive elaboration of painful memories. Adult victims of similar traumatic events may have more limited access to attachment figures, both in the outside interpersonal reality and in the inner representational word. This access will be particularly limited if the adults have been insecurely attached children and have not developed compensatory relationships thereafter; if they have been securely attached, their IWM may exert a protective influence against the potentially dissociating effects of the trauma in their meaning structures (see Yehuda & MacFarlane, 1995, for epidemiological data concerning the percentage of adults reacting with dissociation and with acute posttraumatic stress disorder to different types of acute traumas: The percentage that does not react in this way may conceivably be composed mainly by securely attached people). If the adult victims of traumatic events have previously constructed the IWM of disorganized attachment, then not only will they lack the protective factor related to the IWM of secure attachment but also they may even be actively predisposed, because of their already multiple and dissociated meaning structures, to develop serious dissociative symptoms in response to the adverse event.

DISSOCIATION OF MEANING STRUCTURES: RELATED AND UNRELATED TO TRAUMA

The reflections summarized in the preceding paragraph illustrate the basic assertion of this chapter: People who, because of the cognitive consequences of disorganized early attachments, are prone to construe interpersonal events (implying the activation of the attachment system) according to the roles of the drama triangle, are likely to have dissociative experiences during such a process of meaning making, and are almost surely destined to develop serious dissociative symptoms when faced with adverse life events.

It is almost impossible to achieve a successful mental synthesis of such contradictory, dramatic meanings as those related to the roles of rescuer, persecutor, and victim in an interpersonal relationship, when these meanings are constructed simultaneously or in quick succession. Whichever among these meanings may come to be more steadily processed in consciousness, the others, rather than being actively repressed because of defensive purposes, will *remain* in a subconscious status (which is exactly Janet's view of dissociation and of the relationship between conscious and unconscious mental processing).

The interpersonal events more likely to prime from memory the contradictory meaning structures stemming from disorganized infant attachment are emotional or physical maltreatment inflicted by an attachment figure. It is immediately intuitive how these events, while they activate the child's attachment system, could reactivate the simultaneous meanings of (1) deserving such abuses (self as "persecutor," that is, evil and therefore worthy of violence); (2) being the helpless, innocent target of the maltreatment (self as "victim"); and (3) being bound to the duty of forgiving the maltreating parent or even of understanding and comforting the emotional distress that underpins his or her abusive behavior (self as "rescuer"). However, this threefold dissociated process of attributing contradictory meanings to attachment interactions could also be set into motion by frightening but not directly maltreating parental behavior (Hesse & Main, in press). Babies whose parents, while they are taking care of their children, express fear, pain, and disorientation because of the sudden intrusion in their conscious mental processes of unresolved memories of past losses and traumas, may construe what is happening in the relationship as follows: (1) The self is held responsible for the parent's distress (self as "persecutor"); (2) the parent is the cause of the distress experienced by the child because of the misattunement in the parent–child relationship (self as "victim"); (3) the self is able to provide comfort to the parent (self as "rescuer" in an inverted attachment relationship). Thus, the dissociative process of meaning making according to the three poles of the drama triangle may be set into motion in interpersonal circumstances that do not imply any evident maltreatment of the child, nor any defensive mental process.

The model of the dissociative processes based on disorganization of attachment, thus, explains both those cases of dissociative psychopathology that recognize abuse in the parent–child relationship, and those that do not. Even when no real trauma (in the sense of evident emotional neglect or maltreatment, and of physical or sexual abuse) is traceable back as an antecedent of dissociative symptoms, however, the disordered mental processes are, according to this model, the outcome of real interpersonal events rather than of unconscious fantasies. Models of psychopathology derived from self psychology (see, e.g., Lichtenberg et al., 1992) and from control–mastery theory (Weiss, 1993), insofar as they state the importance of reality-based interpersonal events in the genesis of many psychiatric disorders, seem in substantial accord with the theory of dissociation presented in this chapter.

If disorganized early attachment sets the stage for construing further interpersonal events (particularly, but not only, traumatic events) that imply the activation of the attachment system according to a dissociated set of meaning structures, the final destiny of the developmental processes—toward dissociative psychopathology or toward at least relative mental health—will depend on a complex interplay of risk factors and protective factors.

Among the risk factors that could add to early experience of disorganized attachment resulting in dissociative psychopathology in adult life, we should take into account not only traumatic experiences (including losses), but also temperamental variables, possible neurophysiological dysfunction, and seriously distorted family communication. Grave and frequent misattunements in the interpersonal exchanges (Stern, 1985), or serious empathic failures (Lichtenberg et al., 1992; Wolf, 1988), may hinder the personal synthesis of emotionally ridden information concerning the meaning of one's own and significant others' behaviors and attitudes. Lies, deception, and the systematic distortion in family communication of important emotional information concerning the relationship of children with their attachment figures, however, are likely to exert a much greater dissociating influence than misattunements and empathic failures. Such a distortion of important information within family communication has been masterfully described by Bowlby as a major source of dissociation between semantic and episodic memory storage (Bowlby, 1980, Chap. 4; Bowlby, 1988, Chap. 6). Lies, deceptions, and other sources of seriously distorted family interactions force the growing child to exclude new and potentially meaningful information, already stored in the implicit or in the episodic memory system, from communication, and therefore from semantic processing and from conscious thought.[8] In Janet's terminology, in these circumstances, the personal synthesis of a coherent meaning of one's own and other people's behavior will be further impaired. These adverse interpersonal influences, however, according to the theory hitherto outlined, will not be sufficient causes of dissociative symptoms if they do not impinge upon an already dissociated IWM of attachment, that is, if they are not preceded or accompanied by disorganization of the attachment system.

The primacy attributed to real intersubjective experiences (disorganized early attachment, abusive parenting, deceptive family communications) by this theoretical model does not imply that defensive mental processes play no role in the development of dissociative disorders. Defensive processes do play an important role, according to this model, mainly taking the form of defensive inhibition of the attachment system. In order to protect themselves from the frightening dissociative experience of extreme disorientation and disorganization (in the terminology of self psychology, from the experience of loss of cohesion of the self; e.g., Wolf, 1988), children may defensively inhibit as far as possible the activation of the attachment system to which the dissociated system of meaning structures composing their internal working model of self and others, and ultimately responsible for the dissociative experience, is related. When distressed, frightened, or otherwise feeling vulnerable, disorganized children dealing with interpersonal needs and events may defensively and unconsciously try to rely on inborn motivational systems different from the attachment system (e.g., the sexual system, or the competitive, agonistic system; see Gilbert, 1989, or Lichtenberg, 1989, for two alternative treatises of the basic motivational systems that, together with the attachment system, mediate human interpersonal relationships). This improper activation of different motivational systems may bring forward further difficulties and misunderstandings on the interpersonal level, and further impairments in the construction of a coherent representation of self and others (personal synthesis) on the intrapsychic level. Thus, the growing child will appear to self and others as improperly seductive, or improperly aggressive, while at a not fully conscious level, he or she will intuit that what he or she desperately wishes and fears is protective proximity to another human being.[9] Such a disconnection between one's outward behavior and cognition on the one side, and one's feelings and interpersonal needs on the other, will eventually make impossible any adaptive cognitive regulation of impulses and emotions, and any satisfactory engagement in interpersonal relationships. Explicit psychopathology is then likely to ensue either before or shortly after adolescence. The type of explicit psychopathology that will emerge is represented by syndromes composed by impulse disregulation, interpersonal difficulties, and dissociative experiences (depersonalization, with or without accompanying panic attacks; blank spells or pervasive feelings of emptiness; amnesia; disorganized thought processes). At the base of these syndromes, dissociated meaning structures (rapid shifts among the three roles of the drama triangle in construing one's own and other people's behavior and attitudes) will be evident on close scrutiny by the expert psychotherapist. The theory expounded in this chapter asserts that these dissociated meaning structures are related to the early pattern of disorganized attachment.

Protective factors may also be present during socioemotional development that progressively limit or correct the psychopathological consequences of early disorganized attachment. Secure or at least organized attachment to at least one family member, relatively free and sincere communication with an available significant other, and the progressive recovery of the disorganized caregiver from his or her previously unresolved grief or posttraumatic stress disorder seem to be the more important ones. Thanks to the intervention of these and other protective factors (e.g., temperamental variables), the failure of personal synthesis in infancy may be overcome in the course of a favorable later development, and this may indeed be the case with most disorganized infants. Thus, to assume early disorganized attachment as a model for the study of pathological dissociation across the lifespan does not imply that all or even most of disorganized infants are likely to develop dissociative disorders—or other disorders based on dissociation—later in life. Assuming disorganized attachment as a prototypic model of dissociation implies only that "looking backward from those already suffering from such disorders we may find that a substantial majority has been disorganized with the primary caregiver during infancy" (Main & Morgan, 1996, p. 108).

SUMMARY AND CONCLUSION

To recapitulate, in this chapter, on the basis of phenotypic resemblance with adult dissociative states, clinical observations, and some recent research findings, disorganized attachment is assumed to be the prototypic example and the model of dissociation. According to this model, dissociation, when it is not related to primary neurophysiological disturbances, concerns early, multiple, incoherent, reciprocally incompatible and dramatic representations of the self, mediated by interpersonal relationships with a frightened or frightening caregiver, and based on the inborn human need for protective proximity to another human being when one is in danger or suffering. Subsequent factors of vulnerability for the development of a dissociative disorder (including psychological trauma) should be understood as increasing the risk of pathological dissociation already inscribed in early disorganized attachment; that is, trauma acquires dissociating properties mainly, or perhaps only, when it confirms previously dissociated mental structures constructed on the basis of attachment-related memories. Disorganized attachment is the prototypic, although not necessarily the only, road to the construction of attachment-related memories that form the basis of dissociative processes. Therefore, the link between trauma and dissociation is not to be understood primarily as a defense against painful affects, but rather as a reaffirmation of multiple, incoherent meaning structures involving the representations of self-with-others (where "others" are to be understood as attachment figures rather than as partners in relationships mediated by motivational systems different from the attachment system, for example, competitive or sexual relationships).

According to this theory, then, the subjective experiences that are usually labeled "dissociative" (trance-like states, blank spells, amnesia, flashbacks, depersonalization, out-of-body experiences) should be understood both in terms of painful emotional experiences *and* according to a theory of consciousness and memory in keeping with the type of cognitive processing implied in the construction of the internal working models of attachment. Janet's theory of the working of the mind as aimed at the construction of coherent, unitary meaning structures (the personal synthesis), and Edelman's theory of consciousness and contemporary cognitive models of memory and meaning-making processes seem to converge in outlining such a theory of consciousness and memory.

NOTES

1. The phrase "multiple internal working model" refers to a multiple and contradictory representation of an aspect of reality that ought to be represented as unitary or at least as coherently integrated in its various facets. Thus, the phrase does not apply to the different models a child may construct of the diverse attachment relationships with mother, father, and other caregivers, insofar as these different models of the self and of the caregivers can be contextualized within different relationships with different persons. The phrase does apply to a multiple and incoherent representation of the self, and of the other person, within the single context of a relationship between one body and a single other *body* (e.g., Main, 1991, p. 132).

2. The types of dissociative processes considered in this chapter are those for which no primary neuroanatomical injury, nor any primary toxic cause, can be detected. In classic psychiatric terminology, this chapter is concerned only with the functional dissociative disorders, not with the types of dissociation of consciousness that acknowledge an organic basis. In contemporary psychiatry, many disorders that were classically called "functional" may be interpreted on the basis of their neurophysiological or neurochemical underpinnings, which is not necessarily incompatible with their interpretation in terms of psychological dynamics, and such is also the case with the functional dissociative disorders with which this chapter is concerned. Excluded from the scope of this chapter are only the classic cases of organic disorders of consciousness, such as those of temporal lobe epilepsy and deliriums.

3. Although a coherent theory of dissociation is presented in this chapter, my aim is *not* to review and discuss all the other theories of dissociation that have been

formulated in recent years (for a review, see Putnam, 1995). The theory expounded here may be compatible, or not, with other theories (for instance, neurophysiological theories that postulate changes in the brain microstructure as a consequence of early adverse experiences may not be incompatible with this theory). However, it would be impossible to argue in favor or against the integrability of different models of dissociation within the limited scope of a book's chapter. Also, although the theory outlined here may appear closer to deficit models of psychopathology (such as those expounded by self psychology: see, e.g., Kohut, 1971; Wolf, 1988) than to conflict models (see, e.g., Kernberg, 1992), a discussion on whether this impression is true or not goes beyond the scope of this chapter. Thus, the aim here is simply to outline (so that more people might be interested in testing it) a theory of dissociation based on the consequences of an early construction of multiple representations of the self and of an attachment figure—not to discuss the relative merits and demerits of rival theories. Being focused on *representations*, the theory is admittedly a cognitive one. A forewarning is mandatory in this context. Cognitive theories may appear to relegate the role of affective experience on a secondary level. This is true only insofar as the choice of the focus of discourse is concerned, not with respect to how the overall field of inquiry is considered. To equate focusing on cognitive processes with discarding the relevance of painful, overwhelming emotions in the genesis of psychopathology assumes that the relationship between affect and cognition is one of mutual independence and of relative primacy of one aspect of mental life over the other. This assumption is not beyond question. An alternative view of the relationship between affect and cognition is that of a recursive process where the affective experience feeds the constructive processes of meaning making, while at the same time, cognitive structures continuously modulate the intensity of the ongoing affective experience. In this view, painful affects become overwhelming and dissociative processing of information takes place not just when it is impossible to avoid them through any behavioral or attentional strategy (e.g., avoidance behavior and selective, defensive exclusion of emotional information from conscious processing): To elicit dissociative processing of information, affects should also be not assimilable within any coherent meaning structure. The theory of dissociation outlined in this chapter takes for granted the first reason for traumatic affective experiences becoming dissociated (lack of escape from painful emotions), and focuses mainly on the second reason (lack of coherent meaning structures to which the painful experience could be assimilated).

4. Janet used mostly the French word *desaggregation* in his original writings. Dissociation is the favorite English translation for *desaggregation*, but somehow falls short of the original French term in conveying the meaning of "failed integration," or "disrupted synthesis."

5. In Janet's words: "Memory is an action: it is essentially the action of telling a story" (quoted by van der Kolk and van der Hart, 1989, p. 1534).

6. The idea that psychopathology may be related to quick shifts between the roles of rescuer, persecutor, and victim (the "drama triangle") within important dyadic relationships was originally formulated by Karpman (1968). Karpman stated that everybody in real life, like the hero in fairy tales and in the theater, starts off in one of these three roles, with the other principal figure (the antagonist) in one of the two complementary roles. When a crisis occurs, the two "players" switch roles.

According to Karpman, emotionally intense and very quick switching among these roles usually implies psychopathological disturbances.

7. The relationship between trauma and dissociation has been asserted by a huge literature on the posttraumatic stress disorders (e.g., Horowitz, 1986), the dissociative disorders (e.g., Putnam, 1989, 1995), the borderline personality disorder (e.g., Gunderson & Sabo, 1993), the eating disorders (e.g., Dalle Grave, Oliosi, Todisco, & Rigamonti, 1996; van der Linden, 1993), and the anxiety disorders (e.g., David, Giron, & Mellman, 1995). It would be erroneous, however, to regard dissociation as the necessary consequence of psychological trauma, or traumatic events as the necessary antecedent of dissociative processes. A substantial minority of patients suffering from dissociative symptoms (depersonalization, blank spells, trance-like states, amnesias, etc.) do not report particularly traumatic childhood or later experiences, while many victims of serious traumas do not suffer from dissociative experiences (Paris, 1996; Tillman, Nash, & Lerner, 1996; Yehuda & MacFarlane, 1995; Zweig-Frank, Paris, & Gudzer, 1994a, 1994b). Thus, the relationship between trauma and dissociation needs to be understood within a model that justifies both the statistical association between these two variables and the many cases in which no such an association can be found.

8. Theories that consider higher level consciousness as depending on verbal exchanges between self and others (see, e.g., Edelman, 1989) support the idea that what is excluded from communication acquires a less than optimal representation in the integrative processes of consciousness.

9. The role played by the defensive deactivation of the attachment system in the pathological development of early disorganized attachments may explain why, at least in childhood, the main sequelae to infant disorganization of attachment seem to be hostility and aggression, rather than dissociative symptoms (Lyons-Ruth, 1996; Solomon et al., 1995). On the one hand, dissociative symptoms in children who have been disorganized infants may be less evident, and less easy to assess, than aggressive behavior at home or at school (although they are likely to be present in these samples of children; see Carlson, 1997). On the other hand, disorganized children may try to protect themselves from the painful consequences of the activation of the attachment system (which, according to this theory, implies loss of cohesion in the sense of self) by defensively inhibiting it (Solomon et al., 1995) and by activating instead the competitive (also called adversative or agonistic; Gilbert, 1989, 1992; Lichtenberg, 1989) motivational system. This defensive strategy makes many formerly disorganized children and adolescents appear unduly aggressive or hostile. The defensive strategy is likely to fail, or to be insufficient to prevent the attachment system from becoming active later in life, in the face of losses, major separations, or traumatic events that will bring forth a massive stimulation of attachment needs. With such a reactivation, the dissociated IWM of attachment also becomes operative and facilitates dissociative experiences.

REFERENCES

Ainsworth, M. D. S., & Eichberg, C. (1991). Effects on infant–mother attachment of mother's unresolved loss of an attachment figure, or other traumatic experiences. In C. M. Parkes, J. Stevenson-Hinde, & P. Marris (Eds.), *Attachment across the life cycle* (pp. 160–187). London: Routledge.

Amini, F., Lewis, T., Lannon, R., Louie, A., Baumbacher, G., McGuinnes, T., & Zirker, E. (1996). Affect, attachment, memory: Contributions toward psychobiologic integration. *Psychiatry, 59*, 213–239.

Anderson, C. L., & Alexander, P. C. (1996). The relationship between attachment and dissociation in adult survivors of incest. *Psychiatry, 59*, 240–254.

Bartholomew, K., & Horowitz, L. (1991). Attachment styles among young adults: A test of a four-category model. *Journal of Personality and Social Psychology, 61*, 226–244.

Benoit, D., & Parker, K. C. (1994). Stability and transmission of attachment across three generations. *Child Development, 65*, 1444–1456.

Bernstein, E., & Putnam, F. (1986). Development, reliability and validity of a dissociation scale. *Journal of Mental and Nervous Disease, 174*, 727–733.

Bowlby, J. (1969/1982). *Attachment and loss: Vol. 1. Attachment.* London: Hogarth Press.

Bowlby, J. (1973). *Attachment and loss: Vol. 2. Separation.* London: Hogarth Press.

Bowlby, J. (1979). *The making and breaking of affectional bonds.* London: Tavistock.

Bowlby, J. (1980). *Attachment and loss: Vol. 3. Loss.* London: Hogarth Press.

Bowlby, J. (1988). *A secure base.* London: Routledge.

Carlson, E. A. (1990). *Individual differences in quality of attachment organization in high-risk adolescent mothers.* Unpublished doctoral dissertation, Columbia University, New York.

Carlson, E. A. (1997, April). *A prospective longitudinal study of consequences of attachment disorganization/disorientation.* Paper presented at the 62nd meeting of the Society for Research in Child Development, Minneapolis, MN.

Carlson, E. A., & Sroufe, L. A. (1995). Contribution of attachment theory to developmental psychopathology. In D. Cicchetti & D. Cohen (Eds.), *Developmental psychopathology: Theory and methods* (Vol. 1, pp. 581–617). New York: Wiley.

Cassidy, J. (1988). Child–mother attachment and the self in six-year-olds. *Child Development, 59*: 121–134.

Coe, M. T., Daleenberg, C., Aransky, K. M., & Reto, C. S. (1995). Adult attachment style, reported childhood violence history and types of dissociative experiences. *Dissociation, 8*, 142–154.

Crittenden, P. M. (1995). Attachment and psychopathology. In S. Goldberg, R. Muir, & J. Kerr (Eds.), *Attachment theory: Social, developmental and clinical perspectives* (pp. 367–406). Hillsdale, NJ: Analytic Press.

Dalle Grave, R., Oliosi, M., Todisco, P., & Rigamonti, R. (1996). Dissociation and traumatic experiences in eating disorders. *European Eating Disorders Review, 4*, 232–240.

David, D., Giron, A., & Mellman, T. A. (1995). Panic–phobic patients and developmental trauma. *Journal of Clinical Psychiatry, 56*, 113–117.

Davies, J. M., & Frawley, M. G. (1994). *Treating the adult survivor of childhood sexual abuse: A psychoanalytic perspective.* New York: Basic Books.

Edelman, G. M. (1989). *The remembered present: A biological theory of consciousness.* New York: Basic Books.

Erickson, M. (1964). The confusion technique in hypnosis. *American Journal of Clinical Hypnosis, 6,* 183–207.

George, C. (1996). A representational perspective of child abuse and prevention: Internal working models of attachment and caregiving. *Child Abuse and Neglect, 20,* 411–424.

George, C., & Solomon, J. (1996). Representational models of relationship: Links between caregiving and attachment. *Infant Mental Health Journal, 17,* 198–216.

Gilbert, P. (1989). *Human nature and suffering.* Hillsdale, NJ: Erlbaum.

Gilbert, P. (1992). *Depression: The evolution of powerlessness.* New York: Guilford Press.

Gunderson, J. C., & Sabo, A. (1993). The phenomenological and conceptual interface between borderline personality disorder and post-traumatic stress disorder. *American Journal of Psychiatry, 150,* 19–27.

Hesse, E., & Main, M. (in press). Second-generation effects of trauma in non-maltreating parents: Previously unexamined risk factor for anxiety. *Psychoanalytic Inquiry.*

Hesse, E., & van IJzendoorn, M. H. (in press). Parental loss of close family members and propensities toward absorption. *Developmental Science.*

Hilgard, E. R. (1986). *Divided consciousness: Multiple controls in human thought and action* (2nd ed.). New York: Wiley.

Horowitz, M. J. (1986). *Stress response syndromes* (2nd ed.). New York: Aronson.

Karpman, S. B. (1968). Fairy tales and script drama analysis. *Transactional Analysis Bulletin, 7,* 39–43.

Kernberg, O. F. (1992). *Aggression in personality disorders and perversions.* New Haven, CT: Yale University Press.

Kohut, H. (1971). *The analysis of the self.* New York: International Universities Press.

Kolar, A. B., Vondra, J. I., Friday, P. W., & Valley, C. (1993, March). *Intergenerational concordance of attachment in a low-income sample.* Paper presented at the 60th meeting of the Society for Research in Child Development, New Orleans, LA.

Kotre, J. (1995). *White gloves: How we create ourselves through memory.* New York: Free Press.

Jacobsen, T., Edelstein, W., & Hoffmann ,V. (1994). A longitudinal study of the relation between representation of attachment in childhood and cognitive functioning in childhood and adolescence. *Developmental Psychology, 30,* 112–124.

Janet, P. (1889/1973). *L'automatisme psychologique.* Paris: Alcan (original ed.); Paris: Payot (reprinted).

Janet, P. (1907/1965). *The major symptoms of hysteria.* New York: Macmillan (original ed.). New York: Hafner (reprinted).

Lichtenberg, J. D. (1989). *Psychoanalysis and motivation.* Hillsdale, NJ: Analytic Press.

Lichtenberg, J. D., Lachmann, F., & Fosshage, D. (1992). *Self and motivational systems: Toward a theory of technique.* Hillsdale, NJ: Analytic Press.

Liotti, G. (1992a). Disorganized/disoriented attachment in the etiology of the dissociative disorders. *Dissociation, 5,* 196–204.

Liotti, G. (1992b). Disorganizzazione dell'attaccamento e predisposizione ai disturbi funzionali della coscienza. In M. Ammaniti & D. Stern (Eds.), *Attaccamento e psicoanalisi* (pp. 219–232). Rome: Laterza.

Liotti, G. (1993). Disorganized attachment and dissociative experiences: An illustration of the developmental–ethological approach to cognitive therapy. In K. T. Kuehlvein & H. Rosen (Eds.), *Cognitive therapies in action* (pp. 213–239). San Francisco: Jossey-Bass.

Liotti, G. (1995). Disorganized/disoriented attachment in the psychotherapy of the dissociative disorders. In S. Goldberg, R. Muir, & J. Kerr (Eds), *Attachment theory: Social, developmental and clinical perspectives* (pp. 343–363). Hillsdale, NJ: Analytic Press.

Liotti, G. (in press). Understanding the dissociative processes: The contribution of attachment theory. *Psychoanalytic Inquiry*.

Liotti, G., Intreccialagli, B., & Cecere, F. (1991). Esperienza di lutto nella madre e predisposizione ai disturbi dissociativi della prole: Uno studio caso-controllo. *Rivista di Psichiatria, 26*, 283–291.

Lorenz, K. (1981). *Leben ist lernen*. Munich: Piper Verlag.

Lowenstein, R. J. (1993). Post-traumatic and dissociative aspects of transference and countertransference in the treatment of multiple personality disorder. In R. P. Kluft & C. Fine (Eds.), *Clinical perspectives on multiple personality disorder* (pp. 287–301). Washington, DC: American Psychiatric Association Press.

Lyons-Ruth, K. (1996). Attachment relationships among children with aggressive behavior problems: The role of disorganized early attachment patterns. *Journal of Consulting and Clinical Psychology, 64*, 64–73.

Main, M. (1991). Metacognitive knowledge, metacognitive monitoring, and singular (coherent) versus multiple (incoherent) models of attachment. In C. M. Parkes, J. Stevenson-Hinde, & P. Marris (Eds.), *Attachment across the life cycle* (pp. 127–159). London: Routledge.

Main, M. (1995). Recent studies in attachment: Overview, with selected implications for clinical work. In S. Goldberg, R. Muir, & J. Kerr (Eds.), *Attachment theory: Social, developmental and clinical perspectives* (pp. 407–474). Hillsdale, NJ: Analytic Press.

Main, M., & Cassidy, J. (1988). Categories of response to reunion with the parent at age 6: Predicted from infant attachment classification and stable over a 1-month period. *Developmental Psychology, 24*, 415–426.

Main, M., & Hesse, E. (1990). Parents' unresolved traumatic experiences are related to infant disorganized attachment status: Is frightened and/or frightening parental behavior the linking mechanism? In M. T. Greenberg, D. Cicchetti, & E. M. Cummings (Eds.), *Attachment in the preschool years* (pp. 161–182). Chicago: University of Chicago Press.

Main, M., & Hesse, E. (1992). Disorganized/disoriented infant behavior in the Strange Situation, lapses in the monitoring of reasoning and discourse during the parent's Adult Attachment Interview and dissociative states (Translated into Italian). In M. Ammaniti & D. Stern (Eds.), *Attaccamento e psicoanalisi* (pp. 86–140). Rome: Laterza.

Main, M., Kaplan, N., & Cassidy, J. (1985). Security in infancy, childhood and adulthood: A move to the level of representation. In I. Bretherton & E.

Waters (Eds.), Growing points in attachment theory and research. *Monographs of the Society for Research in Child Development, 50*(Serial No. 209), 66–104.

Main, M., & Morgan, H. (1996). Disorganization and disorientation in infant Strange Situation behavior: Phenotypic resemblance to dissociative states? In L. Michelson & W. Ray (Eds.), *Handbook of dissociation* (pp. 107–137). New York: Plenum.

Main, M., & Solomon, J. (1990). Procedures for identifying infants as disorganized/disoriented during the Ainsworth Strange Situation. In M. T. Greenberg, D. Cicchetti, & E. M. Cummings (Eds.), *Attachment in the preschool years* (pp. 121–160). Chicago: University of Chicago Press.

Paris, J. (1996). *Social factors in the personality disorders.* Cambridge, UK: Cambridge University Press.

Putnam, F. W. (1989). *Diagnosis and treatment of multiple personality disorder.* New York: Guilford Press.

Putnam, F. W. (1995). Development of dissociative disorders. In D. Cicchetti & D. Cohen (Eds.), *Developmental psychopathology: Theory and methods* (Vol. 2, pp. 581–617). New York: Wiley.

Radojevic, M. (1992). *Predicting quality of infant attachment to father at 15 months from prenatal representations of attachment.* Paper presented at the 25th International Congress of Psychology, Brussels, Belgium.

Ross, C. (1989). *Multiple personality disorder.* New York: Wiley.

Semerari, A. (1995). Il modello clinico negli "Studi sull'isteria." *Psicoterapia, 1*(3), 37–55.

Solomon, J., & George, C. (1996). Defining the caregiving system: Toward a theory of caregiving. *Infant Mental Health Journal, 17,* 183–197.

Solomon, J., George, C., & De Jong, A. (1995). Children classified as controlling at age six: Evidence of disorganized representational strategies and aggression at home and at school. *Development and Psychopathology, 7,* 447–463.

Spiegel, D., & Cardena, E. (1991). Disintegrated experience: The dissociative disorders revisited. *Journal of Abnormal Psychology, 100,* 366–378.

Stern, D. (1985). *The interpersonal world of the infant.* New York: Basic Books.

Stolorow, R. D., & Atwood, G. (1992). *Contexts of being: The intersubjective foundations of psychological life.* Hillsdale, NJ: Analytic Press.

Tellegen, A., & Atkinson, G. (1974). Openness to absorbing and self-altering experiences, a trait related to hypnotic susceptibility. *Journal of Abnormal Psychology, 83,* 268–277.

Tillman, J. G., Nash, M. R., & Lerner, P. M. (1996). Does trauma cause dissociative pathology? In S. J. Lynn & J. W. Rhue (Eds.), *Dissociation: Clinical and theoretical perspectives* (pp. 395–414). New York: Guilford Press.

van der Hart, O., & Horst, R. (1989). The dissociation theory of Pierre Janet. *Journal of Traumatic Stress, 2,* 399–411.

van der Kolk, B. A. (Ed.). (1987). *Psychological trauma.* Washington, DC: American Psychiatric Association Press.

van der Kolk, B. A., & van der Hart, O. (1989). Pierre Janet and the breakdown of adaptation in psychological trauma. *American Journal of Psychiatry, 146,* 1530–1540.

van der Linden, J. (1993). *Dissociative experiences, trauma and hypnosis: Research findings and clinical applications in eating disorders*. Amsterdam: Eburon Delft.

van IJzendoorn, M. (1995). Adult attachment representations, parental responsiveness and infant attachment: A meta-analysis on the predictive validity of the Adult Attachment Interview. *Psychological Bulletin, 117*, 382–403.

Ward, M. J., & Carlson, E. A. (1995). The predictive validity of the adult attachment interview for adolescent mothers. *Child Development, 66*, 69–79.

Wartner, U. G., Grossmann, K., Fremmer-Bombik, E., & Suess, G. (1994). Attachment patterns at age six in South Germany: Predictability from infancy and implications for preschool behavior. *Child Development, 65*: 1014–1027.

Weiss, J. (1993). *How psychotherapy works: Process and technique*. New York: Guilford Press.

Wolf, E. S. (1988). *Treating the self: Elements of clinical self psychology*. New York: Guilford Press.

Yehuda, R., & McFarlane, A. (1995). Conflict between current knowledge about post-traumatic stress disorder and its original conceptual basis. *American Journal of Psychiatry, 152*, 1705–1713.

Zweig-Frank, H., Paris, J., & Gudzer, J. (1994a). Psychological risk factors for dissociation in female patients with borderline and non-borderline personality disorders. *Journal of Personality Disorders, 8*, 203–209.

Zweig-Frank, H., Paris, J., & Gudzer, J. (1994b). Dissociation in male patients with borderline and non-borderline personality disorders. *Journal of Personality Disorders, 8*, 210–218.

CHAPTER 12

The Adult Attachment Projective
Disorganization of Adult Attachment at the Level of Representation

CAROL GEORGE
MALCOLM WEST
ODETTE PETTEM

John Bowlby's primary goal in formulating attachment theory was to develop a "new" model of developmental psychiatry that emphasized the role of real-life events, especially childhood experiences with a parent, as potential contributors to "mental ill-health" (Bowlby, 1988). In the first volume of *Attachment and Loss, Attachment,* Bowlby (1969) explicated developmental risk in terms of attachment insecurity, defined as feelings of apprehension, anxiety, and fear that result from experiences of compromised maternal care. By the second edition of this volume (1982), his more generalized concepts regarding insecurity were assimilated into Ainsworth's model (Ainsworth, Blehar, Waters, & Wall, 1978), with insecurity thereafter defined in terms of the avoidant and ambivalent attachment patterns. A decade of research appeared to support Bowlby's hypothesis of a link between attachment insecurity and developmental risk. Early attachment research found that, compared to secure children, insecure children (particularly avoidant children) were more likely to have problems with social competence, aggression, self-esteem, agency, peer popularity, and autonomy (see Thompson, 1999, for a review).

A growing number of researchers and clinicians have become interested in a "new" form of insecurity—disorganized attachment (Main & Solomon, 1986, 1990). Recent research that has differentiated disorganized and organized forms of insecurity suggests that disorganization may be a more serious developmental risk factor than the traditional "organized" patterns of insecurity. An increasing number of studies have reported an association between attachment disorganization and social–emotional and cognitive deficits in children (see Lyons-Ruth & Jacobvitz, 1999, and van IJzendoorn, Schuengel, & Bakermans-Kranenburg, 1999, for reviews). Additionally, attachment disorganization is prevalent in children living in high-risk environments, such as situations where parents are abusive, alcoholic, or depressed (e.g., Carlson, Cicchetti, Barnett, & Braunwald, 1989; Teti, Gelfand, Messinger, & Isabella, 1995; O'Connor, Sigman, & Brill, 1987). Historically, the concept of disorganized attachment emerged from observations of infant behavior in the laboratory (Main & Solomon, 1986, 1990). Compared with infants whose attachments are organized (secure, avoidant, ambivalent), infants judged disorganized lacked a coherent behavioral strategy both during the reunion episode of the strange situation, and sometimes across episodes of this procedure. Studies of attachment in early childhood (Cassidy & Marvin, 1987/1989/1990/1991/1992; Main & Cassidy, 1988; Wartner, Grossmann, Fremmer-Bombik, & Suess, 1994) suggested that the disorganized behavior of the infant is transformed into brittle behavioral control strategies. "Controlling" children act in ways that appear to place the child in control of parent–child interactions. Although the behavior of disorganized children seems to become organized with age, the attachment system nonetheless remains disorganized at the level of representation (Solomon, George, & De Jong, 1995). This observation suggests to us that the key to understanding the meaning of disorganization lies in the close examination of attachment at the representational level.

In this chapter, we describe the mental representations of attachment disorganization in adults. We note that the term "disorganized attachment" is not typically used to describe adult attachment status. Rather, because early research linked infant disorganization to mothers' unresolved loss (e.g., Ainsworth & Eichberg, 1991; Main, Kaplan, & Cassidy, 1985), the adult equivalent of childhood disorganization has typically been described as "Unresolved" attachment.[1] Previously, we have suggested that Bowlby's (1980) concept of segregated systems, a form of defensive exclusion that he linked to pathological mourning and mental health risk, is the defensive underpinning of disorganization in children (Solomon et al., 1995) and Unresolved adults (West & George, in press). We begin this chapter with a discussion of segregated systems and Unresolved adult attachment. We then highlight the discriminating features of mental representations of disorganized attachment in children. Finally, we discuss our work examining attachment disorganization in Unresolved adults.

Until recently, no assessment tools have been available that allowed for direct comparisons between child and adult representations of attachment. Although the Adult Attachment Interview (AAI; George, Kaplan, & Main, 1984/1985/1996) provides access to an adult's current "state of mind" with regard to his or her childhood attachment experiences (Main, 1995), implicit in the AAI classification scheme is the assumption that adults are capable of abstract thinking and metacognitive reasoning, developmental accomplishments that do not achieve mature form until adolescence. The ideas presented here are based on our observations of mental representation using a new assessment measure of adult attachment, the Adult Attachment Projective (AAP; George, West, & Pettem, 1997). This measure is analogous to the projective measures used to assess attachment in childhood and, therefore, allows us to compare mental representations of attachment in adults and children based on their responses to similar measures. We present preliminary data regarding the correspondence between classifications based on our adult projective measure and AAI classifications. We then describe the ways in which representational patterns in the AAP responses of adults who are Unresolved on the AAI parallel the representational patterns of disorganized children.

SEGREGATED SYSTEMS

Bowlby (1980), in his study of the ways individuals adapt to the experiences of attachment trauma (in particular, loss through death), introduced the concept of segregated systems. He postulated that segregated systems were generated as the mental product of complete defensive exclusion. According to this theory, when the pain associated with certain kinds of attachment experience is so great that the memories and feelings associated with these experiences threaten to undermine the individual's ability to function, mental material related to attachment must literally be "housed" elsewhere. Defensive exclusion in its most complete and active form encodes trauma-related attachment memories and emotions in a separate representational model that is kept, as completely as possible, inaccessible to consciousness. Segregated systems, therefore, keep attachment-related information from being integrated into the thoughts and feelings that predominantly influence the individual. Although unconscious and deactivated, Bowlby emphasized that segregated systems are, in and of themselves, organized representational systems that can, when activated, frame and execute plans. Upon activation, however, behavior, feeling, and thought are likely to appear chaotic and disorganized.

Bowlby proposed that the short-term benefits of segregated attachment models (i.e., segregated systems) were outweighed by the risks of the potential long-term maladaptation associated with this extreme form of defensive exclusion. Segregated models cannot be blocked from consciousness indefinitely. Although more research is needed to identify the circumstances that unleash segregated models, recent attachment theorists have suggested that this form of defensive exclusion fails at those moments when the individual needs defenses the most, that is, when the individual experiences certain internal or external events that are appraised as threatening. It is precisely in these circumstances, when the individual's attachment system is intensely activated, that the emergence of segregated feelings is most likely (George & Solomon, 1999; West & George, in press). Upon release of segregated material, the individual is prone to dysregulation, a state in which behavior and thought become disorganized and disoriented by either emotional flooding or attempts to prohibit or block these emotions from consciousness. Vacillation between organized and disorganized states exactly describes the patterns of behavior and thought that have been observed in disorganized children. Under some circumstances, many disorganized children act in a clearly organized manner, seeking to dominate and control attachment-related situations and interactions with the parent. Indeed, as we mentioned earlier, this classification group is labeled "controlling" in childhood. For example, upon reunion in the laboratory, controlling children use punitive (e.g., rude, insulting) or caregiving (e.g., making sure mother is comfortable and happy) strategies to regulate the mother's behavior (Cassidy & Marvin, 1987/1989/1990/1991/1992; Main & Cassidy, 1988). In fact, mothers of controlling children frequently describe their children as trying to dominate them; interviews with the mothers of these children are filled with descriptions of the child engaging the mother in willful battles for power (George & Solomon, 1996). Following the model presented earlier, we believe that the child's controlling behavior in all of these contexts is the result of attempts that may be presumed to be largely unconscious to keep segregated material out of consciousness, thereby preventing the child from becoming emotionally flooded and behaviorally out of control. As discussed in the following section, these attempts are not always successful, and controlling children do become overwhelmed and lose control of their emotions. In adults, the evidence for the role of segregated systems in unresolved states of mind is derived exclusively from the AAI. Empirical investigations of unresolved attachment have been guided by Main and Goldwyn's (1985/1991/1994) operational definition of lack of resolution of mourning and trauma. Based on adults' responses to the AAI, Main and Goldwyn defined lack of resolution as specific states of mind in which the individual demonstrates significant lapses in the metacognitive monitoring of reasoning and discourse when discussing experiences of either loss or physical abuse. This means that regardless of how coherent, idealized, angry, or passive an individual appears to be when describing nontraumatic attachment experiences, his or her interview is characterized by sudden references to the deceased or experiences of abuse, unusual attention to the details regarding circumstances and individuals, or inexplicable passages of incoherent speech in describing these events. Following Bowlby (1980), Main and Goldwyn designated these individuals Unresolved. In our view, Main and Goldwyn's operational definition of "lack of resolution" assesses a form of dysregulation of segregated attachment systems.

MENTAL REPRESENTATIONS OF ATTACHMENT DISORGANIZATION IN CHILDREN

Attachment theory and research suggest that from 3 years of age onward, the internal representations of children become more stable, elaborate, and accessible at the symbolic level (Bowlby, 1969/1982; Bretherton, 1985; Case, 1992; Main et al., 1985). As a result, inferences can now be made about the organization of the attachment system from observations of symbolic play and story scripts regarding attachment-related scenarios. Child attachment researchers have used a wide range of tools to assess attachment at the representational level—most frequently, doll-play enactment of attachment-related story stems (Bretherton, Ridgeway, & Cassidy, 1990; Cassidy, 1988; Oppenheim & Waters, 1995; Shouldice & Stevenson-Hinde, 1992; Solomon et al., 1995) and picture projectives (Jacobsen, Edelstein, & Hoffman, 1994; Kaplan, 1995; Slough & Greenberg, 1990).[2]

Evidence drawn from this body of research indicates that the symbolic representations of children who are classified disorganized are characterized by a unique constellation of story content and process features. Their themes and story scripts depict parents, adults, and children as frightened, frightening, chaotic, abusive, absent, helpless, or abandoned; events and characters are often out of control (sometimes violently), and family members are unable to prevent life-threatening dangers (Kaplan, 1995; Solomon et al., 1995).[3] Solomon et al. (1995) stressed that the most definitive feature of disorganization in the doll-play stories of 6-year-old children was the failure to resolve attachment threats. In their stories, the child or the family were left in a state of disarray or disintegration (e.g., house blows up, family breaks up, child dies, parents abandon the child, wicked witch drives family from their home).

In terms of process, disorganized children characteristically act as if they are overwhelmed or threatened by the attachment task. They typically become dysregulated, as evidenced by flooding and, presumably, losing grasp of the representational rules that guide or "ground" organized children's responses to the task. In family drawings, for example, figures lacked grounding or form. Family members were placed in spatially disoriented postures or positions, such as appearing to float in the air (Kaplan & Main, as reported in Main et al., 1985). In response to doll play, many aspects of the play lost its spatial and temporal orientation. Children whirled family members or materials around the doll house; characters were depicted as clumsy, falling dangerously, reckless, and engaged in endless chaotic activities, including those that ended in destruction or annihilation. The tempo or flow of story events was often interrupted by distractions and cognitive freezing (George & Solomon, 1998; Solomon et al., 1995). By contrast, a small subset of disorganized children were not flooded during doll play; rather, their dysregulation was revealed by shutting down. These children were constricted and unable to complete the attachment scenarios, presumably, as the result of attempting to block segregated material from consciousness (Solomon et al., 1995). This left them literally frozen, preventing the construction of story themes and often preventing children from handling the play materials.

With these descriptions of the symbolic representations of disorganized children as background, we next examine whether or not we can apply the same broad representational markers to identify Unresolved adults. To this end, we describe a new attachment measure that allows us to examine this question more closely.

THE ADULT ATTACHMENT PROJECTIVE

The Adult Attachment Projective (AAP; George et al., 1997) is a method of assessing attachment in adults in a format that is analogous to the representational projective measures used to assess attachment in children. During the procedure, the adult is presented with eight pictures (examples of four of the pictures are provided in the Appendix). The AAP begins with a neutral, warm-up picture of children playing ball, followed by seven attachment scenes: *Child at Window*—a child, with its back to the viewer, looking out of a picture window; *Departure*—an adult man and woman facing each other with suitcases; *Bench*—a youth sitting alone on a bench; *Bed*—a woman and child sitting facing each other at opposite ends of a bed; *Ambulance*—a woman and child looking out a window at a person on a stretcher being put into an ambulance; *Cemetery*—an adult man standing in front of a gravestone; and *Child in Corner*—a child standing laterally in a corner, turned around slightly, with an arm extended outward. Working with a graphic artist, the picture set was developed from such diverse sources as children's literature, psychology textbooks, and "coffee table" books of photographers' work. Pictures were drawn to contain only sufficient detail to identify the event; strong facial expressions and other biasing details were omitted. The picture set was developed carefully to avoid gender or race bias.

The picture set was designed to capture three attachment-related dimensions. The first dimension is activation of attachment. According to Bowlby (1969/1982), behavior and thought that are the products of the attachment system can only be observed when the system is activated. The picture set includes events known to activate attachment, such as illness, separation, solitude, death, and threat. Furthermore, the order in which the pictures are presented is thought gradually to increase activation of the attachment system. The second dimension is availability of a relationship. Bowlby (1973) stated that one of the greatest sources of fear and threat was being alone. The picture set thus includes scenes in which the individual is depicted as alone or in a dyadic relationship. The third dimension is age. Bowlby (1969/1982) conceived of attachment as important across the lifespan. The picture set, therefore, depicts both child and adult attachment situations.

Although the pictures were designed as projective stimuli, the method of administration more closely follows the format of semistructured interviews (e.g., AAI) than the traditional projective format (e.g., Thematic Apperception Test). The interviewer asks the individual to make up a story about what is happening in the picture, what led up to the scene, what characters are thinking and feeling, and what might happen next. The interviewer uses open-ended probes, if necessary, to ensure that individuals address these elements in their scenario.

Classification is based on the verbatim transcription of the individual's stories to the seven attachment pictures. We developed a scheme that encompasses a number of representational variables, or "markers," that are used to evaluate specific content and defensive process characteristics of the interview. We used attachment theory to derive those markers that are unique to our scheme. Others were developed by drawing upon the broad features of three existing attachment representational classification schemes: the AAI (Main & Goldwyn, 1985/1991/1994), Attachment Doll-Play Procedure (Solomon et al., 1995), and the Caregiving Interview (George & Solomon, 1996).

DEVELOPMENT OF THE CLASSIFICATION SCHEME

The AAP classification system was developed to predict the four main attachment groups designated by the AAI (secure, dismissing, preoccupied, unresolved). Work to date has proceeded in two stages. We began with a community sample of 13 men and women recruited through newspaper advertisement. Each individual was given the AAP; 9 individuals were also administered the AAI before the administration of the projective. Verbatim transcripts of their AAP scenarios were examined, noting themes, descriptive images, and discourse patterns that are linked empirically or theoretically to the attachment construct. A classification system was developed by moving back and forth between the AAP and the AAI classifications, guided also by theoretical and empirical criteria regarding the patterns of AAP codes that should discriminate between attachment groups.

We then tested our preliminary classification scheme by examining the AAP interviews of a randomly selected subset of 25 mothers drawn from an ongoing study of infant perinatal risk conducted by Diane Benoit at the University of Toronto.[4] In this data set, mothers were interviewed using the AAP and AAI by Benoit or her research assistants. Administration of the AAP and AAI were counterbalanced. This data set was used to evaluate the system we had developed. We examined interjudge reliability of AAP classifications and the convergence between classifications derived from the AAP and the AAI. AAI's were classified by Benoit, a trained AAI judge, and AAP's were independently classified by the authors. Disagreements on AAP classifications were resolved through consensus. The AAI and AAP judges were blind to risk status and all other information about the mothers in this sample.

AAP CLASSIFICATION SYSTEM

Three categories of variables are used to evaluate an individual's response to each attachment picture: discourse, content, and defensive process (see Table 12.1). All categories are coded to indicate either the qualitative features of the marker or its presence or absence. Discourse codes evaluate *Personal Experience* and *Coherency*. Personal Experience indicates whether or not the individual's stories include statements regarding his or her own life experiences. *Coherency* assesses each story's overall coherence by evaluating quality, quantity, relation, and manner (following coherence ratings for the AAI). These coherency dimensions are collapsed and overall coherency is designated according to a 3-point scale.

Content codes include *Agency of Self, Connectedness,* and *Synchrony. Agency of Self* and *Connectedness* are coded only for the "alone" pictures; *Synchrony* is coded for "dyadic" pictures. *Agency of Self* assesses the degree to which the story character is involved in moving psychologically or behaviorally in the direction of integration, understanding, or empowerment.

TABLE 12.1. Summary of AAP Coding Variables

Variables	Pictures coded	Definition	Specific dimensions
Discourse variables			
Personal Experience	All	Story includes own life experience in response.	Present, absent
Coherency	All	Degree of organization and integration in the story as a whole.	3-point rating scale combining quality, quantity, relation, manner
Content variables			
Agency of Self	Alone	Designates degree to which story character is portrayed as integrated and capable of action.	Internalized secure base, capacity of act, no agency
Connectedness	Alone	Expression of desire to interact with others.	Clear signs of a relationship in the story. Relationship not possible (e.g., someone walks away, someone is dead); engaged in own activity; relationship is blocked or desire for relationship is absent.
Synchrony	Dyadic	Characters' interactions are reciprocal and mutually engaging.	Mutual, reciprocal engagement; failed reciprocity.
Defense variables			
Deactivation	All	Evidence of deactivation and demobilization.	Negative evaluation, rejection, social roles, power, stereotyped scripts, minimization, nullification, shutting down narrative, distancing, neutralizing, derision, demotion.
Cognitive Disconnection	All	Evidence of uncertainty, ambivalence, and preoccupation.	Uncertainty, withdrawal/withhold, anger, busy/distractedness, feisty, entangled, disconnection, passive language, unfinished thoughts, stumbling, glossing over, literal descriptions
Segregated Systems	All	Evidence of dysregulation or disintegration.	Danger/failed protection, helplessness/out of control, emptiness/isolation, odd/disturbing, dissociation, intrusion, constriction

This code takes one of two forms: internalized secure base or capacity to act. Internalized secure base is evidenced by either the character's capacity to make use of solitude (self-reflection, introspection, thoughtfulness) or to appeal to relationships in order to solve a problem. Capacity to act is evidenced when the character is able or confident to effect change in the present or the immediate future. *Connectedness* assesses the desire or the ability of the story character to be in a relationship or to interact with others. *Synchrony* assesses the degree to which the story characters are portrayed in a reciprocal, mutually engaging and satisfying relationship, and is coded for all pictures where characters are depicted in dyadic interaction.

The final category in our coding scheme is defensive processes. These codes identify the forms of defensive exclusion that emerge in response to each attachment stimulus. Research indicates that activation of the attachment system elicits a broad range of defensive processes that, working together, determine how the individual modulates accompanying emotions (Bowlby, 1980; George & Solomon, 1996). Following the classification system developed to identify different patterns of defense assessed in relation to maternal caregiving and child doll play (George & Solomon, 1996; Solomon et al., 1995), the AAP codes for three forms of defensive exclusion: *Deactivation, Cognitive Disconnection,* and *Segregated Systems.* The presence of defensive exclusion is evaluated from both the content of the story and its structure, that is, the mental processes that are revealed during the construction of the story. *Deactivation* is evidenced when the individual diminishes, dismisses, or devalues characters, story events, or the self. Deactivation markers for story content include, for example, negative evaluation of characters or self, rejection, social roles, and appeals to power or intelligence. Deactivation process markers include, for example, minimization, shutting down the narrative, and derision. Both content and process markers reveal an underlying organization of thought that shifts attention away from arousal of attachment or information that is personal or about the character as an individual (as does avoidant behavior in the strange situation, or dismissing discourse during the AAI), allowing the individual to complete the story.

Cognitive Disconnection is evidenced by uncertainty, ambivalence, and mental preoccupation with experiences, individuals, or feelings. Cognitive Disconnection story content markers include, for example, uncertainty, withdrawal, anger, and entanglement. These markers are all forms of behavior, feeling, or thought that have been found by attachment researchers to be associated with expressions of ambivalent attachment in reunion, doll play, and interview contexts (George & Solomon, 1996; Solomon et al., 1995; Main, 1995; Main & Cassidy, 1988). Cognitive Disconnection process markers include, for example, disconnection (i.e., opposing themes), passive language, glossing over (i.e., turning the attachment issue into something positive or simply skipping over it entirely), and literal descriptions (i.e., very detailed) of the scenes portrayed by the pictures. These markers all reveal some attempt to terminate arousal of attachment by splitting "apart" or literally disconnecting the details of the stories or pictures themselves. The result, in some instances, is the focus of mental attention on the relatively meaningless or positive aspects of the story. In other instances, the story shifts back and forth between opposing interpretations. In either case, this defensive process results in marked interference with completion of the task. In some instances, cognitive disconnection results in a story that appears to be somewhat incomplete; in others, the results is the construction of two parallel scenarios.

Of primary interest to the work reported here are the defensive exclusion markers that indicate the presence of *Segregated Systems*. There are two steps in coding Segregated Systems. The first step is to note the presence of content or process markers for Segregated Systems. Four types of story content codes are used to denote activation of Segregated Systems. *Danger/ Failed Protection* markers include images in which story characters are portrayed as vulnerable and unprotected, such as themes or images of physical assault, abuse (physical, sexual, mental), abandonment, threat, crisis (e.g., life-threatening disease or heart attack), catastrophe, or the character's desire to flee or become invisible. *Helplessness/Out of Control* markers include references to or images of characters as frightened, helpless (e.g., being overpowered) or out of control (e.g., drunkenness, emotional outburst, repeated acts or threats of repeated acts of violence). *Emptiness/Isolation* markers include images of characters who are completely inhibited, constricted, or withdrawn, such as being jailed, estranged, extremely withdrawn, or images of characters that lack basic human qualities, such as being described as faceless or lifeless. Finally, story content markers are also noted for *Odd/Disturbing* material, such as completely idiosyncratic descriptions or thoughts (e.g., explaining an event because of its similarity to Van Gogh's bed) and peculiar or illogical explanations for events (e.g., "Parents hit kids because they have nothing better to do").

Three types of Segregated Systems process markers are also coded. Dissociation markers include references to images or thoughts that portray a dissociated, eerie, or magical quality, such as ghosts and spirits, talking to the deceased, or images that connote out-of-body experiences (e.g., being on the outside looking in). These images are, by definition, considered to have a dissociated quality because they reveal dissolution of the boundaries between what is real and not real, or between the living and the dead. *Intrusion* markers (a set of markers that taps Main & Goldwyn's lapses in metacognitive monitoring) include slips of the tongue and the description of the individual's own traumatic experiences (i.e., the inability to keep self and story characters separate in the mind). The third and final process marker for segregated systems is *Constriction,* a mental state that is the product of extreme fear (George & Solomon, 1998; Perry, Pollard, Blakley, & Vigilante, 1995; Solomon et al., 1995). In some cases, Constriction is revealed by mental freezing; here, the individual refuses to, or cannot, tell a story about a picture, and in some situations, the individual may give the picture back to the interviewer or ask to go to the next picture. In other cases, Constriction results in hypervigilance and an attentional obsession with the details of the drawing. By focusing on picture details at this level, the individual can remain minimally involved in the task without becoming flooded.

The second step in coding Segregated Systems is to note if segregated markers are resolved/contained or unresolved/unintegrated. Resolution and containment represent mental strategies used by the individual to organize threatening material that has emerged into consciousness. Stories are considered integrated when characters draw upon internal resources to understand, resolve, or prevent a situation from getting out of hand, or seek assistance, protection, or care from others (described earlier as an internalized secure base); stories are considered contained when characters demonstrate a clear capacity to act (i.e., the character is not left helpless and the situation is not hopeless). Stories in which segregated material is left unintegrated because it is neither resolved nor contained are designated as unresolved (U_d). These stories typically leave characters without protection, describe feelings of extreme mental distress that have not been diminished or transformed, or leave threatening images looming without addressing them further (e.g., simply stating that the event in the Ambulance picture is a terminal illness). Mental constriction and uncontained hypervigilance are also considered indications of failed integration or failed containment and, therefore, designated as U_d.

Upon completion of these six major codes (Personal Experience, Coherency, Agency of Self, Connectedness, Synchrony, Defensive Processing), one of four attachment classifications is assigned by examining the individual's patterns of codes for their responses to the entire attachment picture set (i.e., the neutral warm-up picture is not coded). A complete discussion of the pattern profiles that are used to determine each classification group designation is beyond the scope of this chapter. For the remainder of our discussion, we concentrate on the patterns of AAP responses that are associated with the AAI U_d classification.

AAP PATTERN PROFILE OF UNRESOLVED ATTACHMENT

The determination of whether or not the subject of an interview is Unresolved is the first evaluation made by the judge during the AAP classification process. An individual is judged Unresolved if one or more of the seven attachment stories is designated as Unresolved according to the criteria described earlier. In the discussion below, we first present our findings regarding interjudge reliability and AAI convergence in the perinatal risk sample. We then describe the code profile associated with the AAP U_d classification. We include at the end of this discussion examples of picture scenarios in order to provide the reader with a better understanding of how attachment disorganization is revealed in response to the AAP.

Interjudge reliability and the convergence between measures were calculated by percentage of agreement among judges. AAP interjudge agreement was .81 (kappa = .73, p < .000). Convergence between AAP and AAI secure versus insecure classifications was .84 (kappa = .50, p < .01); convergence between AAP and the four major AAI classifications groups (Secure, Dismissing, Preoccupied, Unresolved) was .72 (kappa = .59, p < .000). Attachment classification distributions for both measures are shown in Table 12.2. Although it is not the purpose of this chapter to discuss the AAP classification system in detail, some discussion of the largest group of

TABLE 12.2. Sample Distribution on the AAP and AAI for Four Classification Groups

	AAI				
AAP	Secure	Detached	Preoccupied	Unresolved	Row total
Secure	3 (60)[a] (60)[b]	1 (20) (50)	0	1 (20) (10)	5
Detached	0	1 (100) (50)	0	0	1
Preoccupied	0	0	8 (73) (100)	3 (27) (30)	11
Unresolved	2 (25) (40)	0	0	6 (75) (60)	8
Column total	5	2	8	10	25

Note. Kappa = .59, p < .000.
[a]Percent within AAP.
[b]Percent within AAI.

"misses" in the perinatal sample is of interest. This group comprised interviews that were judged Enmeshed on the AAP but Unresolved on the AAI. Given that our system was in its earliest form when these classifications were made, these misses may be due to errors in our classification rules. We note, however, that the U_d/Enmeshed confusion is a common error in AAI classification (van IJzendoorn, 1995) and, furthermore, the Enmeshed classification is frequently assigned as the alternate classification in AAI cases judged U_d.[5] The misses on these AAP cases are, therefore, not unlike that errors that appear in AAI classification, suggesting an underlying link at the level of mental processes between enmeshed and unresolved mental states.

In the discussion that follows, we describe qualitatively the code profile of the six major AAP codes for individuals who have been judged U_d on the AAI.[6] The patterns of Connectedness and Synchrony codes indicate that, similar to Secure individuals, the AAP attachment representations of many U_d individuals reveal the desire and capacity for reciprocal, responsive relationships. The contexts in which reciprocal connectedness was expressed, however, appear somewhat paradoxical. Consider first the patterns revealed for Connectedness codes in response to the two alone pictures, *Child at Window* and *Bench*. In Secure individuals, AAP representations of characters as connected in reciprocal relationships were more likely to be revealed in response to the greater attachment stress portrayed in the *Bench* picture than in response to the milder stress portrayed in the *Child at Window* picture. In U_d individuals, however, the AAP Connectedness patterns were generally the opposite. Representations of characters in reciprocal relationships were more typically given in response to the relatively mild attachment stimulus, *Child at Window,* and were notably absent when the attachment system was placed under greater stress in *Bench.*

Consider next the patterns revealed for Synchrony, the analogous code for dyadic pictures that assesses the degree to which the stories depict relationships as reciprocal and goal-corrected. Both Secure and U_d individuals were likely to respond to the *Bed* picture with descriptions of reciprocal partnerships; the contexts where reciprocity was described, however, were likely to be quite different. Secure individuals often responded to the *Bed* picture without clear activation of the attachment system. Scenarios were typically of a mother and child greeting each other in the morning or saying "goodnight" to each other at bedtime. U_d individuals, on the other hand, tended to interpret *Bed* in terms of heightened attachment, such as the child being sick or awakened by a nightmare. The child was then portrayed as needing the mother's comfort or protection, and the mother was portrayed as providing reciprocal care. These different patterns suggested to us that U_d individuals are especially sensitive to AAP pictures that represent mild attachment threats, and their representations of attachment indicate that reciprocal care and protection break down under heightened attachment stress.

The profiles for Agency of Self and Personal Experience codes of U_d individuals were more clearly similar to the patterns of other insecure individuals. Like the characters in the stories of Dismissing and Preoccupied individuals, the characters in the stories of U_d individuals were generally neither able to use solitude for self-reflection, nor did they demonstrate the capacity to act. When characters were not being threatened, they were portrayed as passive and lacking in effectiveness. Characters were described as simply continuing life, walking away, or returning to previous activities. As well, U_d and organized insecure individuals both had difficulty telling stories that did not include references to their own personal lives. This phenomenon was rarely observed in the stories of Secure individuals. In some instances, U_d individuals described their own traumatic experiences, including tales of parental or partner abuse, attempted suicide, alcoholism, and the loss of a parent, child, or spouse.

The code patterns related to mental processing or "states of mind" variables (Coherency and Defensive Processes) were very heterogeneous for U_d individuals. Coherency codes across all seven stories ranged from low to high. When the scene did not unleash segregated material, some of the stories of U_d individuals were highly coherent. Of course, as we have already discussed, the form of defensive exclusion that characterized this group was the individual's inability to resolve or contain segregated material. No other pattern of defensive exclusion was predominant for U_d individuals; their stories revealed patterns of deactivation and cognitive disconnection strategies that were similar to the defensive patterns of individuals in all three organized attachment groups.

EXAMPLES OF STORIES ASSOCIATED WITH U_D AND RESOLVED STATUS

We provide here examples of unresolved and resolved stories in order to demonstrate the differences between resolution/containment and dysregulation. As will be seen in the responses judged unresolved, the story characters and the feelings or images represented in the story remain unintegrated. Markers for segregated systems are noted in *italics* in the text and the type of marker as designated by our coding system is noted on the right. The pictures from which the story examples were taken are provided in the Appendix. We begin with examples of responses to the *Child at Window* picture.

Unresolved

Um, well, this looks kind of depressing. It looks like a kid looking out the window, but. . . . And uh, he just looks like he's, he or she is, looking out, wishing they were out there. [And what do you think led up to this?] Uh, either boredom, or maybe the child's being punished, so they're *in a room by themselves with nothing in there.* [And how is the child feeling or thinking?] It's hard to say.   Emptiness/Isolation
They're obviously *staring out the window and you can't see their face* so. [And what happens next?] I   Dissociation
don't know. Just waiting around.

Unresolved

Uh, moment of contemplation, um, the older boy, could be a girl, um deep in thought, and maybe a momentary lapse where the kid is left alone. Looks like it could be at home, or it could be in um an office, probably not in *an institution*   Emptiness/Isolation
because this looks like long curtains and the scene outside looks like a residential street scene, so I would assume that he's at home, although it looks kind of sparse, so it's kind of strange that way, it adds to the *alienation,* that there's a bit of, there's a sense of *alienation* to the picture. [Any   Emptiness/Isolation
idea what the child is thinking or feeling?] Um, it's contemplative and not necessarily negative or disturbing but because of the uh again the *blankness of the presentation,* like there's . . . it's a *faceless* house across the street and the room is *very empty* aside from the curtains, um, so you get a sense of *alienation or isolation.* Uh, or things aren't quite right, there's, there's, he's lacking, he's *lacking something.* [What happens next?] Um, we turn around and we see a *blank face*—I guess because it got *set up from the previous picture.* Almost expect   Odd Response
that—uh, so there's, there's this, um, there's a   Danger/Failed Protec-
potential kind of *horror or disturbance to it.*   tion

Resolved

This one is harder. . . . Well he probably is in some kind of a room looking outside the window, at a tree and a house. Um, by the way I guess he is standing, he is probably thinking I wish I could be out there doing—oh, God this is so hard, *can I skip it?* [Take your time. Anything that comes to mind?] . . . like depressed, and to me he is like I guess feeling upset or angry and to me he looks like he is wishing he could be outside, amongst these things. [Why do you think that he is thinking and feeling that way? What led up to that?] Um, he is standing there with his hands in his pockets looking out, staring at houses . . . and it's like a dull kind of like looking place where he is at, so to me he is standing there going I wish I could be out there, like he is *trapped* wherever he is. To me it looks like he is *trapped.* [What's going to happen next?] Well, hopefully, *he can get out.*

Constriction

Helplessness/Out of Control
Contained

The *Child at Window* picture tends to elicit segregated systems themes that are related to isolation, helplessness, danger and failed protection, and dissociation. The second example contains other segregated systems markers. The reference to feelings of horror is an extreme response given the quality of the picture and the subject's reference to the previous story comes out of nowhere. The failure to resolve or contain the segregated systems markers in the Unresolved stories is contrasted with the resolution evidenced in the final scenario. In this scenario, the child is depicted as having the capacity to act and, as such, the child will not remain trapped, and the segregated systems markers have been contained.

The next set of examples are responses to the *Bench* picture.

Unresolved

This is definitely negative depiction of emotion. Um definite *alienation and isolation,* it looks outdoors, um, *brick wall* and then the bench and looks like, like, looks like a youngish person who's, um, just found a place to uh *hole up in* and um *bury* him or herself in self pity and uh sadness, depression. [What led up to this?] Um, lack of, uh, *inability to communicate with others and not being able to find anyone* who can mentor him or her, be an emotional crutch, so there's *nobody for him or her to talk to,* there's *no emotional outlet,* so

Emptiness/Isolation

Danger/Failed Protection

Emptiness/Isolation

it's *all internalized.* [And what happens next?] Um well, one of two things, either he or she will continue on this path and become more and *more alienated* from everybody else and become more resentful and *reclusive,* emotionally, or um, he or she will encounter, which I find less likely in terms of this particular depiction because it's less likely he or she would actually go out of their way to find somebody, and less likely that somebody would accidentally stumble on this person and give him or her a helping hand, so probably *continued, or escalated sense of isolation.*

Resolved

Well, this girl looks like she's totally *devastated* by something. And she's crying her eyes out. It's hard to say what led up to it. Something that's really taken her away, or taken her aback, either some bad news or something bad has happened to her or—it's hard to tell her age so it could be a relationship gone bad, she could've failed a test, but something's that's affecting her personally. And she's crying about it, and feeling very alone and *isolated.* [How do you think it's going to turn out?] Well since I don't see anybody else there, I think it's probably something *she'll have to come to terms with herself and she'll have to work it out* on her own. Without any support	Helplessness/Out of Control Emptiness/Isolation Resolution/Integration

In these two examples, segregated systems markers include images or references to isolation, helplessness, and being flooded by potentially devastating emotions. In the story judged resolved, the character coming to terms with her isolation is a clear form of integration; that is, she draws upon internal resources.

The next story examples are responses to the *Cemetery* picture.

Unresolved

Let me see, the anniversary of someone's death and this man came to the graveyard to pay his respects, remember whoever passed away. Um, the outcome will be that he'll pay his respects and leave. [And what do you think he's thinking?] Um, probably sadness and *emptiness* and missing the person who isn't there any longer.

Emptiness/Isolation

Unresolved

This person is visiting the cemetery and it looks like things aren't, sort of, taken care of properly there. This person's probably upset and whoever they love or whatever is sort of just, not *mistreated* but that the grounds and it's not cared for. And probably lonely and wanted to sort of have some sort of um *meeting with this person who's dead.* [Tell me a little bit more about what he's thinking and feeling.] I guess he's thinking he wish he could speak to them and see them again and uh . . . I guess he just *wants to maybe tell them* how things are going in his life or whatever. [And what's going to happen after?] He's gonna leave and go on to his regular life.

Odd [person is dead]

Dissociation

Resolved

This man is visiting a cemetery, someone who has a stone that's tilted, apparently it was some time ago. The man is still very . . . had to look and find where that stone was, there's some grass growing around it. He's thinking and wanted to come, made a deliberate choice to seek out this stone among all of the other ones. It's an important one to him. Important because he wanted to um think about this person who has been in his life previously and honor them somehow in a quiet way. He hasn't brought flowers, that's that's okay. The fact that he's come is the thing that's important, it's that he has sought out this person that he wants to think about and remember or *speak with perhaps. Tell something important to,* some change. The man is grown up, he's all dressed up but it's like this is a break in his normal life and a time when he has to come and do this thing for himself, there's no one else there with him. *He's done it for himself, that's something that he's chosen to do deliberately. And when he's gone, he'll be quietly glad that he did that.*

Dissociation

Resolution/Integration

The segregated systems markers in the *Cemetery* story typically range from feelings of profound emptiness or loneliness to the desire to speak with or be with the deceased [a marker for dissociation]. As compared with unresolved stories, there is no ambiguity in the boundaries between the living and the dead in the resolved/contained stories; feelings of isolation and loneliness are addressed directly, and these stories often describe a personal insight, memory, or integration that is the product of visiting the grave site, as is revealed in the third example provided here.

The final set of examples are in response to the *Corner* picture.

Unresolved

Oh, I don't know how to interpret this one. Well, it looks like, I don't know, it looks like the child is um, oh okay, okay, now this is what I interpret this as is the child putting its hands up and turning its head away because somebody is gonna *hit him*. That's what I interpret there. A parent, or or brother, sister, or whatever. That's that's how I interpret that. [What led up to it?] Maybe nothing, *sometimes parents just hit kids because they got nothing better to do.* Um, I don't know, *I can't . . .*

Danger/Failed Protection

Odd Content
Constriction

Unresolved

I thought of *abuse* right away, *child abuse,* because of the gesture of the left hand, saying stop or *don't hit me* or, and then the gesture of the right hand, covering the face, like the way you know children *cover their face,* and it gives them a sense of self-protection, like if they can't see, then *they can't be seen* and therefore can't be *attacked.* Um, and uh being cornered like that too you know, *as small a figure as possible,* or to *take up the least amount of space as possible,* it looks like the child's being really *victimized.* [And what led up to this?] Uh, I would assume *parent abuse,* because um it looks like it's *not an unfamiliar scene for this child.* His gestures seem kind of automatic. [Does anything else happen?] Um, well, I think the child was was *struck,* not badly, but but *struck* enough to to be *terrified,* uh and still, but still able to somewhat defend him- or herself but uh, but really resigned, you know, he's basically *cor-*

Danger/Failed Protection

(*Note*: The protection is a false sense of protection.)

nered him or herself. [And what happens next?] Um, well he or she is *at the total mercy* of whoever is standing I assume in front, and uh uh at this point, maybe the parent, *abusive parent feels like the child has uh has ... has become submissive enough* that they won't go any further.

Helplessness/Out of Control

Unresolved

Whoa this is a strange picture—I always used to get put in the corner the other way—always. If we were ever to get smacked it wouldn't have been when we were in the corners, it's when we're coming through the doorway, so ... Damn ... *I don't want to do this one.*

Constriction

Resolved

Oh. Um, at first it look like he dropped something and he was gonna, you know, looking over to pick it up, but it can also look like he's in a corner and somebody's *attacking* him. He's *trying to protect himself.* And what's gonna happen—um [Can you follow that up?] Sure—kind-of-looks like he's, he's in the corner of a, of a house and like his older brother or something's picking on him, or a parent, and he is going to get in trouble, like he's, I mean he is there by himself, so. He'll *try to defend himself.* [What's going to happen next?] Um oh, I think he'd get, I think whatever would happen will happen. He won't be able to prevent it, because he's in the corner. [How's he feeling?] Upset. Well *scared. He looks scared.*

Danger/Failed Protection

Containment: Strategy for active attempt to protect self

Danger/Failed Protection

Danger, failed protection, physical abuse, vulnerability, and helplessness are typically the major segregated systems markers that are given in response to this picture. In the Unresolved examples, the child is vulnerable; the conditions are such that the child is left feeling utterly helpless, and it is likely that the abusive behavior will reoccur. Unresolved individuals are unable to introduce any themes of protection and defense into their stories. Without protection, the child is at risk for "disintegration." Contrast these stories with the story of the resolved individual who introduces the idea that the child will try to protect and defend himself. Despite continuing to be afraid and stating that the child will not able to prevent the behavior, based on our analysis of the story scenarios, the theme of self-protection in the story appears to be enough to keep the individual's defensive processes organized.

CONCLUSIONS

Bowlby (1980) proposed behavioral and mental disorganization to be the product of defensive processes that segregate attachment-related experience from access to consciousness. Investigations of mental representations of disorganized children have supported the notion that the underlying mechanism of child attachment disorganization is segregated systems. Guided by Bowlby's view, and expanding on the work already done with children, we developed a coding scheme to identify segregated systems at the representational level in adults. Like disorganized children's responses to projective attachment stimuli, the responses of Unresolved adults to the AAP pictures demonstrate that they have not integrated threatening attachment experiences and fears into organized mental representations of attachment. The stories of Unresolved adults reveal "unmetabolized" emotions through story themes of isolation, helplessness, danger, and failed protection. Furthermore, and similar to some disorganized children, the activation of the attachment system of some Unresolved adults results in constriction and severe inhibition. Constriction appears to be a "desperate" mental strategy that prohibits segregated attachment models from becoming activated and, thus, blocks painful attachment material from flooding consciousness. We also observed AAP interviews in which U_d adults alternated between displays of flooding and constriction, a phenomenon that Bowlby (1980) described as one of the major observable signs characteristic of segregated systems, and that has also been noted in the doll-play scenarios of disorganized/controlling children.

The literature on attachment has traditionally been governed by two sovereign ideas. First, the dimension of secure–insecure attachment has been used to delineate quality of attachment. Second, insecure attachment has been analyzed along a dimension of two organized strategies, avoidant/dismissing and ambivalent/preoccupied attachment. The AAP data presented here on unresolved/disorganized representations of attachment may be viewed as part of a larger current emphasis upon a third dimension that attachment researchers have found necessary to describe attachment relationships. This third dimension is the concept of dysregulation (Solomon & George, Chapter 1, this volume). In contrast to the two dimensions that differentiate the qualities of the traditional organized attachment groups, dysregulation accents the degree to which attachment organization is undermined or made incoherent by the extreme forms of defensive exclusion associated with segregated systems. Our data add to a growing number of studies that suggest that without the inclusion of this third dimension, descriptions of attachment are necessarily incomplete.

Our growing understanding of disorganization in adulthood has important implications for our understanding of pathological risk. According to Bowlby's view of segregated systems, the attachment contribution to understanding mental health risk is based on our developing further understanding of the processes underlying the breakdown or dysregulation of one or more segregated attachment systems. Our work examining adult disorganization at the level of representation suggests similarities in attachment-related pathways for psychopathological risk in adults and children; that is, based on the concepts of segregated systems, disorganization, and dysregulation, the adult forms of psychopathology with which Bowlby was concerned (e.g., dissociated mental states; depersonalization; pathological levels of anxiety or self-blame; aggressive, reckless, and violent and destructive behavior directed toward the self and others; compulsive caregiving; compulsive self-reliance; and euphoria) and, more recently, the forms of psychopathology receiving attention from new attachment researchers (e.g., borderline states—Fonagy et al., 1995; dissociative disorder—Liotti, Chapter 11, this volume) are likely to have strong attachment contributions. The function of the attachment system is to ensure that children, and later, adults, develop a relationship with a "stronger and wiser" individual who will provide protection from danger and threat. Following the model presented here and in other chapters in this volume (e.g., Solomon & George, Chapter 1, this volume), mental "ill health" is likely to result from the emotional flooding and constriction that accompanies dysregulated attachment. Clinical symptomology results when dysregulation of the attachment system leaves the individual overwhelmed by feelings of helplessness, vulnerability, and fear of abandonment.

ACKNOWLEDGMENT

Carol George was partially supported during the preparation of this work by appointment to the Letts—Villard Endowed Chair.

NOTES

1. We use the capitalized form of the word "unresolved" specifically to indicate that individuals are designated as such following the convention of the AAI classification system.

2. See Solomon and George (1999) for a complete discussion of representational assessments of attachment in childhood.

3. Although other investigators, for example, Bretherton and her colleagues (1990), noted these themes in their work, they did not associate these themes specifically with disorganized attachment. Rather, these themes were described more generally as markers for insecurity.

4. The perinatal risk sample included interviews from both mothers whose infants are at risk and their controls.

5. This finding is especially interesting in light of the results of a recent study of adult and child attachment in a middle-childhood sample. This study found that mothers of disorganized/controlling children are more likely to be judged Enmeshed on the AAI than Unresolved (Solomon & George, 1998).

6. This description is based on refinements made to the AAP classification system by incorporating information regarding the misses between AAI and AAP classifications in the perinatal sample. We note that we are about to embark on a construct and discriminant validity study of the AAP with a community sample.

REFERENCES

Ainsworth, M. D. S., Blehar, M. C., Waters, E., & Wall, S. (1978). *Patterns of attachment: A psychological study of the Strange Situation.* Hillsdale, NJ: Erlbaum.

Ainsworth, M. D. S., & Eichberg, C. (1991). Effects on infant–mother attachment of mother's unresolved loss of an attachment figure, or other traumatic experience. In C. M. Parkes, J. Stevenson-Hinde, & P. Marris (Eds.), *Attachment across the life cycle* (pp. 160–186). New York: Routledge.

Bowlby, J. (1969/1982). *Attachment and loss: Vol. 1. Attachment.* New York: Basic Books.

Bowlby, J. (1973). *Attachment and loss: Vol. 2. Separation.* New York: Basic Books.

Bowlby, J. (1980). *Attachment and loss: Vol. 3. Loss.* New York: Basic Books.

Bowlby, J. (1988). *A secure base.* New York: Basic Books.

Bretherton, I. (1985). Attachment theory: Retrospect and prospect. In I. Bretherton & E. Waters (Eds.), Growing points in attachment theory and research. *Monographs of the Society for Research in Child Development, 50*(1-2, Serial No. 209), 3-35.

Bretherton, I., Ridgeway, D., & Cassidy, J. (1990). Assessing internal working models of attachment relationships: An attachment story completion task for 3-year-olds. In M. T. Greenberg, D. Cicchetti, & E. M. Cummings (Eds.), *Attachment in the preschool years* (pp. 273-308). Chicago: University of Chicago Press.

Carlson, V., Cicchetti, D., Barnett, D., & Braunwald, K. (1989). Disorganized/disoriented attachment relationships in maltreated infants. *Developmental Psychology, 25*, 525-531.

Case, R. (1992). The role of frontal lobes in the regulation of cognitive development. *Brain and Cognition, 20*, 51-73.

Cassidy, J. (1988). Child-mother attachment and the self in six-year-olds. *Child Development, 59*, 121-134.

Cassidy, J., & Marvin, R. S. (1987/1989/1990/1991/1992). *Attachment organization in preschool children: Coding guidelines.* Unpublished coding manual, MacArthur Working Group on Attachment, Seattle, WA.

Fonagy, P., Steele, M., Steele, H., Leigh, T., Kennedy, R., Mattoon, G., & Target,

M. (1995). Attachment, the reflective self, and borderline states: The predictive specificity of the Adult Attachment Interview and pathological emotional development. In S. Goldberg, R. Muir, & J. Kerr (Eds.), *Attachment theory: Social, developmental and clinical perspectives* (pp. 233–277). Hillsdale, NJ: Analytic Press.

George, C., Kaplan, N., & Main, M. (1984/1985/1996). *Attachment Interview for Adults.* Unpublished manuscript, University of California, Berkeley.

George, C., & Solomon, J. (1996). Representational models of relationships: Links between caregiving and attachment. *Infant Mental Health Journal, 17,* 198–216.

George, C., & Solomon, J. (1998, July). *Attachment disorganization at age six: Differences in doll play between punitive and caregiving children.* Paper presented at the meeting of the International Society for the Study of Behavioral Development, Bern, Switzerland.

George, C., & Solomon, J. (1999). Attachment and caregiving: The caregiving behavioral system. In J. Cassidy & P. R. Shaver (Eds.), *Handbook of attachment theory, research, and clinical applications* (pp. 649–670). New York: Guilford Press.

George, C., West, M., & Pettem, O. (1997). *The Adult Attachment Projective.* Unpublished attachment measure and coding manual, Mills College, Oakland, CA.

Jacobsen, T., Edelstein, W., & Hofmann, V. (1994). A longitudinal study of the relation between representations of attachment in childhood and cognitive functioning in childhood and adolescence. *Developmental Psychology, 30,* 112–124.

Kaplan, N. (1995). *Patterns of response to imagined separation in six-year-olds judged secure, avoidant, ambivalent and disorganized with mother in infancy: Resourceful, inactive, ambivalent, and fearful.* Unpublished manuscript, University of California, Berkeley.

Lyons-Ruth, K., & Jacobvitz, D. (1999). Attachment disorganization: Unresolved loss, relational violence, and lapses in behavioral and attentional strategies. In J. Cassidy & P. R. Shaver (Eds.), *Handbook of attachment: Theory, research and clinical applications* (pp. 520–554). New York: Guilford Press.

Main, M. (1995). Recent studies in attachment. In S. Goldberg, R. Muir, & J. Kerr (Eds.), *Attachment theory: Social, developmental, and clinical perspectives* (pp. 467–474). Hillsdale NJ: Analytic Press.

Main, M., & Cassidy, J. (1988). Categories of response to reunion with the parent at age 6: Predictable from infant attachment classifications and stable over a 1-month period. *Developmental Psychology, 24,* 1–12.

Main, M., & Goldwyn, R. (1985/1991/1994). *Adult attachment scoring and classification systems.* Unpublished classification manual, University of California, Berkeley.

Main, M., Kaplan, N., & Cassidy, J. (1985). Security in infancy, childhood, and adulthood: A move to the level of representation. In I. Bretherton & E. Waters (Eds.), Growing points in attachment theory and research. *Monographs of the Society for Research in Child Development, 50*(1–2, Serial No. 209), 66–104.

Main, M., & Solomon, J. (1986). Discovery of a new, insecure–disorganized/disoriented attachment pattern. In T. B. Brazelton & M. Yogman (Eds.), *Affective development in infancy* (pp. 95–124). Norwood, NJ: Ablex

Main, M., & Solomon, J. (1990). Procedures for identifying infants as disorganized/disoriented during the Ainsworth strange situation. In M. T. Greenberg, D. Cicchetti, & E. M. Cummings (Eds.), *Attachment in the preschool years* (pp. 121–160). Chicago: University of Chicago Press.

O'Connor, M., Sigman, M., & Brill, N. (1987). Disorganization of attachment in relation to maternal alcohol consumption. *Journal of Consulting and Clinical Psychology, 55*, 831–836.

Oppenheim, D., & Waters, H. S. (1995). Narrative processes and attachment representations: Issues of development and assessment. In E. Waters, B. E. Vaughn, G. Posada, & K. Kondo-Ikemura (Eds.), Caregiving, cultural, and cognitive perspectives on secure-base behavior and working models. *Monographs of the Society for Research in Child Development, 60*(2–3, Serial No. 244), 197–233.

Perry, B. D., Pollard, R. A., Blakley, T. L., & Vigilante, D. (1995). Childhood trauma, the neurobiology of adaptation, and "use dependent" development of the brain: How "states" become "traits." *Infant Mental Health Journal, 16*, 271–289.

Shouldice, A., & Stevenson-Hinde, J. (1992). Coping with security distress: The Separation Anxiety Test and attachment classification at 4.5 years. *Journal of Child Psychology and Psychiatry, 33*, 331–348.

Slough, N. M., & Greenberg, M. T. (1990). Five-year olds' representations of separation from parents: Responses from the perspective of self and other. In I. Bretherton & M. W. Watson (Eds.), *New directions for child development: Vol. 48. Children's perspectives on the family* (pp. 67–84). San Francisco: Jossey-Bass.

Solomon, J., & George, C. (1998). *Caregiving, adult attachment, and child disorganized/controlling attachment in mother–child dyads at age six.* Unpublished manuscript, Mills College, Oakland, CA.

Solomon, J., & George, C. (1999). The measurement of attachment security in infancy and childhood. In J. Cassidy & P. R. Shaver (Eds.), *Handbook of attachment: Theory, research, and clinical applications* (pp. 287–316). New York: Guilford Press.

Solomon, J., George, C., & De Jong, A. (1995). Children classified as controlling at age six: Evidence of disorganized representational strategies and aggression at home and school. *Development and Psychopathology, 7*, 447–464.

Teti, D., Gelfand, D., Messinger, D., & Isabella, R. (1995). Maternal depression and the quality of early attachment: An examination of infants, preschoolers, and their mothers. *Developmental Psychology, 31*, 364–376.

Thompson, R. A. (1999). Early attachment and later development. In J. Cassidy & P. R. Shaver (Eds.), *Handbook of attachment: Theory, research, and clinical applications* (pp. 265–286). New York: Guilford Press.

van IJzendoorn, M. H. (1995). Adult attachment representations, parental responsiveness, and infant attachment: A meta-analysis of the predictive validity of the Adult Attachment Interview. *Psychology Bulletin, 117*, 387–403.

van IJzendoorn, M. H., Schuengel, C. & Bakermans-Kranenburg, M. J. (1999). Disorganized attachment in early childhood: Meta-analysis of precursors, concomitants, and sequelae. *Development and Psychopathology, 11*, 225–249.

Wartner, U. G., Grossmann, K., Fremmer-Bombik, E., & Suess, G. (1994). Attachment patterns at age six in South Germany: Predictability from infancy and implications for preschool behavior. *Child Development, 65*, 1014–1027.

West, M., & George, C. (in press). Abuse and violence in intimate adult relationships: New perspectives from attachment theory. *Attachment and Human Development.*

APPENDIX: EXAMPLES OF PICTURES FROM THE ADULT ATTACHMENT PROJECTIVE

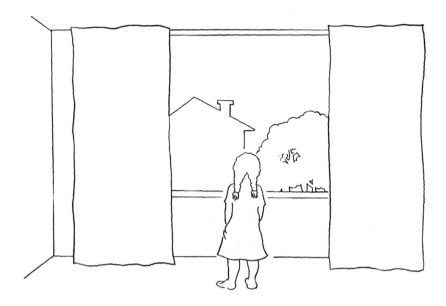

PICTURE 1. Child at Window.

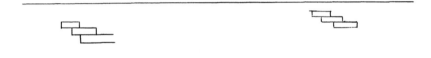

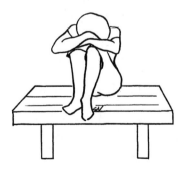

PICTURE 2. Bench.

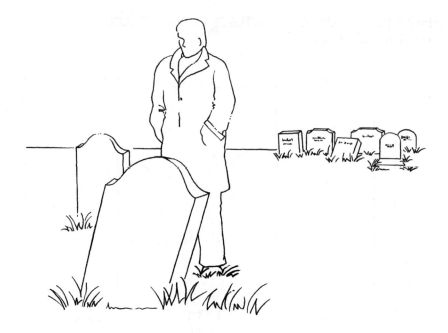

PICTURE 3. Cemetery.

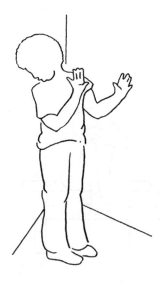

PICTURE 4. Child in Corner.

CHAPTER 13

Attachment Quality in Young Children of Mentally Ill Mothers

Contribution of Maternal Caregiving Abilities and Foster Care Context

TERESA JACOBSEN
LAURA J. MILLER

With the implementation of deinstitutionalization in the 1960s, mental health service delivery for individuals with severe mental disorders was shifted from a primarily inpatient location to outpatient community mental health centers (Appleby, Desai, Luchins, Gibbons, & Hedeker, 1993). This change has had a profound effect on the lives of mentally ill women and their children. An unintended consequence of deinstitutionalization has been a dramatic increase in the number of women with chronic mental disorders who are giving birth to children (Burr, Falek, Strauss, & Brown, 1979). Many of these mothers have serious parenting problems and cannot provide consistent, long-term care for their children (Apfel & Handel, 1993; Nicholson, Geller, Fisher, & Dion, 1993). Studies of clinical samples estimate that about 60% of mothers with major mental illness are not raising their own children (Coverdale & Aruffo, 1989; Miller & Finnerty, 1996).

Mental health professionals are often asked to assess and give opinions on the attachment of a child to a mentally ill mother who is a noncustodial parent, and to assess how the child would be affected if the child were returned to her care. They may also be asked to assess how a child's emotional development is likely to be affected by various placement alternatives. These opinions may weigh heavily in decisions about whether a child should be returned to a mentally ill mother, or whether parental rights should be terminated.

While it is known that both maternal caregiving abilities (e.g., Lyons-Ruth, Connell, Grunebaum, & Botein, 1990) and mother–child separations can profoundly affect a child's attachment security (Bowlby, 1973; Robertson & Robertson, 1989), systematic research on the attachment bonds of children who have been removed from the care of a mentally ill mother is lacking, as is research on factors that contribute to individual differences in the quality of attachment in those children. Such research could be critical in helping mental health professionals and child welfare personnel make better custody decisions and in planning effective parenting rehabilitation when feasible (Herman, 1997; Rutter, 1995). Systematic data of this sort could also guide child welfare policy and program development.

The current chapter reviews literature on the effects of maternal mental illness on children's attachment quality, and on maternal caregiving. It also examines factors that influence mother–child attachment during prolonged mother–child separations. This overview provides a framework for presenting pilot data on the attachment of children who have been removed from the care of a mentally ill mother. The study focuses on the contribution of maternal caregiving abilities and type of substitute care to individual differences in children's attachment bonds to their mothers. The chapter begins with a brief overview of attachment classification.

ATTACHMENT CLASSIFICATION

Attachment classification is based on an infant's reunion responses to the strange situation, a laboratory observation that consists of two brief separation and reunion episodes (Ainsworth, Blehar, Waters, & Wall, 1978). This observation is stressful and activates the infant's attachment system (Bowlby, 1969/1982). It thus provides information about a child's strategy in gaining protection from the caregiver. Patterns of attachment identified in this laboratory procedure have been found to reflect the quality of mother–child attachment interaction as experienced by the child during the first year of life (Ainsworth et al., 1978; Isabella & Belsky, 1991).

Infants who actively seek proximity, or contact with, their caregivers after the brief separations, and who are able to use their mothers as a secure base for exploration, are classified as secure. This pattern has been associated with sensitive and responsive caregiving. Infants who avoid their mothers on reunion, and who do not actively seek her out for comfort or proximity, are classified as insecure–avoidant. This pattern has been linked to a mother's rebuffing of her baby's needs for comfort and closeness. Infants who cannot be settled by their mothers, and who have difficulties with exploration, are classified as insecure–ambivalent. This classification has been associated with inconsistent caregiving.

The traditional attachment groups (secure, avoidant, and ambivalent) involve "organized" strategies for coping with stressful situations in that they help children to achieve the goal of proximity to the caregiver (Main & Solomon, 1990; Solomon & George, 1996). Securely attached infants have the strategy of directly approaching their mother under stress, while infants with an insecure–avoidant or insecure–ambivalent pattern either maintain indirect proximity to their mothers or elicit her attention through angry behavior.

By contrast, infants with an insecure–disorganized attachment classification do not have an organized strategy for obtaining help from their mothers under stress (Main & Solomon, 1990). They display highly contradictory or fearful behaviors toward their mothers in reunion episodes. Some infants with this classification, for instance, may begin to approach their mothers, but then become dazed and wander away. The disorganized pattern has been linked to frightening or frightened parenting behaviors (Main & Hesse, 1990), and to intrusive and hostile maternal interaction quality (Lyons-Ruth, Repacholi, McLeod, & Silva, 1991). Mothers whose children have a disorganized attachment pattern often feel helpless in the mothering role and fail to provide protection (George & Solomon, 1996; Solomon & George, 1996). There is some evidence that some mothers of children with disorganized attachment have a history of unresolved mourning of prior losses or trauma (Main & Hesse, 1990).

By early childhood, children with disorganized attachment often begin to "organize" their mothers' behavior, either by consoling their mothers or by asserting their authority and dominance. Thus, characteristics signs of a disorganized attachment pattern in older children include conspicuously controlling behaviors on the part of the children during reunion, such as punishing or role-reversed behaviors (Main & Cassidy, 1988; Solomon & George, 1996). The disorganized/controlling pattern is prevalent in young children who have been maltreated (Carlson, Cicchetti, Barnett, & Braunwald 1989), which suggests that it may be an important tool for identifying at-risk relationships.

EFFECTS OF MENTAL ILLNESS ON MOTHER–CHILD ATTACHMENT QUALITY

Several studies have utilized Ainsworth's methodology to assess the attachment patterns of infants and children to mothers with severe mental disorders. These studies typically document high rates of insecure attachment patterns (D'Angelo, 1986; Murray, 1992; Radke-Yarrow, Cummings, Kuczynski, & Chapman, 1985; Zahn-Waxler, McKnew, Cummings, Davenport, & Radke-Yarrow, 1984), and particularly high rates of the insecure–disorganized/controlling pattern (DeMulder & Radke-Yarrow, 1991) when young children of mentally ill mothers are compared to index groups of children with nonmentally ill mothers. In high-risk, low socioeconomic status families, the rate of disorganized attachment status in young children of depressed mothers has been estimated to be as high as 60% (Lyons-Ruth et al., 1990). Rates of insecure–disorganized attachment status have been found to be higher in chronically depressed mothers than in mothers who are not chronically depressed (Teti, Gelfand, Messinger, & Isabella, 1995). A high rate of disorganized attachment status has also been documented in studies of children of mothers who have alcoholism (O'Connor, Sigman, & Brill, 1987) and other drug addictions (Rodning, Beckwith, & Howard, 1991). These findings make theoretical sense, given that the disorganized attachment pattern has been specifically linked to frightening experiences with a mother (Main & Hesse, 1990) and to maternal feelings of helplessness (George & Solomon, 1996; Solomon & George, 1996). A mentally ill mother can be unpredictable in interacting with children (Lyden, 1997), or emotionally absent. This can be frightening and, ultimately, disorganizing for young children, especially if their mothers are unable to actively calm or comfort them.

Much less is known about individual differences in the attachment patterns of young children who are removed from a mentally ill mother's care. This is not an uncommon experience for many children of mentally ill parents, who may be raised by others, while receiving only intermittent caregiving from their own mothers (Lyden, 1997). A retrospective study of adult children of parents with schizophrenia found that, during childhood, participants were, on the average, raised in three different settings (Caton, Cournos, Felix, & Wyatt, 1998). Some experienced as many as seven different caregiving environments. All participants also reported being raised by the patient–parent for some time from birth to age 18 years. For about 60% of the participants, however, a grandparent, aunt, or uncle was the most significant nurturing adult. This person provided not only emotional support and companionship, but also material support and shelter to participants.

When child protective service agencies remove children from the custody of mentally ill parents, the children may be placed with relatives, in nonrelative placements, or in a shelter or group home (Solnit, Nordhaus, & Lord, 1992). Some children experience multiple foster care placements until their mothers are capable of resuming their caregiving roles, or until decisions are made about custody.

There is a lack of systematic data on the attachment of children with a mentally ill mother who is currently not a custodial caregiver. Clinical reports suggest that when an infant is separated from a mentally ill mother right after birth, there may be no attachment to the biological mother (Helfer, 1972; Hurd, 1975; Leiderman & Seashore, 1975; Lynch & Roberts, 1977), or the bond may be, at best, highly tenuous (Eliacheff, 1997). Although children who are removed at birth or in the first months of life are likely to form a primary attachment to a foster parent, they may continue to have regular contact with their mother, who is seeking to regain custody of them. A child in these circumstances may grow up with multiple mothers.

Children who are separated from a caregiver after having formed a primary attachment to that caregiver may show grief responses (Bowlby, 1980). When a separation is prolonged, these children may live in a state of uncertainty as to whom they belong (Eliacheff, 1997). This may be exacerbated by pressures from biological and foster parents to declare loyalty, and by a lack of information that children in foster care receive about why they were placed in foster care. In some cases, it can be extremely difficult to ascertain who is the psychological parent for a child (cf. Goldstein, Freud, & Solnit, 1979).

In other cases, children may continue to organize their attachment feelings around a mentally ill mother despite prolonged separations. Jolowicz (1946, see Bowlby, 1963) used the term "Hidden Parent" to describe the influence on children of a parent with whom they have little, if any, contact. This phenomenon was described by Holley (1997), who was raised by relatives for several years after her mother developed schizophrenia. Although Holley lived with her mother only briefly throughout her childhood, many of her thoughts and feelings remained organized around her mother. She idealized her mother and maintained a secret relationship with her in her mind. Little is known about why some children continue to secretly organize their feelings around a parent who is absent, although failure on the part of adults to talk about the absent parent may facilitate this (Bowlby, 1963).

Young children who experience extreme neglect or abuse coupled with care by multiple caregivers may develop an attachment disorder of infancy or early childhood (Zeanah, 1996). At present, there are no systematic data on the prevalence of attachment disorders in infants and young children who have been removed from the care of a mentally ill mother. Disorders of attachment are thought to differ from the standard attachment classifications identified in the strange situation, however, in that they involve pervasive and profound disturbances in a child's feelings of security (Lieberman & Pawl, 1988), but little is known about the relationship between attachment disorders and the insecure–disorganized pattern (see Boris, Fueyo, & Zeanah, 1997, for recent research in this area).

EFFECTS OF SEVERE MENTAL ILLNESS ON MATERNAL CAREGIVING

Parenting ability is often impaired in mothers with major mental disorders (Apfel & Handel, 1993; Lyons-Ruth & Block, 1996; Rogosch, Mowbray, & Bogat, 1992). Several studies document that mothers with severe mental disorders may have more aberrant attitudes about childrearing and children than non–mentally ill mothers (Cohler, Grunebaum, Weiss, Hartman, & Gallant, 1976; Kissane & Ball, 1988). These attitudes can be reflected in potentially dangerous behaviors. Mothers who are hospitalized for postpartum psychoses following childbirth, for instance, may experience a loss of love for their infant, harbor thoughts of killing them, or may actually attempt to injure their infants (Sneddon, Kerry, & Bant, 1981).

Difficulties in adapting to the parenting role often persist in mothers with severe mental disorders. These mothers may feel that their children are too difficult to handle and demand too much attention. Some mothers with mental illness may feel that their children's wills are stronger than their own, and that their children are uncontrollable (Uddenberg & Engelsson, 1978).

Severity and chronicity of a mother's mental illness have been viewed as more important in influencing parenting than specific psychiatric diagnoses (Campbell, Cohn, & Meyer, 1995; Sameroff, Seifer, & Zax, 1982; Teti et al., 1995). Nonetheless, several studies provide some data about potential effects of particular illnesses on parenting. Major depression in a mother, for instance, may promote the belief that she is not a good mother, the belief that there is something wrong with the child (often accompanied by the belief that it is the mother's fault), and/or the belief that the child would be better off with the mother dead (Kissane & Ball, 1988). Behaviorally, severely depressed mothers tend to be less active in interactions with their children, and less able to tend to their children's basic needs (Cohn, Campbell, Matias, & Hopkins, 1990). Some children of chronically depressed mothers begin, at early ages, to parent their mothers and/or their siblings (Zeanah & Klitzke, 1991).

Bipolar mood disorder has a high likelihood of new onset and exacerbation postpartum. Postpartum mania can pose high immediate risk to infants (Sneddon et al., 1981), but not necessarily long-term risk if treatment is effective (McNeil, Persson-Blennow, Binett, Harty, & Karyd, 1988).

Parents with schizophrenia or related psychotic disorders may experience reduced ability to discern nonverbal cues (e.g., recognizing affect from facial expression). They may have reduced ability to foster mutual social interchange, with diminished initiation of behavior (e.g., less touching and playing with babies, and less stimulation of babies or older children) (Persson-Blennow, Naeslund, McNeil, Kaij, & Malmquist-Larsson, 1986; Persson-Blennow, Binett, & McNeil, 1988; Seeman, 1996). Some may have unpredictable, inappropriate, and/or aggressive involvement with children, due to fluctuations in psychotic symptoms. Specific hallucinations and delusions about the child may contribute to this behavior. Antipsychotic medication in itself may affect parenting by reducing affective expression and reducing ability to waken in response to a baby's cries.

Although parenting can be significantly impaired in mothers with severe mental disorders, these mothers usually maintain the desire to have children and care for them (Caton et al., 1998; White, Nicholson, Fisher, & Geller, 1995). The effects of mental illness on parenting are also not uniform across individuals (Apfel & Handel, 1993; Jacobsen & Miller, 1998a). Factors that are likely to influence how a mentally ill mother cares for her children are the mother's experiences with her own caregivers in infancy and childhood (Main & Hesse, 1990), her age, the number of children she is caring for, her relation to her spouse or partner, economic resources, her insight into her mental illness and responsiveness to treatment (Cassell & Coleman, 1995), and the social support she receives in the parenting role (Crittenden, 1985; Fendrich, Warner, & Weissman, 1990). A support network can facilitate a mother's ability to cope with her mental illness, while providing alternate caregivers to her children if needed.

FACTORS AFFECTING ATTACHMENT AND CAREGIVING DURING PROLONGED SEPARATIONS

During a prolonged separation, young children may experience profound changes in their feelings toward their caregivers, especially if they are cared for by unfamiliar substitute caregivers (Robertson & Robertson, 1989). In this situation, a young child who has previously had an adequate relationship to a mother will initially protest by crying and calling for her in the first days. If the separation persists, the child's response may change to one of despair. A child in this phase appears depressed and withdrawn, and refuses friendly overtures or food from others. If the separation persists, a child may become more interested in food and material goods and begin to form indiscriminate and shallow relationships. The child may fail to recognize the caregiver and show other highly detached behavior in his or her presence. In some cases, detachment may persist indefinitely (Bowlby, 1973).

Bowlby (1973) stressed that in understanding the attachment patterns of young children to mothers from whom they are separated, it is important to consider the contribution of two main factors: (1) a mother's caregiving abilities and, in particular, a mother's sensitivity to her child's individuality; and (2) the consistency and quality of care experienced by a child in the interim. Young children who are undergoing a major separation fare better when they experience stable, responsive mothering than if they are handled and cared for by a succession of unknown people (Robertson & Robertson, 1989). It is postulated that care by a responsive substitute caregiver may hold a child's anxiety at a manageable level and thus curtail the deteriorating sequence of protest, despair, and detachment. Little is known, however, about the influences of maternal caregiving abilities and consistency of foster care on the attachment patterns of children who have been living in foster care due to removal from the care of a mentally ill mother.

A child's age at the time of the separation, and the length of time that a child is separated, have also been found to influence the child's relation to the absent mother (Bowlby, 1973; Heinicke & Westheimer, 1965). The effects of separation are generally thought to be greater in the first 3 years of life, due to the vulnerability of young children, their notion of time, and the fragility of their representational abilities (Bowlby, 1980).

During a prolonged separation, a mother's feelings may also undergo change, especially if the child is removed immediately after birth (Bensel & Paxson, 1979; Leiderman & Seashore, 1975; Peterson & Mehl, 1978). A mother's feelings for her child may cool during a prolonged separation (Westheimer, 1970). Family life may become organized along lines that leave little room into which a child can fit upon return home (Bowlby, 1973). In cases where a child is living in foster care, a mother's emotional investment and hope of regaining custody of her children may oscillate, depending on the status of the court case and her relationship to the foster family.

PILOT STUDY: THE ATTACHMENT BONDS OF CHILDREN WHO WERE REMOVED FROM THE CARE OF A MENTALLY ILL MOTHER

The previous review underscores the dearth of studies on the attachment patterns of young children who have been removed from the care of a mentally ill mother, and on factors that condition individual differences in these patterns. Although prior theorizing and research (Bowlby, 1973) underscore that differences in maternal caregiving abilities and in children's foster care placement will contribute to differences in the mother–child attachment bond, these factors have not yet been systematically studied in this population.

A pilot study was conducted to explore the attachment patterns of young children to mentally ill mothers who were noncustodial caregivers at the time of study entry. A major objective of the study was to identify the types of attachment patterns present in children under these circumstances. A second objective was to examine the contribution of maternal caregiving dimensions and foster care contexts to individual differences in attachment patterns. The pilot study was designed to provide preliminary data to inform the design of a larger, ongoing study of parenting capability in mentally ill mothers.

The pilot study examined three general types of mother–child attachment patterns:

Group 1: Traditional (organized) attachment patterns (Ainsworth's secure, avoidant, and ambivalent categories).

Group 2: Disorganized or controlling attachment patterns (Main and Solomon's insecure–disorganized attachment category and Main and Cassidy's controlling category).

Group 3: Tenuous attachment or no attachment.

We tested whether mothers in the three groups differed with regard to their (1) attitudes about childrearing and young children, (2) internal representations of their children and their relationship to them, (3) size of social support networks, (4) insight into the effects of their mental illness on parenting, and (5) treatment compliance, and with regard to their children's (6) stability of foster placement (single vs. multiple) and (7) type of foster placement (relative vs. nonrelative).

Study Sample

The study included 30 mothers and their children. Participants met the following inclusion criteria:

1. The mother had a major mental illness, defined as a DSM-IV diagnosis of schizophrenia, schizoaffective disorder, bipolar mood disorder, severe major depression, chronic posttraumatic stress disorder, dissociative disorder, or personality disorder (American Psychiatric Association, 1994).
2. The mental illness had resulted in a psychiatric hospitalization within the past 5 years.
3. The mother was an alleged perpetrator of child abuse and/or neglect, and had an active case within the child welfare system.

Because the age when a child is separated from its mother and the length of separation can contribute considerably to differences in children's attachment quality (Bowlby, 1973), we controlled for these variables by including only children between the ages of 1 and 4 years, children who were removed from their mother's care before age 3, and children who had been living in foster care for at least 1 year. Thus, the study focused on mothers whose mental disorders were severe enough to require a psychiatric hospitalization and on their young children who had been removed in infancy or early childhood, and who had been out of their mother's care for at least 1 year.

Study Sample Composition

At the time of assessment, 12 children (40%) were between ages 12 and 29 months, and 18 (60%) were between ages 30 and 48 months. Mothers ranged in age from 19 to 44 years (mean age = 31 years), with 15 being of African American (50%), 14 of Caucasian (47%), and 1 of Hispanic (3%) origin. Sixteen mothers (53%) had not completed high school; 12 (40%) had a high school or General Equivalency Degree; 2 (7%) had attended college. Fifteen mothers (50%) were unemployed and living on public aid or social security. Eleven mothers (37%) were employed, most often at low-level temporary jobs; 4 (13%) were supported by a husband, father, or partner. Thirteen mothers (43%) had schizophrenia or schizoaffective disorder; 9 (30%) had a personality disorder; 7 (33%) had a mood disorder (either recurrent major depression or bipolar disorder), and 1 (3%) had a dissociative disorder.

Circumstances Surrounding Custody Loss

Mothers in our study lost custody of their children due to risk of harm ($n = 18$; 60%), actual harm to the target child ($n = 2$; 7%), inadequate supervision of the target child ($n = 6$; 20%), or to combinations thereof ($n = 4$; 13%). Risk of harm had been indicated in one case because the mother had killed an older child, and in one case because the mother had murdered an adult. In other cases ($n = 3$), the mother had harmed an older child in the family. One mother had beaten a daughter, leaving bruises and bite marks. In several cases ($n = 7$), risk of harm was indicated because mothers had come close to harming the target child. One woman, for instance, had been observed shaking her week old infant upside down by the foot and had threatened to bash the baby's head. Several mothers had threatened to kill themselves and their children. Inadequate supervision and neglect were indicated in one case when a mother left her infant alone for several hours as she went to purchase drugs. In other cases ($n = 3$), risk was indicated when a mother abandoned her children in a shopping mall, or when children were discovered alone outside by neighbors. In none of the cases was there evidence for persistent and gross maternal abuse or neglect of the target child, although, in some cases, older siblings had had these experiences. Half of the mothers in our study had one-time involvement with the child welfare system; half had experienced between 2 and 26 involvements. Length of separations ranged from 1 to 2.4 years (average length = 2 years, SD = 1 year). Fifteen children (50%) had been removed from their mothers at birth or in the first few months of life. Seventeen (57%) were placed with relatives; 7 (23%) were in nonrelative foster care; 6 (20%) children experienced two or more foster placements. At the time of the study, all of the children had supervised visits with their mothers.

Methods

The data for this pilot study come from a large, ongoing research project on factors that contribute to child maltreatment risk in mothers with chronic mental disorders. Table 13.1 presents an overview of the main risk and protective factors, and of the specific tools used in the larger study.

The assessment period comprised three sessions, each lasting between 2 and 4 hours. The first session involved a psychiatric interview to determine the mother's psychiatric diagnosis or diagnoses, to assess her insight into her psychiatric condition and adherence to the current psychiatric treatment and its efficacy, and the effect of her psychiatric symptoms on parenting, both at baseline and during acute episodes. In the second session, mothers were interviewed about their own experiences in childhood and their views about how these experiences had influenced their parenting. They were asked about their thoughts and feelings regarding their own parenting capabilities and custody loss, and their views about how their mental illness had affected their parenting. As part of the interview, information was elicited on perceptions mothers had of their relationship to their children and of their children as individuals. During this session, mothers also completed various parenting questionnaires (attitudes about child rearing, parental stress, support network) and were videotaped with their children in a structured attachment observation. An assessment was also made of children's socioemotional functioning and development. The third session involved a home visit, during which mother–child interactions were observed. The home environment was assessed as to its safety and a social assessment was completed. This involved examining the mother's educational background, occupation and financial history, marital status, physical health, and the nature and quality of her support network. Children's perceptions of their family and their foster placement history were also assessed. Collateral historians (mental health professionals,

TABLE 13.1. Assessment and Operationalization of Risk
and Protective Factors

Deficit/strength	Operationalization
Knowledge of child care/development	Parent Opinion Questionnaire (Azar et al., 1984); Home Inventory (Caldwell & Bradley, 1984)
Insight into mental illness and its impact on parenting	Rating of mothers' responses to semistructured interview (David, 1990)
Mother–child attachment quality; ability to read child's cues	Attachment classifications based on videotaped mother–child sessions; record review; observations of mother–child interactions in other settings
Maternal representations of child and relationship	Maternal interview and speech sample
Active psychiatric symptoms	Structured Clinical Interview for DSM-III-R—Patient Edition (SCID-R, Version 1.0) (Spitzer, Williams, Gibbon, & First, 1990); record review
Active drug addiction	SCID-R, record review, interview of therapist; urine drug screen
Childhood trauma that influences current parenting	Childhood Trauma Interview (Fink, Bernstein, Handelsman, Foote, & Lovejoy, 1995), record review; interviewing collateral historians; semistructured maternal interview
Social support	Social Support Inventory (Barrera, 1981); interview of collateral historians
Stress of parenting	Parental Stress Index (Abidin, 1990), pediatric records; developmental assessment of child (Dunn & Dunn, 1996)
Propensity for violent behavior	SCID-R; review of criminal records

foster parents, caseworkers, friends) were interviewed, and available records on the family were reviewed, including records from the child protective agency, medical records, psychiatric and psychological reports, and a Law Enforcement Agencies Data Systems criminal background check. (For a complete description of the assessment, see Jacobsen, Miller, & Kirkwood, 1997).

Measures

Attachment Assessment

A modified Ainsworth paradigm was used to assess differences in mother–child attachment quality. The Ainsworth paradigm provides a structured way both to assess and make sense of individual differences in a child's ability to use a caregiver as a source of comfort or protection, and as a secure base from which to explore. Use of the Ainsworth paradigm allows findings to be related and compared to a large body of theoretical and empirical literature on mother–child attachment quality, and on factors that contribute to individual differences in young children's attachment patterns. A potential drawback in using the Ainsworth methodology for children who have experienced disruptive caregiving, however, is that the four main attachment patterns may fail to adequately capture the variations in the attachment quality of young children to a mentally ill mother with whom they are no longer living. In children who have been in foster care for prolonged periods of time, for instance, there may be a question about whether the child has any attachment to the biological mother, or whether the child has an attachment disorder that is qualitatively distinct from any of Ainsworth's categories. The original Ainsworth methodology may also be problematic for assessing the attachment quality of children who have been separated from their mothers for a prolonged period of time, as it relies only on a brief observation of mother–child interactions in one setting. Without relying on multiple observations and on a review of the child's early attachment history with other caregivers, it may be difficult to understand the meaning of a child's behavior in the strange situation (Boris et al., 1997). For instance, without additional information and observations, a lack of attachment behaviors toward a caregiver in the strange situation could mean that the child is not attached to a caregiver, or that the child has an avoidant attachment pattern.

In the current study, Ainsworth's methodology was adapted to minimize these potential problems. The attachment observation consisted of a 10-minute warm-up period, followed by two brief separation and reunion episodes. The episodes lasted about 3 minutes in length. The observation met the three main criteria proposed by Crittenden (1992) for assessing the attachment relations of young children: It (1) presented children with an unexpected separation that activated the attachment system; (2) allowed mothers to function as attachment figures, and (3) provided opportunities to display strategies of coping with stress, gaining protection, and exploring the environment. Children's responses during the reunion episodes provided the primary basis for the attachment classification. This information was supplemented in each case, however, with observations of children's interactions with their mothers and strangers/examiners in the waiting room, with an extended observation of mother–child interactions at home, with caseworkers' reports about mother–child interactions during visits, and from interviews with relevant collateral historians about the child's attachment history and behaviors. This allowed for a more accurate and comprehensive understanding of the larger meaning of the children's attachment behaviors (see also Zeanah, 1996).

Ainsworth's classification system was used as a framework for classifying the attachment patterns of infants under age 30 months, along with the Main and Solomon (1990) coding for the insecure–disorganized pattern. For older children, comparable attachment classification systems were used, which are analogous to the infant classifications but are based on developmentally relevant behavior (Main & Cassidy, 1988; Cassidy & Marvin, 1990). Children who showed compulsive compliant behavior were placed in the disorganized group, as their behavior seemed to resemble the controlling classification that is a sequel to infant disorganization. These children complied almost unquestioningly to their mothers' demands (Crittenden & DiLalla, 1988; Jacobsen & Miller, 1998b).

Children were assigned to one of the aforementioned main attachment groups when they met the major criteria for the pattern, and when there was clear evidence from observations in other settings, and from collateral historians and records, that they had attachment bonds to their mothers. An additional category was used for children who either were not attached to their mothers or showed a tenuous attachment at best. These children typically showed no attachment behaviors in the structured attachment observation. Across several settings, they consistently failed to seek out their mothers or to cling to them when they were upset. The tenuous nature of the children's attachment was often noted explicitly by their mothers, who stated that their child had either no "bond" to them, or did not know them anymore.

A central focus of this pilot study was to examine factors that contribute to adequate versus risk-related attachment patterns in children who have been removed from the care of a mentally ill mother. Thus, children with secure, avoidant, and ambivalent attachment patterns were combined into a "traditional" attachment group. These children were compared to children with higher-risk attachment patterns, that is, to children in the disorganized and in the tenuous/nonattached groups. Table 13.2 provides brief descriptions of children in the different attachment groups and subgroups.

The attachment classifications were made by an experienced and trained attachment rater and clinician (Jacobsen), who has demonstrated good interrater agreement (kappa = .80–.92) on attachment classifications (Jacobsen, Edelstein, & Hofmann, 1997; Jacobsen, Huss, Fendrich, Kruesi, & Ziegenhain, 1997).

Expectations about Childrearing and Young Children

A modified version of the Parent Opinion Questionnaire (POQ; Azar, Robinson, Hekimian, & Twentyman, 1984) was used to examine whether moth-

TABLE 13.2. Criteria for Assessing Mother–Child Attachment Quality in Infancy and Childhood

	Reunion behaviors in attachment observation	
Attachment group	Infancy	Childhood
Traditional attachment group		
Secure	Infant directly seeks proximity or contact to caregiver; calmed by mother and able to subsequently explore.	Child shows pleasure in seeing mother and is relaxed and natural in her presence; child able to use mother as secure base.
Insecure–avoidant	Infant avoids mother upon reunion and focuses on objects or play	Child's behavior to mother is distant; interactions are largely interpersonal.
Insecure–ambivalent	Infant seeks contact to mother, while angrily resisting her; infant may have marked difficulties with passivity and/or exploration.	Child's shows immature and dependent behaviors during reunion episodes (e.g., child may suck thumb) child may show ambivalent, angry, or avoidant behaviors toward mother.
Disorganized attachment group	Infant shows contradictory or fearful behaviors; or becomes dazed and disoriented in mother's presence	Child's behaviors are highly controlling (either punitive or role reversing); child may show compulsive compliant behaviors with mother; child may also show behavioral signs of disorganization (confusion, apprehension, disordering of expected temporal sequences).
Tenuous/nonattached group	No protesting of separation; minimal or no search behavior; wandering around room during reunion episodes and whimpering; no seeking of mother for comfort or help; oblivious to their mother's comings and goings; did not appear to recognize mother as special person. (Children also showed no attachment behaviors to their mother in other situations.)	

ers had unrealistic expectations about child rearing and children. This questionnaire assesses whether mothers endorse worrisome attitudes and expectations about children's capabilities at different ages. The following are some items that mothers could endorse: "It's all right to bite a 2-year-old back if he bites you so as to teach him a lesson," "It's all right to leave an 8-month-old infant alone on a bed or couch for awhile." The question-naire was shortened for this study by including only questions that referred to children age 6 and younger.

Azar et al. (1984) used an overall score of 16 as a cutoff point to differ-entiate high- versus low-risk mothers. As our revised questionnaire included half the number of original questions, the main outcome mea-sure was whether mothers obtained a score of 8 or above on the POQ.

Maternal Representations

Believed to be derived in part from experiences with the mother's own caregivers in childhood, maternal representations include specific contents (e.g., knowledge of the child as an individual; knowledge of child develop-ment) and information-processing rules that guide maternal feelings and behavior (Bowlby, 1969/1982; Crittenden, 1990; Solomon & George, 1996). Bowlby (1980) likened representational caregiving models to a filter through which the mother–child relationship is organized and understood. A mother's representational caregiving model influences her interactions with, and expectations about, the child, which in turn affect the child's quality of attachment to her (Crowell & Feldman, 1988, 1989). As a brief screening measure of mothers' internal representations of their children, we asked mothers to talk for 5 minutes about their children's characteris-tics and about their relationships with their children. Speech samples of this type have been used in various studies to assess internal representa-tions of caregiving (George & Solomon, 1989; 1996; Zeanah & Benoit, 1995) and the emotional climate of families (Magana, Goldstein, Karno, Miklowitz, & Falloon, 1986). Clinical and empirical research suggests that mothers who are highly critical of their children, who strongly idealize them, or who are unable to differentiate their own needs and wishes from those of their children (Reder & Lucey, 1995) are at increased risk for child maltreatment. Mothers who appear to have little interest in their children as special or unique individuals are also thought to be at heightened risk for maltreatment (Reder & Lucey, 1995).

Drawing on prior research on caregiving representations (Zeanah & Benoit, 1995; George & Solomon, 1996; Main & Goldwyn, 1984), mothers' speech samples were classified into three groups:

1. *Balanced group:* These mothers gave balanced and realistic descrip-tions of their children and of their relationships to them; for exam-ple, they discussed both positive and negative aspects in an objec-tive fashion.
2. *Skewed group:* These mothers gave an unbalanced descriptions. They were overly positive or overly critical about their children and the relationship.

3. *Schematic group:* These mothers gave impoverished, schematic descriptions ("She eats, drinks, and poops"), or descriptions suggesting that they did not know their child's individual needs (e.g., describing a 3-year-old child who could barely utter single words as "fully bilingual in Spanish and English").

Ratings of mothers' internal representations were made on the basis of typed transcripts of mothers' speech samples. Two raters who were blinded as to attachment quality and other measures in the study classified the speech samples into the three groups. Interrater reliability on the threefold classification was high (27/30 = 90%).

Support Network for Parenting

The measure of social support was derived from the Arizona Social Support Inventory (ASSI; Barrera, 1981). This measure assesses the types and numbers of individuals with whom a mother interacts to obtain material aid and advice. For the current study, the ASSI was modified to assess social support that is specifically relevant to parenting. Prior research with high-risk families shows that this tool provides valid information on a mother's support network (cf. Budd & Holdsworth, 1996). For the purposes of this study, the outcome measure was the total number of different persons listed who could provide mothers with direct help with parenting (e.g., babysitting, caring for children if mother needed to go to the hospital). Subjects' reports of their support networks were verified by interviewing collateral historians. Some mothers gave names of persons who could not realistically provide concrete support for parenting (e.g., persons who were no longer living, drinking buddies, infants). These responses were subtracted from the overall number of individuals listed.

Maternal Insight into Effects of Mental Illness on Parenting

The insight rating was based both on therapists' reports and on the Scale for Assessment of Insight (David, 1990). Mothers who denied that they had a mental illness altogether, or who stated that their mental illness had no effect at all on parenting, were in Group 1 (no insight). Those who could see some effects of their illness on parenting were in Group 2 (some insight). These mothers noted, for instance, that their mental illness had made their child worry excessively about them, or that they felt a need to contact others for help with parenting when their symptoms worsened. Maternal insight was coded by a rater who was blinded as to other study measures. A second, blinded rater independently coded 15 therapist reports for insight. Interrater reliability was high (15/15 = 100%).

Treatment Compliance

The compliance measure was based on therapists' reports about the patient's participation in treatment during the past month. Using a 2-point scale (yes/no), a blind rater coded whether mothers had been non-compliant in the past month with whatever treatment they were receiving. Noncompliance meant that they not taking medication, or that they were not attending scheduled therapy programs. A second rater independently coded 15 therapist reports. Interrater reliability was high (15/15 = 100%).

Foster Care Placement

Based on record review, children were grouped according to whether they had (1) experienced a stable foster placement, or (2) changed foster placements two or more times. As an additional factor, we examined whether children were placed in a relative's home (with someone familiar to the mother and, often child) or in a nonrelative placement.

Results

The frequency of children in the three main attachment groups (traditional, disorganized/controlling, tenuous/nonattached) was first calculated. In preliminary analyses, we also examined whether (1) early removal from a mother's care (at birth or in the first few months of life) and (2) maternal psychiatric diagnosis were systematically linked to differences in children's attachment quality, as these were potentially confounding variables. t-tests were subsequently used to compare the attachment groups on continuous variables (e.g., size of support network). To obtain an estimate of significance for qualitative variables, Fisher's exact tests were calculated. The sample size did not permit multivariate analyses.

Sample Characteristics

The overall rate of children who were classified as having a traditional attachment was low in this sample (9/30, 30%). Four children (13%) in the sample showed behaviors that were congruent with secure attachment. Five children (17%) were judged to have an avoidant attachment (4) or ambivalent attachment (1). Eleven children (37%) in the sample were given a disorganized/controlling classification. The behavioral patterning of the remaining 10 children (33%) indicated that they had either a highly tenuous attachment to their caregiver (4) or no attachment at all (6).

Fifteen children were removed from their mother's care at birth or in the first few months of life. Of these, 4 children had a traditional attachment pattern (organized) to their mother, and 11 had a risk-related attachment (6 had a disorganized/controlling pattern; 5 were in the tenuous/nonattached group). There was no significant relation between early removal and attachment status ($p < .90$). There was also no significant relationship between mother–child attachment quality and differences in maternal psychiatric diagnoses ($p < .34$).

Relation between Attachment Patterns and Maternal Attitudes about Young Children and Child Rearing

No mothers in the traditional group obtained a score of 8 or above on the POQ (see Table 13.3). Four mothers in the tenuous/nonattached group and 1 mother in the disorganized/controlling group obtained a POQ score of 8 or above. The finding approached statistical significance ($p < .10$).

Relation between Attachment Patterns and Maternal Caregiving Representations

Mothers' representations of their children varied significantly by attachment group ($p < .001$). Mothers whose children had traditional attachment patterns tended to have balanced representations (see Table 13.4).

As in prior research on caregiving representations, mothers of children with disorganized/controlling attachment were most prone to have skewed and particularly glorified representations of their children (George & Solomon, 1996). They highly idealized their children ("He is my beautiful prince") or talked about them using ephemeral terms ("a tiny, fragile bird"). No mothers in this group were highly critical of their children. Mothers whose children were in the tenuous/nonattached group, on the other hand, were prone to have impoverished representations of their children. The descriptions suggested that they did not know the child's individual needs at all ("The boy gets up the morning, does things, and sleeps").

TABLE 13.3. Children's Attachment in Relation to Maternal Attitudes about Child-Rearing and Young Children

Attachment group	Low score on POQ	High score on POQ
Traditional	9/9 (100%)	0/9 (0%)
Disorganized/controlling	10/11 (91%)	1/11 (9%)
Tenuous/nonattached	6/10 (60%)	4/10 (40%)

Note. Fisher's exact test, $p < .10$.

TABLE 13.4. Children's Attachment in Relation to Maternal Caregiving Representations

Attachment group	Caregiving representations		
	Balanced	Imbalanced	Schematic
Traditional	5/9 (56%)	3/9 (33%)	1/9 (11%)
Disorganized/controlling	1/11 (9%)	7/11 (64%)	3/11 (27%)
Tenuous/nonattached	0/11 (0%)	1/10 (10%)	9/10 (90%)

Note. Fisher's exact test, $p < .001$.

Relation between Attachment Patterns and Social Support

The subjects as a whole had small support networks ($M = 2.0$, $SD = .71$). The average numbers of persons listed for mothers in each group as direct supports for parenting were as follows: Traditional ($M = 3.28$, $SD = .51$); Disorganized/controlling ($M = 2.4$, $SD = .68$), and Tenuous/nonattached ($M = 1.2$, $SD = .46$). There were significant differences between the groups ($F = 6.10$, $df = 2$, $p < .001$).

Relation between Attachment Patterns and Insight into Effects of Mental Illness on Parenting

Only 2 mothers in the traditional attachment group lacked insight into the effects of their mental illness on parenting (see Table 13.5). On the other hand, the majority of mothers in the disorganized/controlling (7/11) and tenuous/nonattached (7/10) groups lacked insight into the effects of their mental illness on parenting. The intragroup differences approached significance ($p < .10$).

Relation between Attachment Patterns and Maternal Compliance with Treatment Recommendations

Over half of the mothers in the disorganized/controlling (6/11) and tenuous/nonattached (6/10) groups were noncompliant with treatment (see

TABLE 13.5. Children's Attachment in Relation to Maternal Insight into Effects of Mental Illness on Parenting

Attachment group	No insight	Some insight
Traditional	2/9 (22%)	7/9 (78%)
Disorganized/controlling	7/11 (64%)	4/11 (36%)
Tenuous/nonattached	7/10 (70%)	3/10 (30%)

Note. Fisher's exact test, $p < .10$.

Table 13.6); one mother in the traditional group was noncompliant. The difference approached statistical significance ($p < .08$).

Relation between Attachment Patterns and Stability of Foster Placement

The relation between attachment quality and stability of foster placement was statistically significant ($p < .02$). Multiple foster placements were most frequent in children in the tenuous/nonattached group (see Table 13.7). Half of the children in this group had experienced multiple foster placements. No child in the traditional group and only one in the disorganized/controlling group experienced multiple foster placements.

Relation between Attachment Patterns and Type of Foster Placement

All of the children with a traditional attachment pattern and all but one of the children with disorganized/controlling attachment were placed in relative foster care (see Table 13.8). Children with a tenuous attachment, on the other hand, were all placed in nonrelative homes. The relation was highly significant ($p < .000$).

Discussion

The Distribution of Different Attachment Types in Children Who Have Been Separated from Mentally Ill Mothers

Prior studies of the attachment patterns of children of mentally ill mothers have documented high rates (50-60%) of disorganized/controlling attachment status (cf. DeMulder & Radke-Yarrow, 1991; Lyons-Ruth et al., 1990). The current study also found a high rate of disorganized/controlling attachment status (35%). In addition, however, this sample showed a high rate of tenuous attachment or no attachment (35%). This finding has not been reported in prior studies of children of mentally ill mothers, but a

TABLE 13.6. Children's Attachment in Relation to Maternal Compliance with Treatment

Attachment group	No compliance	Some/good compliance
Traditional	1/9 (11%)	8/9 (89%)
Disorganized/controlling	6/11 (55%)	5/11 (45%)
Tenuous/nonattached	6/10 (60%)	4/10 (40%)

Note. Fisher's exact test, $p < .08$.

TABLE 13.7. Children's Attachment in Relation to Stability
of Foster Placement

Attachment group	Stable placement	Multiple placements
Traditional	9/9 (100%)	0/9 (0%)
Disorganized/controlling	10/11 (91%)	1/11 (9%)
Tenuous/nonattached	5/10 (50%)	5/10 (50%)

Note. Fisher's exact test, $p < .02$.

lack of affectional bonding has been noted in clinical studies of children in foster care (Eliacheff, 1997) and in a few studies of maltreating mothers who do not keep and nurture their infants (Helfer, 1976; Hurd, 1975; Lynch & Roberts, 1977).

In our study, there was good evidence from reports and collateral interviews that some children who had prior attachments to their mothers showed no current attachment behaviors to their mothers. Their behaviors were consistent with grief reactions observed in some infants and young children (Bowlby, 1973; Lieberman, 1997a; Tidmarsh, 1997). It was difficult to determine, however, if, after a year of separation and seeing their mothers only on visits, these children were showing unresolved grief, or they were detached and had relinquished all emotional investment in their mothers. Longitudinal observations about interactions during visitations will be helpful in making this distinction.

Other children in the tenuous/nonattached group did not appear to have ever had any attachment to their mothers. For most of these children, the foster parent was the primary attachment figure. The history and behavior of one child, however, appeared congruent with reactive attachment disorder (Lieberman, 1997b). This pattern is observed in the context of persistent neglect or abuse from a primary caregiver, frequent changes in caregiving, or other environmental circumstances that seriously interfere with a young child's ability to form an enduring and specific emotional bond to a primary caregiver. This child's frequent changes in placement (an institution followed by two different foster placements) had

TABLE 13.8. Children's Attachment in Relation to Type of Foster Placement

Attachment group	Relative	Nonrelative
Traditional	9/9 (100%)	0/9 (0%)
Disorganized/controlling	11/11 (100%)	0/11 (0%)
Tenuous/nonattached	0/10 (0%)	10/10 (100%)

Note. Fisher's exact test, $p < .000$.

apparently interfered with the child's ability to form a specific and enduring attachment to anyone.

The Contribution of Maternal Caregiving Abilities and Foster Care Contexts to Children's Attachment

The caregiving abilities of mothers whose children had risk-related attachment status differed in important ways from the caregiving abilities of mothers whose children had traditional (organized) attachment patterns. These mothers were significantly more prone than mothers of children with traditional attachment to glorify their children, to have highly incongruous perceptions of them, or to describe them in an impoverished and schematic manner. Mothers of children with risk-associated attachment patterns also tended to have little insight into how their mental illness affected their parenting and to be noncompliant with treatment, although the latter findings did not reach statistical significance. More research is needed to determine whether these trends are upheld in a larger sample of mentally ill mothers and their children.

Some potentially important differences emerged between the two risk-associated attachment groups. Mothers of children in the tenuous/nonattached group had significantly smaller support networks for parenting than mothers in the disorganized/controlling group. They listed, on the average, only one person who could help them with parenting. If this person were not available, these mothers would be stranded. Some of the mothers in this group had no one to turn to for help. The paucity of support could contribute to the helplessness and sense of isolation and loneliness that these mothers likely experience in the role of caregiver (Solomon & George, 1996). Mothers of children in the tenuous/nonattached group were also prone to have highly schematic representations of their children, whereas mothers of children with disorganized/controlling attachment tended to glorify their children and their relationships with them. In some cases, impoverished internal representations appeared to be due to an inability to experience the child as a separate and individual person. For instance, one mother, who could only give a highly schematic description of her child, stated that if she could not have this child, then should would just get pregnant again. Over the years, this woman had relinquished custody of five other children. She appeared to need *a* child to live with her, rather than a specific child.

Lack of sensitivity to their children's individuality was a major way in which mothers in the tenuous/nonattached group differed from mothers of children in the disorganized/controlling group. The idealization of mothers in the latter group suggested that they were investing special emotional significance in their children. This investment may help young children establish or maintain an affectional bond to their mothers. Mothers of children in the tenuous/nonattached groups, on the other hand, did not appear to know their children at all as individuals. Their difficulties in investing emotionally in their child as an individual may have played a critical role in their children not knowing and accepting their mothers as caregivers.

Compared to mothers of children with disorganized/controlling attachment, mothers of children in the tenuous/nonattached group also tended to have more aberrant attitudes about child rearing and about what could be expected of children of different ages. Unrealistic and distorted expectations about children have been noted in prior studies of mentally ill mothers (Cohler et al., 1976; Rogosch et al., 1992), however, and are linked to increased risk of child maltreatment (Azar et al., 1984).

It is important to underscore that about one-third of the mothers in this study had children who showed an traditional attachment patterns. On various measures, these mothers appeared to have adequate, or at least "minimal," caregiving abilities. For instance, these mothers were more realistic and balanced in their appraisals of their children and their relationship, and were thus likely to be more sensitive overall to their children's individuality. These mothers had nonetheless lost custody of their children because they had maltreated a child in the past, or were judged to be at high risk for child maltreatment. As we were not able to assess caregiving before custody loss, it is not known whether their caregiving abilities to begin with were better. More research is needed to address this issue and to determine why some mentally ill mothers might be able to change their caregiving abilities.

Continuity and type of foster care are other variables that are known to profoundly affect individual differences in children's attachment quality to their mothers during a prolonged separation (Robertson & Robertson, 1989). These findings were confirmed in this study. Children in the traditional and disorganized/controlling attachment groups were more prone than children in the tenuous/nonattached group to have experienced a stable foster placement. They were also more likely to have been placed in the home of a relative. These findings underscore the benefits of a stable and familiar placement as factors that can facilitate a bond of attachment (either traditional or disorganized/controlling) of a child to a mother who is currently a noncustodial caregiver (Bowlby, 1973; Robertson & Robertson, 1989).

Although the small sample size precluded multivariate analyses, the findings from these pilot data suggest that different combinations of factors play a role in influencing the particular attachment quality that children had to their mothers. A tentative outline of the different pathways leading to the three attachment groups (traditional, disorganized/controlling, and tenuous/nonattached) is provided in Figure 13.1. Children with traditional attachment patterns experienced stable and familiar foster placements. They also had more positive and sensitive caregiving. Children with disorganized/controlling attachment also experienced a stable and familiar foster placement, but this was coupled with more disturbed caregiving skills of the part of their mothers. Children in the tenuous/nonattached group were prone to have experienced multiple and unfamiliar foster placements, coupled with highly disturbed parenting by their mothers. Overall, it appeared that children with disorganized/controlling attachment experienced less problematic maternal caregiving skills than children in the tenuous/nonattached groups. The relative stability and familiarity experienced by these children in foster care, and their mother's emotional investment in them as individuals, likely helped them to maintain some form of attachment to their mother.

In this study sample, there were no children who experienced multiple placements coupled with more positive caregiving on the part of their mentally ill mothers. In future studies, it will be important to determine which attachment patterns are associated with these caregiving experiences and to examine whether positive caregiving abilities in the child's noncustodial mother can compensate for instability and repeated change in foster care.

The findings presented in this chapter should be viewed as preliminary because of the small sample size, and because of the lack of independent ratings of attachment. As intended, these pilot data raise as many questions as answers. What is the relative influence of maternal caregiving abilities and foster care placements in influencing risk-related versus non-

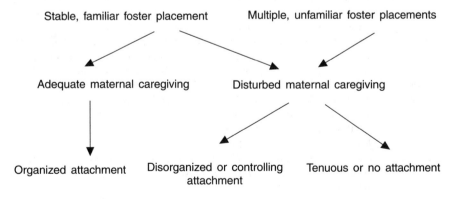

FIGURE 13.1. Posited pathways leading to individual differences in mother–child attachment bonds.

risk-related attachment patterns in this population? What role do different visitation patterns play in influencing the quality of attachment that a child has to a mentally ill mother? What role does a child's attachment quality to substitute caregivers play in influencing attachment quality to their mothers? To which extent do differences in the early attachment patterns of children in foster care affect later behavior, relations, adjustment, and psychopathology? Studies that follow the developmental trajectories and later-life experience of these children will be critical in answering these questions.

Taken as a whole, research and clinical experience to date suggest a profound dilemma: Children of mentally ill mothers may be at high risk when remaining with their mothers, and also when separated from them (Silverman, 1989). Answers to these questions may help families, mental health professionals, and child welfare personnel make better decisions and interventions for each individual mother and child.

REFERENCES

Abidin, R. R. (1990). *Parenting stress index (short form)*. Charlottesville, VA: Pediatric Psychology Press.

Ainsworth, M. D. S., Blehar, M. C., Waters, E., & Wall, S. (1978). *Patterns of attachment: A psychological study of the Strange Situation*. New York: Basic Books.

American Psychiatric Association. (1994). *Diagnostic and statistical manual of mental disorders* (4th ed.). Washington, DC: Author.

Apfel R. J., & Handel, M. H. (1993). *Madness and loss of motherhood: Sexuality, reproduction, and long-term mental illness*. Washington DC: American Psychiatric Association Press.

Appleby, L., Desei, R. N., Luchins, D. J., Gibbons, R. D., & Hedeker, D. R. (1993). Length of stay and recidivism in schizophrenia: A study of public psychiatric hospital patients. *American Journal of Psychiatry, 150*, 72–76.

Azar, S. T., Robinson, D. R., Hekimian, E., & Twentyman, C. T. (1984). Unrealistic expectations and problem-solving ability in maltreating and comparison mothers. *Journal of Consulting and Clinical Psychology, 52*, 687–691.

Barrera, M. (1981). Social support in the adjustment of pregnant adolescents: Assessment issues. In B. H. Gottlieb (Ed.), *Social networks and social support* (pp. 69–95). Beverly Hills, CA: Sage.

Bensel, R. W., & Paxson, C. L. (1979). Child abuse following early postpartum separation. *Journal of Pediatrics, 90*, 490–491.

Boris, N. W., Fueyo, M., & Zeanah, C. H. (1997). The clinical assessment of attachment in children under five. *Journal of the American Academy of Child and Adolescent Psychiatry, 36*, 291–293.

Bowlby, J. (1963). *Child care and the growth of love* (2nd ed.). London: Penguin Books.

Bowlby, J. (1969/1982). *Attachment and loss: Vol. 1. Attachment.* New York: Basic Books.

Bowlby, J. (1973). *Attachment and loss: Vol. 2. Separation.* New York: Basic Books.
Bowlby, J. (1980). *Attachment and loss: Vol. 3. Loss.* New York: Basic Books.
Budd, K. S., & Holdsworth, M. J. (1996). Methodological issues in assessing minimal parenting competence. *Journal of Clinical Child Psychology, 25,* 2–14.
Burr, W. A., Falek, A., Strauss, L. T., & Brown, S. B. (1979). Fertility in psychiatric outpatients. *Hospital and Community Psychiatry, 30,* 527–531.
Caldwell, B. M., & Bradley, R. H. (1984). *Home observation for the measurement of the environment: Administration manual* (rev. ed.). Little Rock: University of Arkansas Press.
Campbell, S. B., Cohn, J. F., & Meyer, T. (1995). Depression in first-time mothers: Mother–infant interaction and depression chronicity. *Developmental Psychology, 31,* 349–457.
Carlson, V., Cicchetti, D., Barnett, D., & Braunwald, K. (1989). Finding order in disorganization: Lessons from research on maltreated infants' attachments to their caregivers. In D. Cicchetti & V. Carlson (Eds.), *Child maltreatment: Theory and research on the causes and consequences of child abuse and neglect* (pp. 494–528). New York: Cambridge University Press.
Cassell, D., & Coleman, R. (1995). Parents with psychiatric problems. In P. Reder & C. Lucey (Eds.), *Assessment of parenting: Psychiatric and psychological contributions* (pp. 169–181). London: Routledge.
Cassidy, J., & Marvin, R. S. (1990). Attachment organization in preschool children: Guidelines for classification. Unpublished scoring manual, MacArthur Working Group on Attachment, Seattle, WA.
Caton, C. L. M., Cournos, F., Felix, A., & Wyatt, R. J. (1998). Childhood experiences and current adjustment of offspring of indigent patients with schizophrenia. *Psychiatric Services, 49,* 86–90.
Cohler, B. J., Grunebaum, H. U., Weiss, J. L., Hartman, C., & Gallant, D. (1976). Child care attitudes and adaptation to the maternal role among mentally ill and well mothers. *American Journal of Orthopsychiatry, 46,* 123–134.
Cohn, J. F., Campbell, S. B., Matias, R., & Hopkins, J. (1990). Face-to-face interactions of postpartum depressed and nondepressed mothers at 2 months. *Developmental Psychology, 26,* 15–23.
Coverdale, J. H., & Aruffo, J. F. (1989). Family planning needs of female chronic psychiatric outpatients. *American Journal of Psychiatry, 146,* 1489–1491.
Crittenden, P. M. (1985). Social networks, quality of child rearing, and child development. *Child Development, 56,* 1299–1313.
Crittenden, P. M. (1988). Relationships at risk. In J. Belsky & T. Nezworski (Eds.), *The clinical implications of attachment* (pp. 136–174). Hillsdale, NJ: Erlbaum.
Crittenden, P. M. (1990). Internal representational models of attachment relationships. *Infant Mental Health Journal, 11,* 259–277.
Crittenden, P. M. (1992). Quality of attachment in the preschool years. *Development and Psychopathology, 4,* 409–441.
Crittenden, P. M., & DiLalla, D. L. (1988). Compulsive compliance: The development of an inhibitory coping strategy in infancy. *Journal of Abnormal Child Psychology, 16,* 585–599.
Crowell, J. A., & Feldman, S. S. (1988). Mothers' internal models of relationships

and children's behavioral and developmental status in mother–child interaction: A study of mother–child interaction. *Child Development, 59,* 1273–1285.

Crowell, J. A., & Feldman, S. S. (1989). Assessment of mothers' working models of relationships: Some clinical implications. *Infant Mental Health Journal, 10,* 173–184.

D'Angelo, E. J. (1986). Security of attachment in infants with schizophrenic, depressed, and unaffected mothers. *Journal of Genetic Psychology, 147,* 421–422.

David, A. S. (1990). Insight and psychosis. *British Journal of Psychiatry, 156,* 789–808.

DeMulder, E. K., & Radke-Yarrow, M. (1991). Attachment with affectively ill and well-mothers: Concurrent behavioral correlates. *Development and Psychopathology, 3,* 227–242.

Dunn, L. M., & Dunn, L. M. (1996). *Peabody Picture Vocabulary Test-III.* Circle Pines, MN: American Guidance Service.

Eliacheff, C. (1997). *Das Kind, das eine Katze sein wollte. Psychoanalytische Arbeit mit Saeuglingen und Kleinkindern.* Munich: Deutscher Taschenbuch Verlag.

Fendrich, M., Warner, V., & Weissman, M. M. (1990). Family risk factors, parental depression, and psychopathology in offspring. *Developmental Psychology, 26,* 40–50.

Fink, L. A., Bernstein, D., Handelsman, L., Foote, J., & Lovejoy, M. (1995). Initial reliability and validity of the Childhood Trauma Interview: A new multidimensional measure of childhood interpersonal trauma. *American Journal of Psychiatry, 152,* 1329–1335.

George, C., & Solomon, J. (1989). Internal working models of caregiving and security of attachment at age 6. *Infant Mental Health Journal, 10,* 222–237.

George, C., & Solomon, J. (1996). Representational models of relationships: Links between caregiving and attachment. *Infant Mental Health Journal, 17,* 198–216.

Goldstein, J., Freud, A., & Solnit, A. J. (1979). *Before the best interests of the child.* New York: Free Press.

Heinicke, C. M., & Westheimer, I. (1965). *Brief separations.* New York: International Universities Press.

Helfer, R. E. (1976). Early identification and prevention of unusual child-rearing practices. *Pediatric Annals, 5,* 91–105.

Herman, S. P. (1997). Child custody evaluation. *Supplement to the Journal of the American Academy of Child and Adolescent Psychiatry: Practice Parameters, 36,* 57S–68S.

Holley, T. E. (1997). *My mother's keeper: A daughter's memoir of growing up in the shadow of schizophrenia.* New York: Morrow.

Hurd, J. M. (1975). Assessing maternal attachment: First step toward the prevention of child abuse. *Journal of Obstetrics and Gynecological Nursing, 4,* 25–30.

Isabella, R. A., & Belsky, J. (1991). Interactional synchrony and the origins of mother–infant attachment: A replication study. *Child Development, 62,* 373–384.

Jacobsen, T., Edelstein, W., & Hofmann, V. (1994). A longitudinal study of the relation between representations of attachment in childhood and cognitive functioning in childhood and adolescence. *Developmental Psychology, 30,* 112–124.

Jacobsen, T., & Hofmann, V. (1997). Children's attachment representations: Longitudinal relations to behavior and competence in middle childhood and adolescence. *Developmental Psychology, 33,* 703–710.

Jacobsen, T., Huss, M., Fendrich, M., Kruesi, M. J., & Ziegenhain, U. (1997). Children's ability to delay gratification: Longitudinal relations to attachment patterns from infancy to early childhood. *Journal of Genetic Psychology, 158,* 411–426.

Jacobsen, T., & Miller, L. J. (1998a). Mentally ill mothers who have killed: Three cases addressing the issue of future parenting capability. *Psychiatric Services, 49,* 650–657.

Jacobsen, T., & Miller, L. J. (1998b). Compulsive compliance in a young maltreated child. *Journal of the American Academy of Child and Adolescent Psychiatry, 37,* 462–463.

Jacobsen, T., Miller, L. J., & Kirkwood, K. P. (1997). Assessing parenting competency in individuals with severe mental illness: A comprehensive service. *Journal of Mental Health Administration, 24,* 189–199.

Kissane, D., & Ball, J. R. B. (1988). Postnatal depression and psychosis—a mother and baby unit in a general hospital. *Australian and New Zealand Journal of Obstetrics and Gynecology, 28,* 208–212.

Leiderman, P. H., & Seashore, M. J. (1975). Mother–infant neonatal separation: Some delayed consequences. *Ciba Foundation Symposium, 33,* 213–239.

Lieberman, A. (1997a). Mood disorder: Prolonged bereavement/grief reaction. In A. Lieberman, S. Wieder, & E. Fenichel, E. (Eds.), *DC:0-3 Casebook* (pp. 61–67). Washington, DC: National Center for Infants, Toddlers, and Families.

Lieberman, A. (1997b). Reactive attachment deprivation/maltreatment disorder of infancy and early childhood. In A. Lieberman, S. Wieder, & E. Fenichel (Eds.), *DC:0-3 Casebook* (pp. 167–179). Washington, DC: National Center for Infants, Toddlers, and Families.

Lieberman, A. F., & Pawl, J. (1988). Clinical applications of attachment theory. In J. Belsky & T. Nezworski (Eds.), *Clinical implications of attachment* (pp. 327–351). Hillsdale, NJ: Erlbaum.

Lyden, J. (1997). *The daughter of the Queen of Sheba.* Boston: Houghton Mifflin.

Lynch, M. A., & Roberts, J. (1977). Predicting child abuse: Signs of bonding failure in the maternity hospital. *British Medical Journal, 1,* 624–626.

Lyons-Ruth, K., & Block, D. (1996). The disturbed caregiving system: Relations among childhood trauma, maternal caregiving, and infant affect and attachment. *Infant Mental Health Journal, 17,* 257–275.

Lyons-Ruth, K., Connell, D. B., Grunebaum, H., & Botein, S. (1990). Infants at social risk: Maternal depression and family support services as mediators of infant development and security of attachment. *Child Development, 61,* 85–98.

Lyons-Ruth, K., Repacholi, B., McLeod, S., & Silva, E. (1991). Disorganized attachment behavior in infancy: Short-term stability, maternal and infant correlates, and risk-related subtypes. *Development and Psychopathology, 3,* 377–396.

Magana, A. B., Goldstein, M. J., Karno, M., Miklowitz, D. J., & Falloon, I. R. (1986). A brief method for assessing expressed emotion in relatives of psychiatric patients. *Psychiatric Research, 17,* 203–212.

Main, M., & Cassidy, J. (1988). Categories of response to reunion with the parent at age six: Predicted from infant attachment classifications and stable over a one-month period. *Developmental Psychology, 24,* 415–426.

Main, M., & Goldwyn, R. (1984). Predicting rejection of her infant from mother's representation of her own experience: Implications for the abused–abusing intergenerational cycle. *Child Abuse and Neglect, 8,* 203–217.

Main, M., & Hesse, E. (1990). Parents' unresolved traumatic experiences are related to infant disorganized attachment status: Is frightened and/or frightening parental behavior the linking mechanism? In M. T. Greenberg, D. Cicchetti, & M. E. Cummings (Eds), *Attachment in the preschool years* (pp. 161–182). Chicago: University of Chicago Press.

Main, M., & Solomon, J. (1990). Procedures for identifying infants as disorganized/disoriented during the Ainsworth Strange Situation. In M. T. Greenberg, D. Cicchetti, & E. M. Cummings (Eds.), *Attachment in the preschool years* (pp. 121–160). Chicago: University of Chicago Press.

McNeil, T. F., Persson-Blennow, I., Binett, B., & Harty, B., & Karyd, U. B. (1988). A prospective study of postpartum psychoses in a high-risk group: 7. Relationship to later offspring characteristics. *Acta Psychiatrica Scandinavica, 78,* 613–617.

Miller, L. J., & Finnerty, M. (1996). Sexuality, pregnancy, and childrearing among women with schizophrenia-spectrum disorders. *Psychiatric Services, 47,* 502–506.

Murray, L. (1992). The impact of postnatal depression on infant development. *Journal of Child Psychology and Psychiatry, 33,* 543–561.

Nicholson, J., Geller, J. L., Fisher, W. H., & Dion, G. L. (1993). State policies and programs that addresses the needs of mentally ill mothers in the public sector. *Hospital and Community Psychiatry, 44,* 484–489.

O'Connor, M. J., Sigman, M., & Brill, N. (1987). Disorganization of attachment in relation to maternal alcohol consumption. *Journal of Consulting and Clinical Psychology, 55,* 831–836.

Persson-Blennow, I., Binett, T. F., & McNeil, T. (1988). Offspring of women with nonorganic psychosis: Antecedents of anxious attachment to the mother at one year of age. *Acta Psychiatrica Scandinavica, 78,* 66–71.

Persson-Blennow, I., Naeslund, B., McNeil, T. F., Kaij, L., & Malmquist-Larsson, A. (1986). Offspring of women with nonorganic psychosis: Mother–infant interaction at one year of age. *Acta Psychiatrica Scandinavica, 73,* 207–213.

Peterson, G. H., & Mehl, L. E. (1978). Some determinants of maternal attachment. *American Journal of Psychiatry, 135,* 1169–1173.

Radke-Yarrow, M., Cummings, M., Kuczynski, L., & Chapman, M. (1985). Patterns of attachment in two and three year olds in normal families and families with parental depression. *Child Development, 56,* 884–893.

Reder, P., & Lucey, C. (1995). Significant issues in the assessment of parenting. In P. Reder & C. Lucey (Eds.), *Assessment of parenting: Psychiatric and psychological contributions* (pp. 3–17). London: Routledge.

Robertson, J., & Robertson, J. (1989). *Separation and the very young.* London: Free Association Books.

Rodning, C., Beckwith, L., & Howard, J. (1991). Quality of attachment and home environments in children prenatally exposed to PCP and cocaine. *Development and Psychopathology, 3*, 351–366.

Rogosch, F. A., Mowbray, C. T., & Bogat, A. (1992). Determinants of parenting attitudes in mothers with severe psychopathology. *Development and Psychopathology, 4*, 469–487.

Rutter, M. (1995). Clinical implications of attachment concepts: Retrospect and prospect. *Journal of Child Psychology and Psychiatry, 36*, 549–571.

Sameroff, A. J., Seifer, R., & Zax, M. (1982). Early development of children at risk for emotional disorder. *Monographs of the Society for Research on Child Development, 47*(7, Serial No. 199), 1–82.

Seeman, M. V. (1996). The mother with schizophrenia. In M. Goepfert, J. Webster, & M. V. Seeman (Eds.), *Parental psychiatric disorder: Distressed parents and their families* (pp. 290–200). Cambridge, UK: Cambridge University Press.

Silverman, M. M. (1989). Children of psychiatrically ill parents: A prevention perspective. *Hospital and Community Psychiatry, 40*, 1257–1264.

Sneddon, J., Kerry, R. J., & Bant, W. P. (1981). The psychiatric mother and baby unit: A three year study. *Practitioner, 225*, 1295–1300.

Solnit, A. J., Nordhaus, B. F., & Lord, R. (1992). *When home is no haven.* New Haven, CT: Yale University Press.

Solomon, J., & George, C. (1994, August). *Disorganization of maternal caregiving strategies: An attachment approach to role reversal.* Paper presented at the 102nd meeting of the American Psychological Association, Los Angeles, CA.

Solomon, J., & George, C. (1996). Defining the caregiving system: Toward a theory of caregiving. *Infant Mental Health Journal, 17*, 183–197.

Solomon, J., & George, C. (1997). *The development of attachment in separated and divorced families: Effects of overnight visitation, parent, and couple variables.* Unpublished manuscript.

Spitzer, R. L., Williams, J. B. W., Gibbon, M., & First, M. B. (1990). *Structured clinical interview for DSM-III-R–Patient edition* (SCID, Version 1.0). Washington, DC: American Psychiatric Association Press.

Teti, D., Gelfand, D. M., Messinger, D. S., & Isabella, R. (1995). Maternal depression and the quality of early attachment: An examination of infants, preschoolers, and their mothers. *Developmental Psychology, 31*, 364–376.

Tidmarsh, L. (1997). Mood disorder: Prolonged bereavement/grief reaction. In A. Lieberman, S. Wieder, & E. Fenichel (Eds.), *DC:0-3 Casebook* (pp. 69–79). Washington, DC: National Center for Infants, Toddlers, and Families.

Uddenberg, N., & Engelsson, I. (1978). Prognosis of post partum mental disturbance: A prospective study of primiparous women and their 4½ year old children. *Acta Psychiatrica Scandinavica, 48*, 201–212.

Westheimer, I. J. (1970). Changes in response of mother to child during periods of separation. *Social Work, 26*, 3–10.

White, C. L., Nicholson, J. Fisher, W. H., & Geller, J. L. (1995). Mothers with severe mental illness caring for children. *Journal of Nervous and Mental Disease, 183*, 398–403.

Zahn-Waxler, C., McKnew, D. H., Cummings, M., Davenport, Y. B., & Radke-Yarrow, M. (1984). Problem behaviors and peer interactions of young children with a manic–depressive parent. *American Journal of Psychiatry, 141,* 236–240.

Zeanah, C. H. (1996). Beyond insecurity: A reconceptualization of attachment disorders of infancy. *Journal of Consulting and Clinical Psychology, 64,* 42–52.

Zeanah, C. H., & Benoit, D. (1995). Clinical applications of a parent perception interview in infant mental health. *Child and Adolescent Clinics of North America, 5,* 539–554.

Zeanah, C. H., & Klitzke, M. (1991). Role reversal and the self-effacing solution: Observations from infant–parent psychotherapy. *Psychiatry, 54,* 346–356.

CHAPTER 14

Resolving the Past and Present

Relations with Attachment Organization

ROBERT C. PIANTA
ROBERT S. MARVIN
MARIA C. MOROG

Two parents were asked to describe their reactions to having a child with a diagnosis of cerebral palsy. Both children have fairly serious cases of cerebral palsy. Although they both perform above the mean on cognitive testing, they are lagging in gross motor development and have difficulty in independent locomotion. Diagnoses were delivered by physicians. The first mother received the diagnosis 4 years prior to the interview, the second 2 years prior. The first mother, A, broke into tears immediately. The second, B, responded calmly.

> Mother A: "When she came in the room and told us, it was so awful. . . . You see your baby there and you wonder, 'Will she live?' and then you think about the walker and the wheelchair. . . . All the way home we cried and I still cry every time it comes up. . . . It was 4 years ago but it's like it happened yesterday. . . . You'd think it'd go away but it doesn't. . . . I try not to think about it. . . . I just tell myself we're going to overcome it somehow. . . . You bet I push her, you have to. . . . If there's anything in the way, we're going through it."

> Mother B: "It was hard, almost like I lost my little girl . . . and you kind of go through a grieving process. . . . I still tear up sometimes, like this summer when I realized she won't be able to take dance lessons . . . but you know I feel like she's doing so well, and we've learned to live with it. . . . I just focus on doing what it is she needs and I read a lot on what to expect for the future."

These are two quite different accounts. Mother A is struggling to handle the strong emotions she experiences when this topic comes up, and she admits to trying to suppress these feelings. She copes by deflecting her attention away from these feelings and toward pushing her daughter to succeed. Mother B also struggles but is more calm and accepting of her experiences, focusing on her daughter's needs and her own responses to them. What these accounts have in common is parents' current and ongoing experiences with loss or trauma in raising a child who has a serious disability. In this chapter, we suggest that parents' resolving these ongoing experiences is an important factor in relation to attachment organization.

As George and Solomon (1999) have reminded us, Bowlby (1969/1982) hypothesized two complementary behavioral systems—the attachment system and the caregiving system—that function as a self-regulating dyadic system to keep the child safe from harm (Bowlby, 1969, 1980; George & Solomon, 1989, 1996, 1999; Solomon & George, 1996). In this chapter, we present information relating mothers' resolution of their child's diagnosis, coded from interviews such as the preceding ones, with child–mother attachment organization and the mothers' adult attachment representations. From our perspective, the child's attachment behavior system can be disorganized by trauma to *either* to the mother's caregiving system, as in the case of raising a child with a disability or serious illness, or to the mother's attachment system, as in the case of unresolved loss of an attachment figure (Main & Hesse, 1990). By examining these relations, we hope to illuminate the ways in which attachment organization is multiply determined and that resolution of mothers' ongoing reactions to their child's condition is a particularly important process in relation to developing an organized attachment.

RESOLUTION OF PAST LOSS AND TRAUMA TO THE ATTACHMENT SYSTEM

Since the identification of the disorganized/disoriented attachment pattern, many investigators have been concerned with the correlates and antecedents of this pattern of child–parent attachment (Main & Solomon,

1986; 1990; Main, 1996). Risks for attachment disorganization have been of particular interest given suggested links between disorganized child–mother attachment and social and emotional maladaptation (Lyons-Ruth, 1996; Solomon, George, & De Jong, 1995; see also Solomon & George, Chapter 1, this volume).

Main (Main & Goldwyn, 1985/1991/1994; Main & Hesse, 1990) discussed two sources of unresolved states of mind in the parent that pose a risk for disorganization in child–parent attachment. The first involves the parent's loss of an attachment figure by death, and the second involves the parent's history of physical maltreatment at the hands of an attachment figure. It has been suggested that parents' experiences of loss and trauma affect the caregiving–attachment dyadic system in part through alteration of the psychological processes that regulate caregiving behavior (Main, 1991; Main & Hesse, 1990; 1992; Main & Solomon, 1990). The conceptualization of the link between loss of a caregiver's attachment figure and the child's attachment disorganization relies on a pathway linking *past* experiences of loss or trauma to caregiving behavior in the present via the adult's *current* state of mind.

There is considerable evidence to support this connection. Unresolved loss or trauma experiences show a strong correlation with disorganized/disoriented attachment of the child to parent (e.g., Ainsworth & Eichberg, 1992; George & Solomon, 1999; Lyons-Ruth, 1996; van IJzendoorn, 1995). The mechanism accounting for this relation is thought to involve a process whereby the child's attachment behavior evokes painful memories in the parent of the loss or trauma that has not been adequately resolved (Main, 1991; Main & Hesse, 1990, 1992). Reactivation of these memories by the child's attachment behavior is thought to be disorienting to the parent. In turn, the parent may not act to comfort the child, may behave in a frightened or frightening way toward the child, and the child is confused by the parent's behavior, thus lacking an organized behavioral strategy for such situations.

It is important to note that Main and Goldwyn (1985/1991/1994) clearly assert that losses in the present or recent past are expected also to have a disorganizing effect on the caregiving–attachment system. This is evident in their recommendation that responses of individuals with recent (within 12 months) losses are to be coded but set aside from analysis, largely because of the assumption that this is a period of crisis during which the individual is expected to be in a state of disorganization and reorientation (Main & Goldwyn, 1985/1991/1994). Thus, with respect to loss or trauma involving an attachment figure, it is clear that such experiences in the *present* pose a risk for attachment disorganization.

CHILD DISABILITY AS A CURRENT AND ONGOING TRAUMA TO THE CAREGIVING SYSTEM

Bowlby (1969/1982) and others (George & Solomon, 1996; Solomon & George, 1996, 1999) have also discussed the role of caregiving in the dyadic caregiving–attachment system and posit both representational and behavioral aspects of a *caregiving* system. Although this caregiving system is most readily identified in terms of observable behaviors such as maternal sensitivity (Ainsworth, Blehar, Waters, & Wall, 1974; Cohn & Tronick, 1989; Isabella, Belsky, & von Eye, 1989), psychological (or representational) processes are also involved in the ongoing regulation and functioning of these behaviors. Parents' beliefs, attributions, perceptions, and expectations for and about the child are cognitive processes that can be hypothesized to affect a parent's behavior toward the child (Bugenthal, Mantyla, & Lewis, 1989; Dix, Ruble, & Zamborano, 1989; Kochanska, 1990; Melson, Ladd, & Hsu, 1993). Likewise emotional experience and caregivers' emotional states, such as depression or anger, also affect behavior toward the child (Cohn, Campbell, Matias, & Hopkins, 1990; Field, 1989). When these representational aspects of the caregiving system become disordered, distorted, or stressed, the caregiver's behavior and the quality of the child's attachment may in turn be affected.

Parents associate learning of their child's diagnosis with a sense of loss or trauma and report grief reactions similar to individuals who experience the loss of someone through death (Blacher, 1984; Burden & Thomas, 1986; Trout, 1983; Waisbren, 1980). In previous papers, we have suggested that parents' ongoing struggles to resolve feelings and beliefs associated with their child's having a serious disability or medical condition are a trauma to the caregiving system that has consequences for the child's attachment (Marvin & Pianta, 1996; Pianta, Marvin, Britner, & Borowitz, 1996). Parents routinely report learning of, and coping with, their child's condition to be a period of considerable crisis and trauma. The family's routines are disrupted, expectations and hopes for developmental outcomes may be dashed or challenged, and parents may feel guilty or responsible, or they may seek to know the reason for this happening to their child; their sense of themselves as providers and protectors is challenged.

Importantly, this is a present and ongoing concern: Caregivers are constantly reminded *in the present* of the child's disability or illness, and, in fact, the provision of sensitive care often requires a direct response to these conditions. The strategies caregivers use to cope with these experiences of the child's condition can negatively influence caregiving because experience may be distorted, filtered, ignored, or amplified in such a way so as to prevent sensitive, balanced caregiving responses (Marvin & Pianta, 1996; Pianta et al., 1996; Sheeran, Marvin, & Pianta, 1997). Because this experience appears to be a traumatic disruption for caregivers and has ongoing consequences for their emotions, beliefs, and behaviors toward their child, reaction to diagnosis represents a possible risk for child–parent attachment disorganization that is based in the present and specifically involves the caregiving system. Our hypothesis is that resolution of this trauma is important for the organized functioning of the caregiving–attachment dyadic system.

METHODOLOGICAL ISSUES

It is important to clarify differences in the conceptualization and assessment of resolution from the Adult Attachment Interview (AAI; George, Kaplan, & Main, 1984/1985/1996) and from the Reaction to Diagnosis Interview (RDI; Pianta & Marvin, 1992a). There are differences between these methodologies that may affect the interpretation of results. First, Main and Goldwyn (1994) operationalize lack of resolution of mourning in terms of signs of disorganization or disorientation in discourse, reasoning, or behavior as indicated in text (verbatim transcriptions of the AAI). These signs are noted and a rating is made (on a 9-point scale) of the degree to which the presence of lapses indicates evidence of lack of resolution of mourning. A rating of 5 or higher is typical of those cases in which there is judgment of an unresolved state of mind.

We developed the RDI (Pianta & Marvin, 1992a) to examine resolution of loss/trauma associated with parents' experiences with raising a child with a disability or chronic illness. Similar to resolution of loss or other attachment-related traumas (Main & Hesse, 1990), resolution of the experience of serious illness or disability in one's child is characterized by integration of this experience into parents' representations of their child and their relationship with the child. This in turn allows for a reorientation and refocus of attention and problem solving on present reality (Main & Hesse, 1992). This refocus on the present and future is critical for supporting caregiving behaviors that relate to organized attachments (e.g., the parent does not act fearfully or frighteningly toward the child in attachment-related situations).

However, at a more specific level, our application of the construct of resolution is somewhat different than Main's original derivation and method. We cast a wider net for signs of resolution. Our operationalization utilizes nonverbal information obtained from videotapes of the RDI. Thus, information on affective expression, crying, depression, facial gestures or grimaces, and so forth, is available to the coder. Although, like Main, we rely on what the parents say, how their narratives indicate active processes of monitoring of the quality of discourse and reasoning, we also utilize the content of what parents report. For example, content of the interview is utilized for the parent acknowledging a change in emotional state, or beliefs about what causes the condition. These diverse data sources (video, narrative) and constructs (beliefs, lapses, nonverbal behaviors) are combined and coded at an overall organizational level into two categories: resolved and unresolved (with associated subcategories coded next).

In this way, our codes for lack of resolution reflect a broadband conceptualization and operationalization of resolution that was not intended as isomorphic to Main's somewhat more narrowband conceptualization of lack of resolution of mourning. These approaches do share many aspects and constructs, including a fundamental tenet that resolution reflects an orientation to the present. Our approach has resulted in strong relations between resolution of the diagnosis and the child's attachment security (Marvin & Pianta, 1996), but we have not yet examined reaction to diagnosis as a correlate of attachment organization.

DIAGNOSTIC ISSUES

Finally, it is critical to note that not all disabilities or serious medical conditions present the same psychological or behavioral challenges to the caregiving system. In our sample of children with disabilities, we have data on two distinct conditions that reflect different presentations: cerebral palsy and epilepsy. Cerebral palsy is a fairly static condition that affects the motor, language, and cognitive development of children. Children typically require assistance in many of the basic functions of life, and the course of their development in major domains is typically slow, although in some domains, it may proceed normally. Difficulties with motor development are a central source of functional impairment.

Epilepsy is different from cerebral palsy in a number of ways and poses an interesting contrast with respect to the construct of resolution. For children with epilepsy, development may proceed typically in many areas, especially when epilepsy is not secondary to other disabling or disease conditions. Children with epilepsy in the moderate and less severe ranges are capable of a level of nonassisted functioning that many children with cerebral palsy may not achieve. But unlike the fairly static condition of cerebral palsy, where developmental course is quite predictable, epileptic seizures are often very unpredictable, and parents are often told that child may "grow out of it" when they inquire about prognosis.

Because these two conditions differ on functional dimensions that are relevant for caregiving, we examined them separately, when possible, in order to discern whether the type of child condition played a role in resolution and attachment organization. For parents of children with cerebral palsy, there is evidence that resolution is most frequently related to actual direct care of the child and acquiring information that enables the parents to focus on skilled care of the child and knowledge of the condition (Pianta et al., 1996). Thus, a focus on the present seems not inconsistent with coping with a child's cerebral palsy. Parents of children with epilepsy report the unpredictability of the condition to be a serious stressor, something that likely undermines a clear and direct focus on the present state of the child. Thus, we expect that the link between resolution and attachment organization may be more evident and strong for parents of children with cerebral palsy.

In summary, this chapter examines resolution of loss or trauma in terms of timing (past or present), relationship affected (an attachment figure or one's child), and the child's condition (cerebral palsy or epilepsy) in relation to child attachment organization. In separate analyses of children with cerebral palsy and with epilepsy, we examine the relations between attachment organization and (1) mothers' state of mind with respect to loss coded from the AAI, or (2) resolution of ongoing trauma to the caregiving system, assessed in the RDI. Relatedly, we examine whether resolution with respect to attachment-related loss is related to resolution of trauma to the caregiving system.

METHODS

Sample

The sample for this study consisted of 73 children ages 15–50 months, who had a diagnosis of cerebral palsy or epilepsy, and their primary caregivers. Numbers of subjects available for particular analyses vary slightly due to missing information. Children were recruited from clinics at university medical centers, community hospitals, and early intervention programs in Virginia, West Virginia, North Carolina, Maryland, and Washington, DC. Forty of the children had a diagnosis of mild-to-moderate cerebral palsy, and 33 were diagnosed with mild-to-moderate severity epilepsy.

The children with cerebral palsy were functionally locomotor. This means they could follow their caregiver around the house in a functional manner. They could crawl, scoot, roll, or walk easily enough to locomote across a room. These children could be considered, as a group, to be mildly-to-moderately impaired. The diagnosis of cerebral palsy was made for each child approximately 12 months prior to data collection, and all diagnoses were made by physicians associated with the cases. Medical chart review showed a diagnosis of cerebral palsy in 100% of the cases. All children met a minimum criterion of an 8- to 10-month level of cognitive development as assessed by the Bayley Scales of Infant Development, the Vineland Adaptive Behavior Scales, and clinic staff and parent reports of functional levels. All children demonstrated minimal competencies in communicating with their mothers (verbal or nonverbal), object permanence, and distinguishing between strangers and familiar persons. There were 28 males and 12 females. Median age of the children was 37 months (range = 18–53 months). Two children were African American, one Hispanic American, the remainder were Caucasian.

Mothers were the primary caregivers for all children with cerebral palsy, except for two cases in which the primary caregiver was the grandmother. In the remainder of this chapter, primary caregivers are referred to as mothers. Mean level of mothers' education was 12.5 years (range = 8–18 years). Seventy-five percent of the mothers were married or had a live-in partner at the time of data collection. Father's education ranged from 4 to 19 years (mean = 12 years).

The 33 children with epilepsy had an average age of 30.6 months, and all had been diagnosed with epilepsy at least 12 months prior to data collection. None of the children in the epilepsy group had a motor impairment or cerebral palsy. The degree to which the children's seizures were controlled varied. Only 3 children were not receiving medication for seizures. In 60% of cases, seizure control was described by parents as fair to good, indicating some breakthrough seizures or complete control. The other cases reported poor or no control of seizures, reflecting daily seizures or several seizures a week. Type of seizures varied, with absence, generalized, and partial complex seizures all represented in the sample. Parents of 12 of the children with epilepsy indicated that the child's seizures were mild, suggesting that they were not disruptive of the child's functioning, and the child could return to normal functioning soon after the occurrence of a seizure. On the whole, the sample of children with seizures represents a mild-to-moderate level of epilepsy severity.

All of the children in the epilepsy sample were cared for by their biological mothers. Seventy-eight percent of the mothers of children with epilepsy were married at the time of data collection. The average number of years of education for the mothers was 14 (range = 10–20), and the average for fathers was 13 (range = 9–19). Twenty-one of the children were Caucasian; two were African American.

There were no significant differences between these two groups in race of the child, marital status at the time of data collection, mothers' education, or fathers' education.

Measures and Procedures

Families were recruited through medical clinics and contacted by the principal investigators in person or by mail. Mothers and children (and usually fathers or live-in partners) traveled to the laboratory to participate in the study. All data were collected at the laboratory site. Depending on child age and severity of motor impairment, parents and children participated in either the standard infant strange situation (Ainsworth et al., 1978) or the Preschool Strange Situation (Cassidy & Marvin, 1987/1990/1991/1992). Parents were administered the RDI (Pianta & Marvin, 1992a), and the AAI (George et al., 1985) as part of an extended interview session.

Reaction to Diagnosis Interview

RDI (Pianta & Marvin, 1992a) was designed specifically to assess parents' resolution of loss/trauma associated with receiving a diagnosis of serious disability or chronic medical condition for their child. Questions elicit the parent's memories, feelings, and beliefs regarding their learning of their child's disability or medical conditions, and their reasons and explanations for it. The RDI was administered by one of the authors or a trained graduate student. The RDI takes approximately 15 minutes to administer.

Subjects' responses to the RDI were coded using the Reaction to Diagnosis Classification System (Pianta & Marvin, 1992b). This system consists of a list of elements of resolution and lack of resolution, a set of two major categories (resolved and unresolved), and two sets of subcategories associated with each of the major categories. The process of classifying an interview involves judgments about the organization of the elements present in a given interview, and the extent to which the elements, at the organizational level, fit the resolved or unresolved category (and an associated subcategory).

Persons classified as resolved with respect to the experience of their child's diagnosis demonstrate a number of integrative strategies for coping with the information regarding the diagnosis and experience. Prominent among these are a reorientation to the present and future, a realistic view of their child's condition and skills, a balanced view of the impact on themselves, and a sense of coherence and autonomy during the interview. These individuals are focused on recounting their story, and they do so with clarity and without enlisting sympathy or anger from the interviewer. Their affect is balanced and the story is realistic, with appropriate detail.

Individuals classified as unresolved demonstrate one, or several, of the many mental strategies consistent with dissociation of traumatic experience. These include cognitive distortions or other attempts to distort reality, an active search for reasons why the experience occurred, unbalanced perceptions of the impact on the self (denial or victimization), and selective attention on past experience to the neglect of present reality. Also included among persons classified as unresolved are those for whom no organized mental strategy is evident. The interviews of these individuals are marked by confusion and mental disorganization with respect to their discussion of the diagnostic experience. As in the case of individuals classified resolved, one or more of these strategies may be evident in the interview.

All interviews were double-coded by at least two coders who were blind to the others' classification decision(s). At the major category level across all cases, the rate of agreement was 92%. Within the locomotor cerebral palsy group, agreement was 96%. Within the nonlocomotor group, agreement was 88%. Within the epilepsy group, agreement was 93%. The rates of agreement did not differ across diagnostic group. All levels of agreement were tested against chance agreement using a χ^2 test and exceeded levels of agreement expected by chance at the $p < .001$ level.

Attachment Assessment and Classification

CHILD–MOTHER ATTACHMENT

Each mother–child dyad was videotaped using either the original, Infant Strange Situation (Ainsworth et al., 1978) or the Preschool Strange Situation (Cassidy & Marvin, 1987/1990/1991/1992). Each *infant's* attachment pattern was classified using the original Ainsworth system (Ainsworth et al., 1978). Each *preschooler's* attachment pattern was classified using the Cassidy–Marvin Preschool Attachment Classification System (Cassidy & Marvin, 1987/1990/1991/1992).

For purposes of this study, each child was classified as either "organized" or "disorganized" with respect to his or her attachment pattern. The organized category included classifications of avoidant, secure, or resistant/ambivalent. The disorganized category included classifications of disorganized, controlling, or insecure–other. Note that the classifications of controlling and insecure–other are from the Cassidy–Marvin Preschool System (Cassidy & Marvin, 1987/1990/1991/1992) and include patterns of behavior that are hypothesized to be the more advanced developmental analogue of the forms of disorganized/disoriented attachment described by Main and Solomon (1990).

All strange situations were classified by coders blind to other results. Seventy-five percent ($N = 83$) were classified by two coders, with an agreement level of 93%. Agreement using the infant system was 88%; agreement using the preschool system was 91%. All levels of agreement were tested against chance agreement using a χ^2 test and exceeded levels of agreement expected by chance at the $p < .001$ level.

ADULT ATTACHMENT

Mothers in the cerebral palsy group and the epilepsy group were administered the AAI by a trained interviewer as part of an extended interview session. The AAI (George et al., 1984/1985/1996) is a semistructured interview in which respondents are asked for descriptions and evaluations of childhood attachment relationships, loss of attachment figures, and effects of childhood attachment experiences on present relational functioning. The interview lasts approximately 1 hour and, in the case of the present study, was videotaped. Audiotapes were dubbed from the video and transcribed; transcriptions were proofed against the video and then subject to coding. The reliability and validity of the AAI have been tested in numerous studies and found to be adequate (see Main, 1996, for a brief summary).

Two trained AAI coders analyzed the transcripts. Both coders also underwent the first stage of systematic reliability assessment using the procedures developed by Main to test the reliability of independent coders of the AAI. The primary coder of AAIs for this study (Morog) passed this first reliability screen at the Group II level, indicating moderate reliability, while the second coder (Pianta) passed at the Group I (highest) level of agreement with Main and Hesse.

Of interest in this study were the four main classification groups of dismissing, autonomous, preoccupied, and unresolved. Coder agreement was tested in two phases (all $p < .05$). First, the second coder double-coded 30% of the cases (randomly selected). The two coders demonstrated significant agreement for the four-way classifications on these cases (kappa = .84). Disagreements were conferenced; however, they occurred most often in cases in which there was a question of scoring unresolved loss (the unresolved classification). So in the next phase, because the unresolved classification was of specific interest for this study and disagreements occurred most often in the cases in which this class was suspected, the second coder double-coded all cases in which the first coder scored the transcript as unresolved. For these transcripts, agreement was significant for the four-way classification (kappa = .76) and for whether the individual fit the unresolved class or not (kappa = .77). All classifications of unresolved were conferenced.

Data Analysis Plan

We examined *bivariate* relations involving mothers' resolution of loss/trauma in their attachment history, resolution of the child's diagnosis, and organization of child–mother attachment behavior. The relation of resolution (from the AAI and from the RDI) to attachment organization was examined in two ways. Chi-square tests examined the significance of the overall bivariate relations among AAI status (unresolved/resolved), RDI status (unresolved/resolved) and attachment status (disorganized/organized). Then, one-way chi-square tests examined the specific prediction of a relation between resolution (from the AAI and RDI) and organized attachment. The cerebral palsy and epilepsy samples were treated separately.

RESULTS

Descriptive results were as follows. For adult attachment status, 70% of the cerebral palsy sample were classified as resolved, while 55% of the epilepsy sample were classified as resolved. On the RDI, 43% of mothers of children with cerebral palsy were classified as resolved, while 50% of mothers of children with epilepsy were classified resolved. With respect to attachment organization, 68% of the cerebral palsy sample were classified as organized, while 70% of the epilepsy sample were classified with organized attachments.

For the sample of mothers with children with cerebral palsy, in the overall analyses of the associations involved, there was no relation between resolution of attachment-related loss or trauma from the AAI and the child's attachment ($\chi^2 = .190$, $df = 1$, $p = .663$) or resolution of child diagnosis ($\chi^2 = 1.627$, $df = 1$, $p = .201$). At the level of one-way predictions from classification as resolved on the AAI to organized attachment status or resolved status on the RDI, the association between AAI–resolved and organized was nonsignificant ($\chi^2 = 2.462$, $df = 1$, $p = .117$), as was the association between AAI–resolved and RDI–resolved ($\chi^2 = 1.000$, $df = 1$, $p = .317$). Thus, resolution with respect to loss in mothers' attachment history was not correlated with the child's organized attachment, nor did it predispose these mothers of children with mild cerebral palsy to be resolved with respect to their child's diagnosis.

For the mothers of children with epilepsy, in the overall test of association, there was no relation between AAI status and attachment status ($\chi^2 = .120$, $df = 1$, $p = .730$). This was also the case in the one-way analysis for the predicted relation between resolved–AAI and organized attachment ($\chi^2 = .068$, $df = 1$, $p = .794$). There was a trend in the overall test of association ($\chi^2 = 3.394$, $df = 1$, $p = .063$) in the expected direction of AAI status to be related to RDI status. However, in the one-way test, there was not a significant result for the predicted association between classification as resolved on the AAI and resolved on the RDI ($\chi^2 = 1.471$, $df = 1$, $p = .225$). Thus, for both forms of diagnosis, epilepsy and cerebral palsy, there was little evidence that *resolution* of loss in the mothers' attachment history was related either to *resolution* of their child's diagnosis, or *organization* of the child's attachment, although in the epilepsy sample, there was a trend toward a relation between adult attachment status and status with regard to the child's diagnosis.

A second set of analyses examined the relation between mothers' status with respect to resolution of their children's medical condition and attachment organization. These results are presented first for the sample of children with cerebral palsy and then for the sample of children with epilepsy.

The overall relation between status on the RDI and child–mother attachment organization for mothers of children with cerebral palsy approached significance ($\chi^2 = 2.973$, $df = 1$, $p = .085$). The specific prediction from resolution on the RDI to organized attachment was significant ($\chi^2 = 7.118$, $df = 1$, $p = .008$). See Table 14.1. The vast majority (82.4%) of mothers who were classified as resolved with respect to the child's disability of cerebral palsy had children who showed organized (secure, avoidant, resistant) attachment behavior. Thus, there was strong prediction of organized attachment classification from mothers' status as resolved with regard to the child's cerebral palsy.

For the sample of children with epilepsy, the overall relation between RDI status and strange situation classification was nonsignificant ($\chi^2 = .414$, $df = 1$, $p = .520$). See Table 14.2. For the specific prediction from RDI-Resolved to Organized, the relation was also nonsignificant ($\chi^2 = .529$, $df = 1$, $p = 467$).

DISCUSSION

These analyses suggest that, for mothers of children with a disability or serious medical condition, resolution of past attachment-related loss was not a predictor of attachment organization or resolution of the child's medical condition or disability. On the other hand, resolution of ongoing experience related to the child's condition was a correlate of organized attachment behavior for the sample of children with cerebral palsy, but not for the children with epilepsy. These data underscore that when trying understand and predict attachment organization, assessing the parent's

TABLE 14.1. Resolution of Diagnosis and Attachment Organization: Cerebral Palsy Sample

Reaction to diagnosis	Attachment		Total
	Organized	Disorganized	
Resolved	14	3	17
Unresolved	13	10	23
Total	27	13	40

TABLE 14.2. Resolution of Diagnosis and Attachment Organization: Epilepsy Sample

Reaction to diagnosis	Attachment		Total
	Organized	Disorganized	
Resolved	12	4	16
Unresolved	11	6	17
Total	23	10	33

current state of mind with respect to loss or trauma involving their representations of their child may be an important source of information. The findings also suggest the possibility that prediction from caregivers' current state of mind may be different for different states: Resolved states may be more regularly associated with attachment organization than unresolved states are associated with disorganization.

It is not possible to overemphasize the importance of the fact that these mothers were raising a child with a serious, often life-threatening, and definitely future-threatening, condition. Thus, from a developmental psychopathology perspective, this was an opportunity to examine whether the expected rules regarding associations between a history of loss and current attachment disorganization (Main & Hesse, 1990) would apply in this special case.

In the context of having to raise a young child with a disability or chronic medical condition, resolution of past loss or trauma to the mothers' attachment system did not predict to the child's attachment organization or to resolution of the child's disability or medical condition. Thus, psychological processes related to integrating loss of an attachment figure from the past did not predict current, day-to-day caregiving–attachment processes *for dyads in which the child has a serious disability*. Nor did unresolved loss predispose mothers to be less resolved with respect to their child's diagnosis.

However, for the cerebral palsy sample, mothers' resolution of the child's diagnosis was a strong correlate of the child's organized attachment. We know from other work with these mothers that the child's disability appears in some, but not all, cases to elicit a strong focus on practical, nonemotional aspects of caregiving—feeding, providing movement for the child, fostering communication—such that psychological concerns (especially those about the past) may recede (Pianta et al., 1996). In fact, the focus of many of these mothers on practical caregiving of the child is singular—they often redefine parenting success in terms of whether they can successfully feed their child or facilitate communication or movement.

Their focus is on helping the child *do* things, and their narratives regarding their child are often devoid of references to emotion or psychological processes. These contemporaneous, ongoing conditions that foster such an intense focus on direct, physical care may, to some extent, override resolution of past circumstances (such as loss of an attachment figure).

Importantly, for this and a larger sample of children with more severe cerebral palsy, the attachment status of the majority of the children of mothers coded as resolved is organized–secure (Marvin & Pianta, 1996). This attests to the likelihood of concordance between these maternal representational and behavioral outcomes *under circumstances of this particular disability*. In our sample of even more severely impaired children with cerebral palsy, there is a higher incidence of attachment security than in the present sample, and its relation with resolution of the child's diagnosis is very strong (Marvin & Pianta, 1996; Pianta et al., 1996). As we suggested earlier, it is possible that a mother's psychological reactions to the disability (e.g., depression, anger) may be addressed through small successes in day-to-day physical care of the child and provide a means for focusing on caregiving in a way that fosters organized attachment behavior under difficult circumstances (i.e., raising a child with a disability). Finally, it is important to note that all of the mothers (and children) in this sample were enrolled in a variety of early intervention programs that were, at least in part, focused on enhancing sensitive caregiving and providing family support.

For mothers of children with epilepsy, the story is different. Their focus is less on physical care than for mothers of children with cerebral palsy, and more on the unpredictable and constant threat of a seizure, which could induce a course of life-threatening *status epilepticus*. For these mothers, this threat is active, ongoing, and real—oftentimes regardless of the degree to which medication may offer control of seizures. This threat is a direct challenge to caregivers' sense of themselves as protector. Parents also report being unsure how firm a stance to take in the face of, for example, a child's tantrum, for fear of "inducing" another seizure. Coupled with this threat is the hope that the seizures may relent over time, and that the child may "grow out of" the epilepsy. There is also the stress of often unpredictable states of the child associated with epilepsy itself, and the treatment of seizures, such that the child's own attachment-related signals can be unpredictable. For example, attentional states of children with epilepsy are often quite unregulated, and motor tremors and lack of coordination can be commonplace. In other words, for reasons having to do with the parents' concerns and the child's neurobiological status, it may be more difficult for parents of children with epilepsy (than for cerebral palsy) to select an appropriate caregiving response when faced with a child's cues. Thus, the psychological, neurological, and behavioral sequelae of epilepsy pose a considerable challenge for understanding links between adult attachment, parents' representations and caregiving behaviors, and child attachment. Interestingly, although, as was the case for cerebral palsy, the majority of attachments for children with epilepsy were organized; unlike for cerebral palsy, most of these attachments were insecure (Marvin, Pianta, & Britner, 1999). This fact may attest to the great difficulty these dyads face in meeting the challenges posed by epilepsy.

For both cerebral palsy and epilepsy, resolution of the child's condition is more strongly related to attachment security (Marvin & Pianta, 1996; Marvin, Pianta, & Britner, 1999) than to attachment organization. This is most likely a function of the fact that classification on the RDI involves a broadband conceptualization and assessment of resolution. This is in contrast to Main and Goldwyn's (1994) focus on very specific lapses in behavior, thought, and discourse that are putatively linked to specific aspects of caregiving behavior that undermine attachment organization. We did not code the RDIs of these mothers for the kind of lapses that Main and colleagues assert are related to attachment organization. Thus, it is possible that we have actually underestimated the link between resolution of the child's condition and attachment (dis)organization by not having an equivalent operationalization of resolution as has been demonstrated to be linked to attachment organization.

Clearly, the different pattern of findings for cerebral palsy and epilepsy suggests that further research in this area consider a range of diagnostic conditions, and variables associated with these conditions. We suspect that parameters, such as whether the condition is progressive or static, mild or severe, predictable or unpredictable, can play very important roles in the level of risk for lack of resolution associated with a condition. This is for the very reason that these factors lead to differences in the parents' sense of whether or not the set goal of their caregiving system is being achieved. To the extent that the course of a medical condition or disability can be predicted, the data suggest that resolution is more likely to be attained (Pianta et al., 1996), whereas conditions that are unpredictable, or offer hopes for an abatement, are somewhat more problematic for parents still in crisis. Furthermore, the implications of this research also suggest that it would be a mistake to use subject groups of varying diagnoses, or widely heterogeneous symptoms patterns within a given diagnosis, in research of this type. Thus, the nature of the loss or trauma may be an important source of variation in resolution and whether ongoing resolution of the child's diagnosis overrides risk for attachment disorganization due to past attachment-related loss.

Finally, it is important to emphasize that we chose to examine the link between adult attachment status and attachment organization in children with special needs because the proximal caregiving challenges posed by these disabilities represented a special case of the relation between resolution (on the AAI) and attachment organization. Although the evidence for resolution on the AAI and attachment organization was not strong, there was evidence that resolution of a different form (on the RDI) predicted attachment organization. Thus, the general link between resolution of loss or trauma and attachment organization received some support in this study.

The implications of the present study seem fairly straightforward. First, in examining antecedents of attachment (dis)organization, ongoing loss or trauma related to the caregiving system appears to be a reasonable focus, especially in circumstances in which the child has special health and/or disability needs. Second, due to the fact that resolution of ongoing caregiving-related concerns could be related to attachment organization, it may be useful for investigators to reexamine data sets for cases in which there was not concordance between AAI-related resolution and attachment (dis)organization. Our data suggest that one explanation for a lack of relation between resolution of loss from the AAI and attachment organization may be resolution of ongoing concerns related to the child. In short, the data presented in this chapter open the possibility for new understandings of the role of resolution of past and present loss and trauma in relation to attachment processes.

ACKNOWLEDGMENT

The research described in this chapter was supported by grants from the National Institute of Child Health and Human Development (No. R01HD26911) and the National Institute of Disability and Rehabilitation Research (No. H133G20118) to Robert C. Pianta and Robert S. Marvin.

REFERENCES

Ainsworth, M. D. S., Blehar, M. C., Waters, E., & Wall, S. (1974). *Patterns of attachment: A psychological study of the Strange Situation.* Hillsdale, NJ: Erlbaum.

Ainsworth, M. D. S., & Eichberg, C. (1992). Effects on infant-mother attachment of mother's unresolved loss of an attachment figure or other traumatic experience. In P. Marris, J. Stevenson-Hinde, & C. Parkes (Eds.), *Attachment across the life-cycle* (pp. 160–183). New York: Routledge.

Blacher, J. (1984). Sequential stages of parental adjustment to the birth of a child with handicaps: Fact or artifact? *American Journal of Mental Deficiency, 89,* 653–656.

Bowlby, J. (1969/1982). *Attachment and loss: Vol. 1. Attachment.* New York: Basic Books.

Bowlby, J. (1980). *Attachment and loss: Vol. 3. Loss.* New York: Basic Books.

Bugenthal, D. B., Mantyla, S. M., & Lewis, J. (1989). Parental attributions as moderators of affective communication to children at risk for physical abuse. In D. Cicchetti & V. Carlson (Eds.), *Child maltreatment: Theory and research on the causes and consequences of child abuse and neglect* (pp. 254–279). New York: Cambridge University Press.

Burden, R., & Thomas, D. (1986). A further perspective on parental reaction to handicap. *Exceptional Child, 33,* 140–145.

Button, S., Pianta, R. C., & Marvin, R. S. (1997). *Psychometric properties of the Parent–Development Interview.* Manuscript in preparation, University of Virginia, Charlottesville, VA.

Cassidy, J., & Marvin, R. S., with the MacArthur Working Group on Attachment. (1987/1990/1991/1992). *A system for classifying individual differences in the attachment-behavior of 2½ to 4½ year old children.* Unpublished coding manual, University of Virginia, Charlottesville, VA.

Cohn, J., Campbell, S., Matias, R., & Hopkins, J. (1990). Face to face interactions of postpartum depressed and non-depressed mother–infant pairs at 2 months. *Developmental Psychology, 26,* 15–23.

Cohn, J. F., & Tronick, E. (1989). Specificity of infants' response to mothers' affective behavior. *Journal of the American Academy of Child and Adolescent Psychiatry, 28,* 242–248.

Dix, T. H., Ruble, D. N., & Zamborano, R. J. (1989). Mothers' implicit theories of discipline: Child effects, parent effects, and the attribution process. *Child Development, 60,* 1373–1391.

Field, T. (1989). Maternal depression effects on infant interaction and attachment behavior. In D. Cicchetti (Ed.), *The Rochester Symposium on Developmental Psychopathology* (pp. 139–164). Hillsdale, NJ: Erlbaum.

George, C., Kaplan, N., & Main, M. (1984/1985/1996). *Adult Attachment Interview.* Unpublished manuscript, University of California, Berkeley.

George, C., & Solomon, J. (1989). Internal working models of caregiving and security of attachment at age six. *Infant Mental Health Journal, 10,* 222–237.

George, C., & Solomon, J. (1993, March). *Internal working models of caregiving.* Paper presented at the Biennial Meeting of the Society for Research in Child Development, New Orleans, LA.

George, C., & Solomon, J. (1999). Attachment and caregiving: The caregiving behavioral system. In J. Cassidy & P. R. Shaver (Eds.), *Handbook of attachment: Theory, research, and clinical applications* (pp. 649–670). New York: Guilford Press.

Isabella, R. Belsky, J., & von Eye, I. (1989). Origins of mother–infant attachment: An examination of interactional synchrony during the infant's first year. *Developmental Psychology, 25,* 12–21.

Kochanska, G. (1990). Maternal beliefs as long-term predictors of mother–child interaction and report. *Child Development, 61,* 1934–1943.

Lyons-Ruth, K. (1996). Disorganized/disoriented attachment in the etiology of dissociative disorders. *Dissociation, 4,* 196–204.

Main, M. (1990). Cross-cultural studies of attachment organization: Recent studies, changing methodologies and the concept of conditional strategies. *Human Development, 33,* 48–61.

Main, M. (1991). Metacognitive knowledge, metacognitive monitoring, and singular (coherent) vs. multiple (incoherent) models of attachment: Findings and directions for future research. In C. M. Parkes, J. Stevenson-Hinde, & P. Harris (Eds.), *Attachment across the life cycle* (pp. 127–159). London: Routledge.

Main, M. (1995). Attachment: Overview with implications for clinical work. In S. Goldberg, R. Muir, & J. Kerr (Eds.), *Attachment theory: Social, developmental and clinical perspectives* (pp. 467–474). Hillsdale, NJ: Analytic Press.

Main, M. (1996). Introduction to the special section on attachment and psychopathology: 2. Overview of the field of attachment. *Journal of Consulting and Clinical Psychology, 64,* 237–243.

Main, M., & Goldwyn, R. (1985/1991/1994). *Adult attachment rating and classification systems.* Unpublished manuscript, University of California, Berkeley.

Main, M., & Hesse E. (1990). Is fear the link between infant disorganized attachment status and maternal unresolved loss? In M. Greenberg, D. Cicchetti, & M. Cummings (Eds.), *Attachment in the preschool years* (pp. 161–182). Chicago: University of Chicago Press.

Main, M., & Hesse, E. (1992). Disorganized/disoriented infant behavior in the Strange Situation, lapses in the monitoring of reasoning and discourse in the parent's Adult Attachment Interview, and dissociative states. In M. Ammaniti & D. Stern (Eds.), *Attachment and psychoanalysis* (pp. 86–140). Rome: Gius, Laterza, & Figli.

Main, M., & Solomon, J. (1986). Discovery of a new, insecure-disorganized/disoriented attachment pattern. In T. B. Brazelton & M. Yogman, (Eds.), *In support of families* (pp. 95–124). Norwood, NJ: Ablex.

Main, M., & Solomon, J. (1990). Procedures for classifying infants as disorganized/disoriented during the Ainsworth Strange Situation. In M. Greenberg, D. Cicchetti, & M. Cummings (Eds.), *Attachment in the preschool years* (pp. 121–160). Chicago: University of Chicago Press.

Marvin, R. S., Pianta, R. C., & Britner, P. A. (1999). *Attachment security in children with epilepsy.* Manuscript in preparation, University of Virginia, Charlottesville, VA.

Marvin, R. S., O'Connor, T. G., & Pianta, R. C. (1994). *Procedures for classifying attachment of children with severe motor impairments.* Unpublished materials, University of Virginia, Charlottesville, VA.

Marvin, R. S., & Pianta, R. C. (1989). *The Strange Situation adapted for children with motor impairments.* Unpublished materials, University of Virginia, Charlottesville.

Marvin, R. S., & Pianta, R. C. (1996). Parents' reaction to their child's diagnosis: Relations with security of attachment. *Journal of Child Clinical Psychology, 25,* 436–445.

Melson, G. F., Ladd, G. W., & Hsu, H. C. (1993). Maternal social support networks, maternal cognitions, and young children's social and cognitive development. *Child Development, 64,* 1401–1417.

Pianta, R. C., Marvin, R. S., Britner, P., & Borowitz, K. (1996). Mothers' resolution of their children's diagnosis: Organized patterns of caregiving representations. *Infant Mental Health Journal, 17,* 239–256.

Pianta, R. C., & Marvin, R. S. (1992a). *The Reaction to Diagnosis Interview.* Unpublished materials, University of Virginia, Charlottesville.

Pianta, R. C., & Marvin, R. S. (1992b). *The Reaction to Diagnosis Classification System.* Unpublished materials, University of Virginia, Charlottesville.

Sheeran, T. F., Marvin, R. S., & Pianta, R. C. (1997). Mothers' resolution of their child's diagnosis and self-reported measures of parenting stress, marital relations, and social support. *Journal of Pediatric Psychology, 22,* 197–212.

Solomon, J., & George, C. (1996). Defining the caregiving system: Toward a theory of caregiving. *Infant Mental Health Journal, 17,* 183–197.

Solomon, J., & George, C. (in press). The caregiving behavioral system: Implications for infant mental health. In J. Osofsky & H. Fitzgerald (Eds.), *Handbook of infant mental health: Volume 3. Parenting and child care.* New York: Wiley.

Solomon, J., George, C., & De Jong, A. (1995). Children classified as controlling at age six: Evidence for disorganized representational strategies and aggression at home and at school. *Development and Psychopathology, 7,* 447–463.

Trout, M. D. (1983). Birth of a sick or handicapped infant: Impact on the family. *Child Welfare, 62,* 337–348.

van IJzendoorn, M. (1995). Adult attachment representations, parental responsiveness, and infant attachment: A meta-analysis on the predictive validity of the Adult Attachment Interview. *Psychological Bulletin, 117,* 387–403.

Waisbren, S. E. (1980). Parents' reactions after the birth of a developmentally disabled child. *American Journal of Mental Deficiency, 84,* 345–351.

Summary of Procedures for Identifying and Rating Attachment Disorganization

TABLE A.1. Indices of Disorganization and Disorientation
(For Infants 12–18 Months Observed with Parent Present)

---

1. Sequential Display of Contradictory Behavior Patterns

Very strong displays of attachment behavior or angry behavior suddenly followed by avoidance, freezing, or dazed behavior. For example:

—In the middle of a display of anger and distress, the infant suddenly becomes markedly devoid of affect and moves away from the parent.

—*Immediately following strong proximity seeking and a bright, full greeting with raised arms, the infant moves to the wall or into the center of room and stills or freezes with a "dazed" expression.*

—*Infant cries and calls for the parent at the door throughout separation: immediately upon reunion, however, the infant turns about and moves sharply away from the parent, showing strong avoidance.*

Calm, contented play suddenly succeeded by distressed, angry behavior. For example:

—*Infant calm and undistressed during both separations from the parent, but becomes extremely focused upon the parent, showing highly distressed and/or angry behavior immediately upon reunion.*

Note. Italics mark very strong indices, which in themselves are usually sufficient for *D* category placement. From Main and Solomon (1990). Copyright 1990 by University of Chicago Press. Reprinted by permission.

2. Simultaneous Display of Contradictory Behavior Patterns

The infant displays avoidant behavior simultaneously with proximity seeking, contact maintaining, or contact resisting. For example:

—While held by or holding onto parent, infant shows avoidance of parent such as the following: (a) infant sits comfortably on parent's lap for extended period but with averted gaze, ignoring parent's repeated overtures; (b) infant holds arms and legs away from the parent while held, limbs stiff, tense, and straight; (c) infant clings hard to parent for substantial period while *sharply* averting head/gaze. (Note: Disorganized only if infant is clinging hard while sharply arching away. Many infants look away or turn heads away while holding on lightly after a pick-up.)

—Infant approaches while simultaneously creating a pathway which avoids and moves away from parent, and this cannot be explained by a shift of attention to toys or other matters. Thus, from its inception the infant's "approach" seems designed to form a parabolic pathway.

—*Movements of approach are repeatedly accompanied by movements of avoidance such as the following: (a) infant approaches with head sharply averted, (b) infant approaches by backing toward parent, (c) infant reaches arms up for parent with head sharply averted or with head down.*

—*Distress, clinging, or resistance is accompanied by marked avoidance for substantial periods, such as the following: (a) infant moves into corner or behind item of furniture while angrily, openly, refusing or resisting parent; (b) infant cries angrily from distance, while turning in circles and turning away from parent.* (Note: Arching backward with flailing arms, and throwing self backward on floor are part of normal infant tantrum displays and are not necessarily considered disorganized.)

—*Extensive avoidance of parent is accompanied by substantial distress/anger indices, such as: infant slightly averts head and body away from parent who is offering or attempting pick-up but makes stiff, angry kicking movements and hits hands on floor.*

Simultaneous display of other opposing behavioral propensities. For example:

—Infant's smile to parent has fear elements *(very strong index* if marked, see no. 6).

—*While in apparent good mood, infant strikes, pushes, or pulls against the parent's face or eyes. (These usually subtle aggressive movements are sometimes immediately preceded by a somewhat dazed expression, or may be accompanied by an impassive expression.)*

3. Undirected, Misdirected, Incomplete, and Interrupted Movements and Expressions

Seemingly undirected or misdirected movements and expressions. For example:

—Upon becoming distressed, infant moves away from rather than to parent. (Note: Do not consider brief moves away from parent disorganized when an infant has been crying and displaying desire for contact for a long period, and parent has failed to satisfy infant. Infant may briefly move away while crying in response to frustration in these circumstances, coming back to parent to try again, without being disorganized.)

—Infant approaches parent at door as though to greet parent, then attempts instead to follow stranger out of the room, perhaps actively pulling away from the parent. (This pattern seems more misdirected or redirected than undirected; see no. 7 for similar behavior.)

—Initiation of extensive crying in parent's presence without any move toward or look toward the parent. (Note: This is not necessarily disorganized if parent is already nearby and attentive. It also is not disorganized if the infant, having already been crying and focused on the parent for an extended period, simply does not look at or move closer to the parent for a few seconds.)

—Any marked failure to move toward the parent when path is not blocked and infant is clearly frightened.

—Similarly, expression of strong fear or distress regarding an object while staring at it, without withdrawing from it or looking toward parent.

—*Extensive or intense expressions of fear or distress accompanied or followed by moves away from rather than to parent, as, infant appears frightened of stranger in parent's presence, moves away and leans forehead on wall.*

—*Infant cries at stranger's leave-taking, attempts to follow her out of room. (This behavior pattern may be more misdirected or redirected than undirected; see also no. 7.)*

Incomplete movements. For example:

—Movements to approach parent are contradicted before they are completed, for example, infant moves hand toward parent and withdraws hand quickly before touching parent, without rationale. Or repeated, hesitant, stop-start approach movements (or reach movements) toward parent.

—Exceptionally slow or limp movements of approach to parent, as though the infant is resisting the movements even while making them ("underwater" approach movements).

—*Exceptionally slow, limp, movements of striking at, pushing at, or pulling at the par-*

ent's face, eyes, or neck ("underwater" movements). The subtle but definite aggressive intent is almost indiscernible because of the incomplete, slow nature of the movements. See also 5.

Interrupted expressions or movements. For example:

—After a long period of contented play, sudden out-of-context crying or displays of distressed anger without rationale.

—*Infant interrupts approach to parent on reunion with a bout of angry behavior, directed away from the parent, then continues approach. As, begins strong approach upon reunion but interrupts approach to look away and strike hand on floor with angry sounds, then completes full approach.*

—*Infant rises or begins approach immediately upon reunion, but falls prone in "depressed" (huddled) posture.*

---

4. Stereotypies, Asymmetrical Movements, Mistimed Movements, and Anomalous Postures

---

Asymmetries of expression or movement. For example:

—Asymmetries of movement on approach to parent (asymmetrical creeping, heavy or fast on one side only), with or without sudden, unpredictable changes of direction.

—Asymmetries of facial expression directly upon the appearance of the parent, for example, an extremely swift "tic" which lifts only the left side of the facial musculature.

Stereotypies. For example:

—Extended rocking, ear pulling, hair twisting, and any other rhythmical, repeated movements without visible function. (Note: Do not include "stereotypies" that make sense in the immediate context, as rubbing eyes in a tired infant, or some initial ear pulling or hair pulling in the stranger's presence).

—Marked stereotypies while held by the parent. (Do *not* include rubbing eyes if infant has been crying, or brief continuation of previous stereotypies while in arms in an infant who showed the same stereotypies during separation.)

Assumption of anomalous postures. For example:

—*Repeated assumption uninterpretable postures, as, head cocking with arms crooked over head.*

—*Assumption of huddled, prone, depressed posture for more than twenty seconds, unless infant is clearly tired.*

—Any posture stereotyped for a particular baby, as, closing eyes and holding hands forward at shoulder height for several seconds in response to each reunion.

Mistimed movements. For example:

—Unpredictable bouts of activity or movement which seem to lack normal preparation time for initiation, and/or which have a jerky, automaton-like (unmonitored) quality. For example, a sudden burst of jerky arm and leg activity in an infant who had been sitting tense and immobilized a second prior.

---

5. Freezing, Stilling, and Slowed Movements and Expressions

Freezing is identified as the holding of movements, gestures, or positions in a posture that involves active resistance to gravity. For example, infant sits or stands with arms held out waist-high and to sides. *Stilling* is distinguished from freezing in that infant is in comfortable, resting posture which requires no active resistance to gravity. Freezing is considered a stronger marker of disorientation than stilling.

Freezing and stilling suggestive of more than momentary interruption of activity. For example:

—*Freezing lasting twenty seconds or more, and stilling lasting thirty seconds or more, accompanied by dazed or trance-like facial expression. For example, freezing accompanied by tense, smooth closing of the lids or by lifeless stare.*

—*Interrupting a bout of resistant or stressed behavior, freezing (ten or more seconds) or stilling (twenty or more seconds) is accompanied by a dazed or trance-like expression.*

—*Freezing lasting twenty-five seconds or more, and stilling lasting thirty-five seconds or more, while held by parent unless infant has recently been engaged in hard crying (below).* (Notes: [1] Context should be considered. [2] Do not consider stilling during the first thirty seconds of reunion if the infant is being held by parent, has been crying hard, and is clearly simply in transition from crying. [3] Infant should not be considered to be freezing or stilling if infant is watching something with lively interest, as, watching stranger demonstrate working of a toy. [4] The C2 infant is passive by definition: general passivity should not be confused with stilling.)

Slowed movements and expressions suggesting lack of orientation to the present environment. For example:

—Markedly apathetic or lethargic movements, as though infant is without purpose in moving forward.

—Slack, depressed, dazed, or apathetic facial expression especially when unexpected, as accompanying approach to parent on reunion ending in raised arms. (Note: Consider only expressions specified above. Neutral or impassive expressions are not considered indicative of disorientation with respect to the current environment.)

---

6. Direct Indices of Apprehension Regarding the Parent

Expression of strong fear or apprehension directly upon return of parent, or when parent calls or approaches. For example:

  —*Immediate responses to noting parent's entrance such as the following:* (a) *jerking back, with fearful expression;* (b) *flinging hands about, over, or in front of face, or over mouth, with fearful expression;* (c) *dashing away from the door/parent upon reunion, with hunched or tucked head and shoulders.*

  —Other expressions of fear or apprehension soon following reunion, such as *fearful facial expression on pick-up.*

Other indices of apprehension regarding the parent. For example:

  —Moving behind chair or behind furniture without immediate rationale (pursuit of toy, interest in object behind chair, or brief exploration), especially when infant is then out of reach or out of sight of parent.

  —Following a hesitant, seemingly cautious approach to the parent with a rapid, tense "away" movement.

  —Offering objects to the parent with tense arm and over an unusual distance, as though avoiding parental "reach" space.

  —Raising or tensing shoulders when approaching or in contact with parent.

  —Highly vigilant posture or appearance when in presence of parent. Movements or posture tense, infant gives impression of being hyperalert to parent even or especially when parent positioned behind her.

---

7. Direct Indices of Disorganization or Disorientation

Any clear indices of confusion and disorganization in first moment of reunion with the parent. For example:

  —Raising hand or hands to mouth directly upon the return of the parent without accompanying confused, wary, or fearful expression. (Do not include thumb or finger sucking, putting objects in mouth, or removing objects from mouth. Do not include if hands already near face.)

  —*"Greeting" stranger brightly at the moment of reunion with parent, that is, approaching stranger with raised arms immediately as parent enters.* (Note: Distinguish from the bright or happy look to stranger made by many infants at the moment of the parent's return, often accompanied by pointing to parent to further mark the event.)

—*Flinging hands over, about, or in front of face directly, upon return of the parent and in clear response to return of the parent.*

—*Raising hand or hands to mouth directly upon the return of the parent with a clearly confused or wary expression.*

—*Confused or confusing sequences of very rapid changes of affect in first few seconds of reunion with parent, as,* (a) *rapid movement of withdrawal* (b) *accompanied by confused cry-laugh* (c) *succeeded by approach movement.*

Direct indices of confusion or disorientation beyond the first moments of reunion with the parent. For example:

—Fall while approaching parent when infant is good walker. Similar unexplained falls when parent reaches for infant, or when parent calls from outside of door.

—Disorganized wandering, especially when accompanied by disoriented expression.

—Rapidly pursuing parent to door, protesting departure, then smiling at door as though in greeting as door closes.

—Disoriented facial expression. Sudden "blind" look to eyes, where infant has previously used eyes normally.

TABLE A.2. Directions for Determining Whether an Infant Is to Be Assigned to Disorganized/Disoriented Attachment Status

---

This system is applied to samples of normal infants 12–18 months of age, and to episodes of the strange situation in which the parent is present. It is presumed that the worker is already reliably trained in the traditional, A, B, C system; that a clear video recording sufficient to permit study of infant facial expression and small-motor movements is available; and that nothing within the conduct of the situation itself is likely to produce disorganization.

1. Attempt to assign an "Ainsworth" (A, B, C) classification and subclassification. If the infant is unclassifiable (U_{ABC}), two or more best-fitting A, B, or C attachment classifications will be assigned in order of descending fit (priority).

2. Review Table A.1: Can the infant's strange-situation behavior be described as fitting to one of several of the thematic headings, or to one of the behavior examples?

3. Make a written record of all behaviors seeming to qualify as indices of disor-

ganization or disorientation, specifying social, behavioral, and temporal context.

4. If any of these are "very strong" indicators (shown in italics in Table A.1) occurring without immediate explanation or rationale, the infant is assigned to *D*.

5. If there are no italicized indicators, the worker must decide whether the recorded indices are sufficient to warrant placement in the *D* category on the basis of the following categorical decisions. Thus, *D* attachment status is assigned if strange-situation behavior appears *inexplicable with respect to the immediate context in which it is observed;* and/or if the infant appears to the observer to be *without a behavioral "strategy"* for dealing with its immediate situation; and/or if the behavior can be explained only by the assumption that the infant is either *fearful of the attachment figure, or is fearful of approaching the attachment figure.*

6. Assign a rating to the infant for degree of disorganization, utilizing a simple nine-point rating scale.

7. If the infant has been assigned to *D* attachment status because of only one type of behavioral display, the worker may elect to assign a tentative *D* subcategory, as, "stilling/freezing of movement," "apprehensive movements and expressions," "depressed/apathetic," or "*A/C.*"

8. Review the final classification assignment. Each tape will ultimately be assigned to one of five major categories (*A, B, C, D,* or *U*), in conjunction with other best-fitting categories where necessary. With respect to infants who cannot be directly classified using the traditional *A, B, C* system, note that some infants will be *D* while being otherwise classifiable (e.g., *D/A*1); many will be *D* as well as being unclassifiable (e.g., *D/UA*1/*B*4); and a few still will be simply unclassifiable (*U/A*1/*B*4).

TABLE A.3. A Rating Scale for Disorganization in the Strange Situation

---

For the above reasons, no exhaustive list of *D* behaviors can be constructed, and because *D* behaviors follow an exclusion principle rather than serving an obvious single function, a satisfactory interactive scoring system comparable to those devised by Ainsworth cannot yet be constructed. Nevertheless, an infant who leans her forehead against the wall and cries in the parent's presence, rises and then falls prone on reunion, and later interrupts her avoidance with tantrum behavior seems more disorganized than an infant who freezes briefly at the stranger's entrance. Note, however, that while avoidance can be scored without knowledge of the full classification system, and without the judge having yet decided upon *A*/not-*A* as a categorical judgment, suggestions for scaling D behavior as given below depend upon a complete consideration of the suitability of the tape for D classification. We may then recognize a simple ordering which presupposes that the nature of the behavior, the context of the behavior being considered, its potential rationale or explanation, and its sequelae have already been taken into account:

1. No signs of disorganization/disorientation. Any behaviors that initially seemed to be indices of disorganization or disorientation have been explained in other terms.

3. Slight signs of disorganization/disorientation. There are some indices of disorganization or disorientation, but the worker does not even begin to consider placement in a D category.

5. Moderate indices of disorganization/disorientation which are not clearly sufficient for a D category placement. No very strong (italicized) indicators are present, and the indices that are present are not frequent enough, intense enough, or clearly enough lacking in rationale for the worker to be certain of a D category placement. The worker using a 5 will have to "force" a decision regarding whether the infant should be assigned to a D category. (Note: Ratings below a 5 [e.g., 4.5] mean the infant is not to be assigned to the D category, and ratings above a 5 [e.g., 5.5] indicate assignment to the D category.)

7. Definite qualification for D attachment status, but D behavior is not extreme. There is one very strong indicator of disorganization/disorientation, or there are several lesser indicators. There is no question that the infant should be assigned to D status, even though exhibition of D behavior is not strong, frequent, or extreme.

9. Definite qualification for D attachment status: in addition, the indices of disorganization and disorientation are strong, frequent, or extreme. Either several very strong indicators are present, or one very strong indicator and several intense exhibitions of one or several other indices.

REFERENCE

Main, M., & Solomon, J. (1990). Procedures for identifying infants as disorganized/disoriented during the Ainsworth Strange Situation. In M. Greenberg, D. Cicchetti, & M. Cummings (Eds.), *Attachment in the preschool years: Theory, Research, and Intervention* (pp. 121–160). Chicago: University of Chicago Press.

Index